Wildlife Ethics

The Universities Federation for Animal Welfare

UFAW, founded in 1926, is an international independent, scientific and educational animal welfare charity and membership society. UFAW's vision is a world where the welfare of all animals affected by humans is maximised through a scientific understanding of their needs and how to meet them. UFAW aims to discover what matters to animals, develop scientific solutions to animal welfare problems and disseminate evidence-based animal welfare information by:

- Funding scientific research
- Supporting the careers of animal welfare scientists
- Disseminating animal welfare science knowledge both to experts and the wider public
- Providing expert advice to government departments and other bodies, helping to draft and amend laws and guidelines

You can help make even bigger strides in animal welfare science by donating, leaving a legacy, or becoming a member of UFAW. For further information about UFAW and how you can help promote and support our work, please contact us at the following address:

Universities Federation for Animal Welfare
The Old School, Brewhouse Hill,
Wheathampstead, Herts AL4 8AN, United Kingdom
Phone: +44 (0) 1582 831818
Website: www.ufaw.org.uk
Email: ufaw@ufaw.org.uk

UFAW's aim with the UFAW/Wiley-Blackwell Animal Welfare book series is to promote interest and facilitate debate on the subject of animal welfare, whilst disseminating information relevant to improving the welfare of kept animals and those affected by human activities in the wild. The books in this series are the works of their authors, and the views they express do not necessarily reflect the views of UFAW.

Wildlife Ethics

The Ethics of Wildlife Management and Conservation

Clare Palmer
Texas A&M University
College Station, TX, USA

Bob Fischer
Texas State University
San Marcos, TX, USA

Christian Gamborg
University of Copenhagen
Frederiksberg, Denmark

Jordan Hampton
University of Melbourne
Parkville, Victoria, Australia

Peter Sandøe
University of Copenhagen
Frederiksberg, Denmark

UFAW

WILEY Blackwell

This edition first published 2023

Series Editors: Huw Golledge and Birte Nielsen.

Registered Offices
John Wiley & Sons, Inc., 111 River Street, Hoboken, NJ 07030, USA
John Wiley & Sons Ltd, The Atrium, Southern Gate, Chichester, West Sussex, PO19 8SQ, UK

For details of our global editorial offices, customer services, and more information about Wiley products visit us at www.wiley.com.

Wiley also publishes its books in a variety of electronic formats and by print-on-demand. Some content that appears in standard print versions of this book may not be available in other formats.

Library of Congress Cataloging-in-Publication Data
Names: Palmer, Clare, 1967- author. | Fischer, Bob (Robert William), author. | Gamborg, Christian, author. | Hampton, Jordan O., author. | Sandøe, Peter, author.
Title: Wildlife ethics : the ethics of wildlife management and conservation / Clare Palmer, Bob Fischer, Christian Gamborg, Jordan Hampton, Peter Sandøe.
Description: Hoboken, NJ : Wiley-Blackwell, 2023. | Series: UFAW/Wiley-Blackwell animal welfare | Includes index.
Identifiers: LCCN 2023003666 (print) | LCCN 2023003667 (ebook) | ISBN 9781119611219 (paperback) | ISBN 9781119611295 (adobe pdf) | ISBN 9781119611264 (epub)
Subjects: LCSH: Wildlife management–Moral and ethical aspects. | Wildlife conservation–Moral and ethical aspects.
Classification: LCC SK355 .P35 2023 (print) | LCC SK355 (ebook) | DDC 333.95/416–dc23/eng/20230602
LC record available at https://lccn.loc.gov/2023003666
LC ebook record available at https://lccn.loc.gov/2023003667

Cover Design: Wiley
Cover Image: © Sourav Dasgupta/Shutterstock

Set in 9.5/12pt Sabon LT Std by Straive, Pondicherry, India

Contents

Foreword

We are delighted to publish this important book by some of the foremost thinkers in animal ethics. It fills a significant gap both in the UFAW/Wiley-Blackwell Animal Welfare book series and in the animal welfare and ethics literature as a whole. There are numerous books covering the ethics of veterinary practice, the use of animals for food, scientific research, and animals as companions or for entertainment, but comparatively little has been written about the ethics of managing and conserving animals in the wild.

At first glance the ethical issues associated with wild animals may seem rather simple compared with those concerning the animals we keep in captivity. Many of us treasure the natural world and would hope that human impacts on wild animals can be minimized. As an animal welfare charity, UFAW was established to protect the welfare of animals through a scientific understanding of their needs and how to meet them. Therefore, as an organization, when we consider wild animals, our concern is for the welfare of each individual with the aim of maximizing the welfare of as many animals as possible. As an example, we support research to establish the welfare consequences of practices that impact wild animals and advocate for the elimination of those that are detrimental to welfare. For instance, we recently funded research to assess which methods of controlling rats when they come into conflict with humans were least humane. When this research confirmed, unsurprisingly, that glue traps are extremely inhumane, we campaigned for their use to be restricted. UFAW has the luxury of being concerned only about the welfare of animals. Conservation of species, the impact of animals on humankind, and many other issues lie outside our purview. However, in the world at large all these concerns and more are just as valid as animal welfare when we consider how we interact with wild animals. Many laudable human aims for animals in the wild are contradictory, raising complex questions. For instance, how can we simultaneously protect animals in the wild from anthropogenic impacts upon their welfare, protect humans from wild animals which spread zoonotic disease and threaten food supplies, preserve natural habitats, and conserve species? The simple answer is that we cannot achieve all these highly desirable outcomes, which raises complex questions about where we should make compromises when there is no single "right thing to do."

How and where we make these compromises is an issue of ethics, and this excellent book is one of the first to consider these ethical issues in relation to wild animals. Careful ethical consideration is needed to allow us to come to conclusions about whether the benefits of our actions toward animals in the wild outweigh the harms. These are rarely simple or obvious judgments. Indeed, some of the proposed solutions to wildlife issues are counter-intuitive and profoundly controversial such as the idea that licensed trade in wildlife products or organized trophy hunting can contribute to species conservation and minimize illegal hunting. It is with complex issues such as these that thoughtful ethical debate is vital if we are to avoid kneejerk reactions before we have considered whether less obvious approaches might be more beneficial.

In this book the authors take real-world scenarios such as those mentioned above to illustrate ethical issues and approaches, some of them longstanding such as the conflict between humans and animals when wild animals threaten human health or food security, and others that have recently risen to prominence such as re-wilding and the impacts of wind turbines on welfare.

This book will be invaluable to all those with an interest in the welfare of wild animals, and the authors have done an excellent job of keeping the material accessible to a general audience whilst tackling complex ethical concepts. This is crucial since those who can use the concepts in the book to bring about positive change for wildlife and the natural world will not, largely, be trained in ethics or philosophy.

I congratulate the authors for producing this important book that I hope will become required reading for those studying wildlife biology or animal welfare as well as those who make policy and guidance about our interactions with animals in the wild.

Huw Golledge

Chief Executive and Scientific Director,
Universities Federation for Animal Welfare

Acknowledgments

We, the authors, received a good deal of help, support, and feedback in writing this book, for which we are most grateful.

First, we would like to thank all who provided very helpful comments on one or more chapters, at different stages of the book (listed in alphabetical order): Dr Pierre-Yves Daoust, Professor Emeritus, University of Prince Edward Island, Canada; Dr Tim Doherty, Discovery Early Career Researcher Award Fellow, University of Sydney, Australia; Dr Claire Haggett, Senior Lecturer, University of Edinburgh, Scotland; Dr John Linnell, Senior Researcher, Norwegian Institute for Nature Research, and Professor, Inland University of Applied Science, Norway; Dr James Russell, Professor, University of Auckland, New Zealand; Dr Craig Stephen, Clinical Professor, University of British Columbia, Canada; Dr Amanda Stronza, Professor, Texas A&M University, USA; Dr Bruce Warburton, Science Team Leader, Wildlife Ecology and Management Team, Manaaki Whenua-Landcare Research, New Zealand.

We would also like to thank the following people who kindly donated photographs (listed in alphabetical order): Jeff Benson, Laura Brannelly, Graeme Coulson, Michael Jackson, Dave Kenny, Laszlo Kupi, Leith Meyer, David Mudge, Alvin Trusty, J.C. Winkler, and Sarah Winnicki-Smith.

Some organizations also donated photographs, for which we are very grateful: Max Pixel, the Royal Zoological Society of Scotland, the University of Washington Libraries, and the University of Wisconsin-Madison.

Thanks to the following individuals who allowed us to reproduce their diagrams: Markus Gusset, David Mellor, and Susan Hunt; Sandra Baker, Trudy Sharp, and David Macdonald; Emmie de Wit and Vincent Munster; Michael Manfredo, Tara Teel, Andrew Don Carlos, Leeann Sullivan, Alan Bright, Alia Dietsch, Jeremy Bruskotter, and David Fulton; Hannah Richie and Max Roser.

At various points in the process, graduate students or research assistants provided very helpful research. We'd like to extend our thanks to Kristian Cantens, Texas A&M University; Eliza Ruiz Izaguirre, University of Copenhagen; and Catarina Kissinger, Texas State University.

We would also like to thank the editors we worked with at Wiley-Blackwell, in particular Loan Nguyen and Monica Rogers, for their help, flexibility, and willingness to answer questions.

Finally, the authors would like to acknowledge that Chapter 18 is a substantially revised and updated version of Palmer, C. (2021) Should we provide the bear necessities? Climate change, polar bears and the ethics of supplemental feeding. In: Bovenkerk, B. & Keulartz, J. (eds) Animals in Our Midst: The Challenges of Co-Existing with Animals in the Anthropocene. Cham, Switzerland: Springer, The International Library of Environmental, Agricultural and Food Ethics, pp. 377–398, licensed under the terms of the Creative Commons Attribution 4.0 International License (http://creativecommons.org/licenses/by/4.0/).

In addition, we have the following acknowledgments as individual authors:

Clare Palmer thanks the Glasscock Center for Humanities Research at Texas A&M University for a one-semester residential fellowship enabling time to be freed from teaching. She also thanks the George T. and Gladys H. Abell Professorship at Texas A&M University for funding that covered travel, accommodation, and food for an author meeting in Texas. Jordan Hampton thanks the McKenzie Fellowship Program at the University of Melbourne for funding that covered author time. Christian Gamborg and Peter Sandøe thank the Department of Food and Resource Economics, University of Copenhagen, for covering the costs of travel for a meeting in Texas with all authors and for paying for a number of the photos used in the book.

PART

1

THE THEORY OF WILDLIFE ETHICS

Introduction

1

1.1 Introduction

The Amazon rainforests of South America are famously home to some of the most beautiful parrots in the world. Not surprisingly, there's demand, both locally and globally, to keep these birds as pets. This has led to a market in which parrots are trapped and traded even as, in many cases, wild populations decline. In Peru, for instance, although the parrot trade was banned in 1973, even in the year 2000 roughly 80 000–90 000 parrots were illegally captured annually (Gastañaga et al. 2011). Declining populations lead to rising prices, creating a positive feedback loop where parrot trapping is further incentivized. Indeed, researchers have found a significant positive correlation between the most profitable species in the wildlife markets of Amazonian Peru and those that are becoming increasingly rare (D'Cruze et al. 2021). Similar practices occur in other parts of South America (Figure 1.1).

Given the serious impact that the pet trade has had on parrot populations, there's been much discussion about how to discourage such practices (Ribeiro et al. 2019). Such discussion raises complex ethical questions. At the most fundamental level, the question is why, exactly, such practices *should* be discouraged. Aren't parrots just another resource, like oil or timber? Why shouldn't humans capture and sell them?

Wildlife Ethics: The Ethics of Wildlife Management and Conservation, First Edition. Clare Palmer, Bob Fischer, Christian Gamborg, Jordan Hampton, and Peter Sandøe.

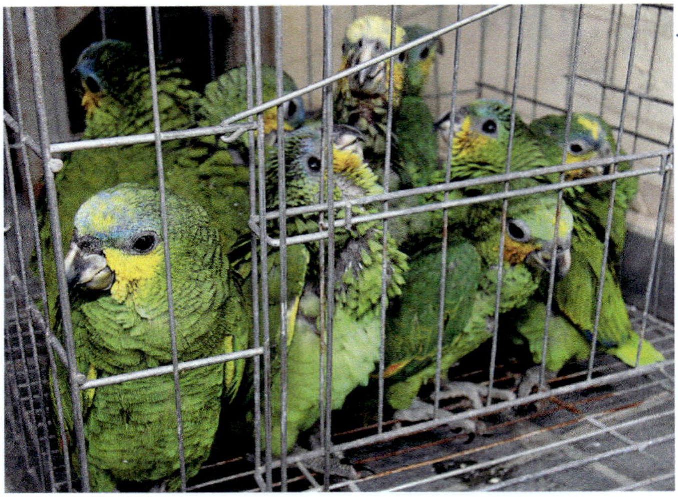

Figure 1.1 A cage full of wild parrots destined for the pet trade, seized by the Police in Brazil. *Source:* Joa Souza/dreamstime LLC/, reproduced with permission.

Granted, some populations and whole species of parrot are becoming scarce. But why does it matter whether parrot species decline or disappear? What's so concerning about the loss of species?

It's also worth asking whether it's fair to deny the many Indigenous parrot trappers of their income. After all, the Indigenous people who trap the parrots aren't responsible for the extensive habitat loss that's primarily causing the decline in parrot populations. Why should they bear the burden of actions from which other, often richer, people benefit?

Taking a different perspective, while trapping parrots may have consequences for populations, species, and the ecosystems of which they form a part, it also affects the welfare of *individual* parrots. There's considerable evidence that being captured and smuggled over long distances is highly stressful for wild parrots, and, despite the efforts of their handlers, birds regularly die in the process (Baker et al. 2013). Being kept in captivity also has welfare consequences; despite being highly social animals, parrots are often kept in small cages and confined alone. But then, how important is the welfare of wild animals? How far – if at all – should welfare be factored into decisions about how to manage populations of animals such as parrots, both in the wild and in captivity?

This book, *Wildlife Ethics: The Ethics of Wildlife Management and Conservation*, has been written to assist in thinking through questions like these. To explain what this book is about, it's helpful to look more closely at what the terms in our title mean. We'll start with "wildlife", for there's certainly no universally agreed definition of what's meant by the term. Most generally, "wildlife" is usually taken to refer to wild *animals* rather than to wild plants, fungi, bacteria, and so on (though these are obviously forms of wild life). Until the 1970s, wildlife was generally used as a synonym for "game" – animals hunted by people – but this use is in decline. Now, the term "wildlife" is most commonly applied to undomesticated animals living free in a natural environment.

However, there are obvious exceptions and boundary cases (and different interpretations of both "natural" and "domestication," which we'll discuss later in the book).

In this book, then, wildlife refers to free-living animals in natural environments, as well as in urban, suburban, and rural areas. We'll also include zoo animals since they are kept as representatives (and sometimes as potential saviors) of their free-living relatives and are generally bred to retain "wild" traits. We'll also include animals that belong to species generally thought of as wildlife but that live at the borderline of being farmed. Some game management practices, for instance, come close to animal husbandry in that the animals are given supplemental feed (e.g., feeding corn to white-tailed deer in North America). Some "wild" animals are even farm reared (e.g., civets and bear species kept in captivity for bile production in East Asia and gamebirds bred to be released for hunting in Europe). There are also "feral" animals, such as cats, pigs, and dogs/dingoes in Australia, which were once farmed or kept as companions but now live outside human support. And sometimes domesticated or "de-domesticated" animals are released to perform ecological functions as part of rewilding projects, such as cattle and horses in northern Europe.

All these borderline cases suggest that there's a wide gray area where animals are more or less wild, including feral, captive-bred, and heavily managed populations. These questions aren't simply terminological; they may well have legal and ethical implications. For instance, it's often thought that human responsibilities toward animals (such as whether sick animals should be treated) are partially determined by the kinds of relationships that humans have with them (Gamborg et al. 2016). However, for the purposes of this book, we'll adopt a broad understanding of wildlife that includes all these animals and untangle the details as we go through them.

In another sense, though, our use of the term "wildlife" in this book is less broad than it could be; we use the term to refer to *sentient* vertebrates (which is also the most common interpretation) for reasons we'll say more about below. By sentient, we mean animals with subjective experiences and inner lives: they can, for instance, consciously experience pleasure and pain, fear, hunger, and excitement. (Note that "consciously" here doesn't mean "reflectively." We assume that animals can have conscious experiences without the more sophisticated metacognitive abilities that humans possess.) This means that as we use the term, wildlife includes at least mammals, birds, reptiles, amphibians, and fish. While we recognize that some invertebrate animals are now widely agreed to be sentient – especially the cephalopod mollusks (such as octopods, cuttlefish, and squid) and decapod crustaceans (crabs, crayfish, etc.) – we won't focus on them in this book. The sentience of other invertebrates – such as insects – is not currently widely accepted, although there's uncertainty here (Lacalli 2022).

One reason for limiting the discussion to sentient animals is that they have a *welfare*, and animal welfare has become an important and complicating ethical consideration in recent discussions of wildlife ethics (Baker et al. 2013). We think that the focus on wild animals as individuals with their own welfare is an important new emphasis that this book brings to debates about wildlife management and conservation. Given the interest that both the public and many decision makers have in animals as individuals, it's increasingly difficult to settle controversies about wildlife by insisting only on the value of species, biodiversity, or ecosystems.

Two other things should be noted: by using the term "animals," we're not intending to imply that humans are *not* animals. They obviously are. However, it would have been clunky to refer to "other animals" or "nonhuman animals" throughout the book. For similar reasons, we have reduced the use of Latin species names to a minimum for ease of reading, including them only where there may be ambiguity about the wildlife species to which we are referring.

So much for wildlife; what about *ethics*? Most generally, ethics deals with questions about what one *should* or *ought* to do, ideas about what's right and wrong or good and bad, using terms such as values, duties, rights, responsibilities, and virtues. While the law often incorporates ethical standards, being ethical isn't the same as following the law; after all, many actions are ethically questionable but still legal. For example, using explosives to catch fish (blast fishing) was legal in Indonesia until 1985 (Fox et al. 2005). Moreover, being ethical isn't just about following one's feelings or intuitions, though both can indeed play important roles. In this book, we take ethics in a wide and inclusive way to involve reasoning about values and the rationales for holding those values, about the possible consequences that might follow from actions, about the interests and rights that might be at stake in a given situation, about individual virtue and character, and about people's aspirations for their societies.

We further take it that decision making about issues such as wildlife management and conservation should depend on being able to give justifying reasons that other people can understand and make sense of, even if they disagree, for reasons that they too can explain. Essentially, we understand wildlife ethics as reasoned dialogue about human management of, and relations with, wildlife that involves bringing to the surface values and ethical commitments that are otherwise often not made explicit. We attempt to be pluralistic in discussing these values and ethical commitments in this book. Thus, we acknowledge that there are many ideas about what's right and wrong, good and bad, which may not be compatible with our personal ethical stances (which also differ between us as authors). Our goal here is to be as even-handed as possible to clarify and analyze different ideas, theories, views, and beliefs – not to defend particular ethical positions.

Finally, then, what about "wildlife management and conservation"? Wildlife management can refer to two kinds of practices. It may involve *actively* manipulating factors such as species population size and density (abundance); location, habitat, and food supply; interactions between wildlife species; and interactions between wildlife and humans (Giles 1978). Or it may refer to more *passive*, hands-off forms of nonintervention, such as setting land aside, where that strategy has been deliberately chosen among alternatives (sometimes called "preservation").

Wildlife management can try to protect present or future levels of use, whether this involves consumptive practices (such as hunting and fishing, which, historically, were of primary importance) or nonconsumptive practices (such as making wild animals more visible for tourists). It can attempt to control unwanted wildlife, whether that means individual animals or entire populations. It can aim at protecting biodiversity in one of its many forms. More recently, wildlife management goals have expanded to include other environmental purposes, such as managing wildlife populations with the goal of influencing carbon cycling (Schmitz et al. 2018).

Let's focus a bit more closely on the idea of wildlife *conservation*, which we take to be a form of wildlife management. This term is important but confusing; in fact, there's no single, widely accepted definition of conservation (Soulé 1985). In its most general use, conservation – a word first recorded in the fourteenth century – has two broad meanings, nicely captured in the *Oxford English Dictionary* (OED 2021): "to prevent the wasteful overuse of a resource" and "to protect from harm or destruction." This double sense carried over into wildlife conservation. However, in the early twentieth century, one of these two meanings became associated with a different term: *preservation*. So, *conservation* meant something like using wildlife wisely, such that stocks could renew for the future (thereby "preventing wasteful overuse of a resource"), while *preservation* meant something like setting land aside entirely and protecting wildlife independently of its use (thereby protecting "from harm and destruction"). Now, however, this distinction is made less frequently; the term "conservation" is commonly used to cover both these senses.

Managing for wildlife conservation, then, might mean actively managing wildlife such that the wildlife can continue to be used in the long term. Or it might mean preserving wildlife more passively by setting land aside, deliberately not allowing wildlife to be used (or at least, not consumptively) in designated reserves, wilderness areas, and so on. More recently, though, as human impacts on wildlife have become more intense, both kinds of conservation have involved more active practices, such as habitat and ecosystem restoration, species reintroduction, and relocation for threatened species, and nonlethal population reduction methods such as fertility control for hyperabundant species.

Let's return briefly to parrot trapping in Peru. It's clear that multiple values are at stake in this case, including social justice, Indigenous groups' rights, the protection of biodiversity and species (since nontarget animals are also affected by the parrot trade), the value of animal lives and animal welfare, the flourishing of ecosystems, the esthetic value of the birds in and outside their natural habitats, and other humans' responsibility for extensive habitat destruction (Gastañaga et al. 2011). By making the parrot trade illegal, specific values, such as species protection, were prioritized over other values. In cases where wildlife use (e.g., hunting) *is* legal, other ways of managing a similar array of values will still need to be chosen. And although decision making about such cases will include social, political, and economic factors, the identification and prioritization of values are of central importance for wildlife management; this is likely to determine, for instance, whether the goal in any particular case should be something closer to sustained use or to complete protection. Questions about what matters, what's valuable, how to weigh these values, and how these values should be put into practice lie at the heart of wildlife management and conservation. We hope this book will be useful for those reflecting on such questions.

1.2 The Scope of the Book

While there are numerous books exploring ethical issues about animals in agriculture (e.g., Schlottmann and Sebo 2018), in research (e.g., Beauchamp and DeGrazia 2019), and a few about companion animals (e.g., Sandøe et al. 2015), this is the first book to attempt to develop a systematic account of the ethical issues related to decisions about managing and conserving wildlife. We recognize, of course, that such decisions are not only about ethics; they also involve economics, ecology, psychology, environmental science, politics, history, and so on. Ethics is just one piece of the puzzle. Still, it's an important piece that deserves a more thorough examination than has been common in the past. Our main aim is to explore the most important ways wild animals can be valued (or disvalued), different theories about how those values can guide practice and policy making, and to think through how these ethical perspectives could be applied to cases in practice.

As such, this book is designed to be useful to many constituencies. We've written it for students and scholars in many fields, including wildlife management, conservation biology, conservation social science, ecology, animal science, and veterinary medicine. We've also written it for wildlife professionals, practitioners, and stakeholders – people who manage, use, control, or protect wild animals or who are affected by those practices. Finally, we've written it for those who are simply interested in wildlife, and we've tried to ensure that the book is accessible. (For instance, we refrain from citing complex quantitative evidence relating to trends in wildlife populations.)

While the role of ethics is becoming increasingly important in wildlife conservation and management, few wildlife managers, conservation biologists, or veterinarians have any formal ethics training and may feel that they lack the tools to respond to these growing ethical concerns and to communicate about ethical issues. There are, of course, related books on specific wildlife controversies and on the problem of trade-offs in conservation (e.g., Woodroffe et al. 2005), some on politics and conflicts in conservation (e.g., Redpath et al. 2015), and some on particular values, including biodiversity and species values (e.g., Newman et al. 2017). However, there is no other book that looks at all these kinds of concerns through an ethical lens.

Trying to produce a book that aims to be helpful across so many different disciplines and professions is, of course, a huge project, especially given the number of wild animal species, the diversity in human cultures and societies, the number of different ecosystems and habitats, the many ways in which humans interact with them, and the multiplicity of values and ethical theories at stake. We therefore needed to restrict the scope of the project to make it more manageable.

To do this, we took our lead from some key ideas that have emerged from recent psychological research about human attitudes to animals – attitudes that have also influenced the shape that wildlife management and conservation has taken in practice. For instance, a significant body of psychological research suggests that, in general, people are much more positive about animals, particularly mammals, that they perceive to be more human-like and much less positive about animals perceived to be very unlike humans. An early (1980s) study, for instance, found that people were much more willing to pay to protect mammalian and bird species than they were to protect fish and spiders (Kellert 1986). There are generally ambivalent or negative responses to species perceived as threatening, such as large mammalian carnivores and venomous snakes.

The perceived cognitive capabilities of animal species also seem important; research suggests that the more cognitively developed an animal species is perceived to be, the less acceptable people consider it to be for humans to use or harm it (Knight and Barnett 2008). Esthetic features, broadly construed, are also important; indeed, researchers have found a strong correlation between esthetic preferences for a particular animal and willingness to protect it. Perceived ugliness seems to have a strong negative effect, while cuteness has a positive effect, especially mammalian facial traits: a round face, big eyes, and a small nose and mouth (Prokop and Randler 2018).

Such psychological research into responses to kinds of species aside, evidence is also mounting that broad changes in some societies – increasing modernization, urbanization, higher levels of education, and less direct reliance on wild animals for items such as food and fur – have led to substantial shifts in attitudes toward wildlife, especially among urbanites and suburbanites, particularly those located in western postindustrialized countries. These countries have seen a popular shift from the idea of human domination over wildlife and the belief that wildlife exists to serve human interests to the idea that wild animals are worthy of care and respect, an attitude called *wildlife mutualism* (Manfredo et al. 2016). Of course, care and respect for wild animals also have long histories in Indigenous communities around the globe. Still, because citizens of industrialized countries have an outsized degree of influence on the shape of contemporary wildlife use, management, and conservation, shifts in their attitudes are significant for present purposes.

This extremely brief summary of some important attitudes to wildlife tells us that while there are highly divergent public attitudes toward wildlife species, some factors are widely found across the populations interviewed, such as a bias in favor of cognitively sophisticated and esthetically pleasing animals, especially mammals, with some human-like features. These attitudes partly explain why there has been a taxonomic bias toward mammals in conservation practice (e.g., Clark and May 2002). Our book, to some degree at least, reflects these attitudes; we took the practical decision, given space limitations, to focus on mammals. To a lesser degree, however, we do also discuss the management of birds, such as the parrots with which we began this chapter, as well as reptiles and amphibians.

This narrowing of focus toward mammals has also, regretfully, led us to emphasize terrestrial rather than aquatic or marine wildlife conservation and management (with a few exceptions). There's much significant popular and scientific concern about marine wildlife conservation and management, of course, but including substantial material on marine ethical issues here would have made the book even more unwieldy than it is already. Marine wildlife ethics deserves its own volume. Likewise, invertebrate ethics would also make a fascinating book. While many of the same considerations would prove relevant, aquatic animals and invertebrates raise a host of questions of their own, including the difficulties of assessing fish and invertebrate welfare (and which invertebrates can be said to have welfare); the complex history and politics of industrial fishing; and the challenge of responding to the "invisible" problems of aquatic animal and invertebrate population decline (Cooke and Cowx 2004). Especially fish, but also increasingly insects, are now being farmed on a large scale, while insects such as mosquitoes are in the front line of research on genetic modification to reduce their capacity to carry disease. All these issues deserve ethical scrutiny; we hope others will develop texts that tackle the many significant questions that, unfortunately, must remain beyond the scope of the one we've written.

1.3 Structure of the Book

This book has two parts. In Part 1, we survey the values, ethical theories, and major value-laden frameworks and movements that have emerged throughout the history of wildlife management and conservation, concluding with a chapter on the challenge of navigating moral disagreement. In Part 2, we turn to a series of real-life wildlife case studies where we put the ideas of Part 1 to work (Figure 1.2).

Part 1 begins properly with Chapter 2, where we distinguish the range of ways in which people value and disvalue wildlife. Many of these values are what are called *instrumental values*: they are values derived from the *uses* that humans have for wildlife. There are also *disvalues*: some animals are seen as threats rather than resources (though, of course, some animals are both). Finally, some people argue that wild species, ecosystems, and/or animals have *intrinsic value* or *moral status* – value in themselves, apart from any use to humans.

Chapters 3–5 consider specific values associated with wildlife. In Chapter 3, we consider the value of the *wildness* of wild animals. That is, their wildness may itself be one reason why they matter. Next, also in Chapter 3, we examine the role of wild animals as contributors to and members of *ecosystems*. In Chapter 4, we look at two closely related ways of valuing wild animals: where they are valuable due to their contribution to biodiversity; and/or because of their embodiment of, or membership in, a particular

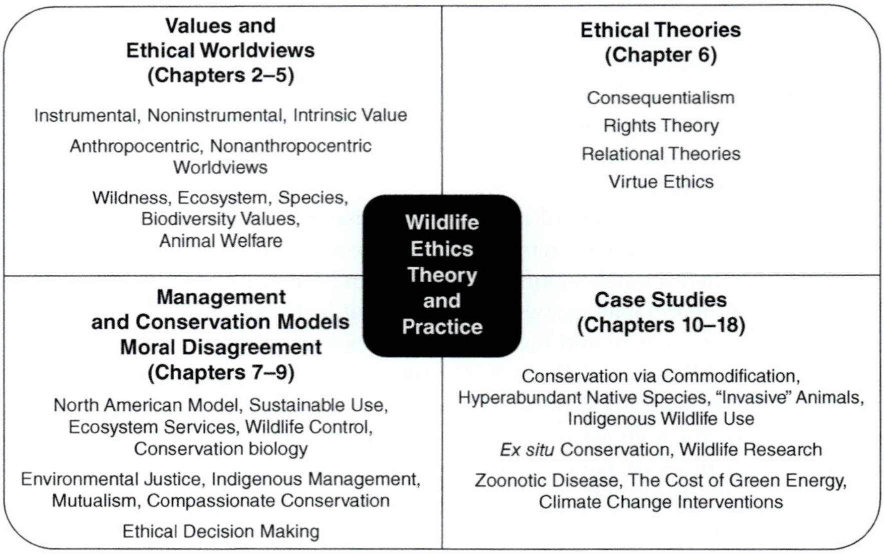

Figure 1.2 The book has two main parts: (a) the theory and (b) the practice of wildlife ethics. The first part examines values, ethical worldviews and theories, management frameworks, and how to deal with moral disagreements. All chapters in Part 1 include short, real-life examples to illustrate concepts and theories. In Part 2, a number of paradigmatic ethical case studies from around the world and across different wildlife species are developed to explore the ethical complexity of specific problems and controversies.

species. In Chapter 5, we consider the importance of animals as *individuals* (rather than as manifesting wildness, contributing to biodiversity, or being members of valuable ecosystems or species). Here, value is located in the *welfare* of wild animals and the significance that can be ascribed to their lives.

Chapter 6 turns toward ethical theory. Values are what *matter* – what's relevant to moral deliberations. Ethical theories take the next step by providing guidance about what to *do* with these values, including how to prioritize these values when making decisions. Here, we discuss consequentialist, rights-based, relational, and virtue-ethical theories.

Chapters 7 and 8 explore broader, value-laden management and conservation frameworks and movements that have been, or may become, particularly relevant to wildlife professionals. These frameworks and movements include a range of values and ethical commitments, not all of which are obvious at first glance, about how humans ought to relate to wildlife in various circumstances. Chapter 7 considers the development of the idea of conservation of wildlife as resources (in particular, the North American model of wildlife conservation); the control of unwanted wildlife ("pest management"); and conserving wildlife primarily to protect species and ecosystems, an approach found in conservation biology. Chapter 8 explores the growth of the environmental justice movement, its intersection with what's become known as the "new conservation" movement supporting Indigenous peoples' wildlife management, and the emerging "compassionate conservation" movement.

We close Part 1 in Chapter 9 by introducing some ways of approaching ethical decision making and dealing with moral disagreement. We consider how individuals might think through specific issues to make their own judgments. We then turn to the even more complex task of justifying decisions to others and making collective decisions that are sensitive to ethical concerns.

Part 2 comprises a series of case studies that go into much more depth than the shorter cases used to ground discussions in Part 1. Thus, in the second part of the book, we apply and develop the concepts, values, ethical theories, and management frameworks discussed in Part 1. We work at disentangling key values and ethical theories at stake and consider what they look like on the ground. Of course, we've had no option here but to be highly selective. Still, we have tried to demonstrate geographical breadth, think through a variety of different ethical problems, and take into account varied wildlife species. We have cases from all continents (except Antarctica) and include geographical regions such as tropical South America, southern Africa, Southeast Asia, northeastern North America, northern Europe, New Zealand, and the Arctic. We look at examples involving (in no particular order) rhinos, frogs, rats, parrots, bats, deer, pandas, whales, and polar bears. Here's a brief look at some of the issues we address in these case studies.

- Rhinos are threatened with extinction. If by establishing a legal, commercial rhino horn market in sub-Saharan Africa, the rhino species could be saved, would it be right to do so? (Chapter 10).
- When native species, such as white-tailed deer in North America, reach high densities in suburban areas, controversies about lethal management frequently arise. What values are at stake here? How should factors such as human convenience, ecological impact, and animal welfare be weighed against one another in the suburbs? (Chapter 11).

- Introduced animal species can have major negative effects on ecosystems, leading to systematic eradication campaigns, as in New Zealand. Should the protection of biodiversity and wildlife species take priority over individual animal lives and welfare? (Chapter 12).
- Ethical tensions arise when traditional practices of wildlife use, especially by Indigenous peoples, appear to conflict with other wildlife values such as species protection and animal welfare. Yet, isn't it a matter of justice for Indigenous groups, such as the Makah people in the US Pacific Northwest, to be able to continue traditional practices that predated colonialism, especially when they are not responsible for broader threats to wildlife species? (Chapter 13).
- Captive breeding and display in zoos are sometimes claimed to contribute to so-called *ex situ* wildlife conservation. One prominent example is the captive breeding of giant pandas in China and their display in selected zoos across the world. However, do captive breeding and display in zoos really achieve conservation goals – and in any case, do the conservation goals justify using captivity as the means? (Chapter 14).
- Wildlife research is an important activity that contributes to human understanding and may help work out ways to better protect species from extinction. But it can involve invasive means and technologies that negatively affect wild animals' welfare, such as clipping the digits of threatened frog species to reidentify them later. Can such practices be ethically justified by the conservation benefits they allegedly bring? (Chapter 15).
- Wild animals are not only of positive value to humans but can also affect human societies negatively through the interspecific spread of infectious diseases, such as Ebola, rabies, and HIV. How should this risk of disease spillover affect our ethical relationship with wild animals? Is the concept of One Health helpful here? (Chapter 16).
- Worldwide, energy demand is increasing while worries about climate change are becoming ever more acute. Most people welcome the fact that an increasing share of energy is produced by means of renewable energy such as wind power, rather than fossil fuels. However, the expansion of wind power can have significant impacts on wildlife, especially bats and birds. In these "green-on-green" dilemmas, where do ethical concerns about wildlife fit? (Chapter 17).
- Climate change is already having significant impacts on wildlife. While some species can adapt, others – especially specialist species or those in places where the climate is changing very fast, such as polar bears in parts of the Arctic – may need human assistance to survive. Should humans intervene to help such animals (especially given that people cause climate change)? Or would it be better to let nature take its course? (Chapter 18).

We end the book with an overall conclusion looking at the future of humans and wildlife, taking stock of current threats, trends in societal views, and emerging technological developments (Chapter 19).

1.4 The Authors

The authors of this book came together somewhat serendipitously and at a point when we were less fully aware of the range of expertise for which this project calls. We come from a variety of academic backgrounds. Peter Sandøe and Bob Fischer studied philosophy at both undergraduate and graduate levels; Clare Palmer studied theology and then completed a DPhil in environmental ethics; Christian Gamborg trained as a forester before taking a PhD in bioethics; Jordan Hampton trained as a veterinarian, developed a research portfolio in wildlife biology, and completed a PhD in animal welfare, spending five years subsequently as the Director of Ecotone Wildlife Veterinary Services.

We have subsequently come to specialize in different areas relevant to wildlife ethics. Bob Fischer is an Associate Professor at Texas State University, USA, where he focuses on animal ethics. Clare Palmer is a Professor at Texas A&M University, USA, where she works in environmental and animal ethics; both are based in Departments of Philosophy. Christian Gamborg is an Associate Professor in the Department of Environment and Natural Resources at the University of Copenhagen, where he specializes in ethical questions related to the environment, wildlife, rewilding, and land use. Peter Sandøe is a Professor at the University of Copenhagen, where he divides his time between the Department of Food and Resource Economics and the Department of Veterinary and Animal Sciences. He works on various issues relating to animal welfare, animal ethics, and veterinary ethics. Jordan Hampton focused his veterinary interests on wildlife, in particular on wildlife welfare and managing unwanted animals, and is currently a McKenzie Research Fellow at the University of Melbourne.

These backgrounds provide a strong foundation for working on a book on wildlife ethics. However, in other ways, our backgrounds and perspectives are clearly limited. We are all white. Four of us are male. Though we live across three continents – Europe, Australasia, and North America – we all come from postindustrial, relatively affluent countries. Our perspectives, then, inevitably reflect a Euro-American-Australian approach to wildlife management and conservation (though this is not, as we'll discuss in this book, by any means a unified approach). Moreover, our on-the-ground engagement with wildlife management and conservation is somewhat limited. Jordan Hampton has worked extensively with Australian wildlife, including programs that cull and use fertility control measures on wild and feral animal populations. Clare Palmer co-owns a 200-acre ranch in Texas that's being restored and managed for wildlife conservation. Peter Sandøe has advised the Danish government on a broad range of issues relating to animal welfare and animal ethics and currently serves as an expert advisor on animal welfare in rewilding projects to the Danish Minister for the Environment. Christian Gamborg has advised the wildlife management council in Denmark on issues related to the management of wolves and wild boars. Bob Fischer works with a think tank, Rethink Priorities, which assesses what causes should be prioritized for urgent funding, including causes involving wild animals. However, it remains the case that only one of us, Jordan Hampton, has done wildlife management or conservation work full time.

There are some fairly significant differences of views about the ethics of wildlife management and conservation between us, though we have not generally made our disagreements visible in the text. Although we take animal welfare seriously, this book largely takes a pluralistic form, not defending one particular value or theory. We aim to present a range of possible views and to explore what these look like when applied to different contexts. We have opted to be as even-handed as possible, only defending particular points of view when they are squarely within our expertise and not widely contested. We hope, therefore, that this book serves to improve discussions about wide-ranging ethical dimensions of wildlife use, management, and conservation. Writing it has certainly improved our own understanding.

1.5 How this Book Might Be Used

We have tried to write this book in an accessible style; it's aimed at those with no formal training in ethics (though we hope it also offers something to those with an ethics background who want to think more systematically about wildlife). We have tried to keep the discussion grounded by using case studies throughout, not just in the second half of the book but also within the chapters in the first half of the book. We hope that the accessibility and grounded nature of the book will encourage readers from very different backgrounds to engage with it, which makes it likely that the book will be approached in different ways and used for different goals.

Of course, some readers may want to sit down and read the whole book, but we imagine that most people will have specific interests in particular chapters or sections. So, for instance, someone wanting to explore the nature of animal welfare and its relevance to conservation could focus on Chapter 5; someone who wants to think about wildness value in the context of rewilding projects might focus on Chapter 3. For classroom use, individual case studies from the later sections of the book could be used for discussion, with relevant chapters from the first half of the book set as background reading.

We hope that *Wildlife Ethics* will help readers to reflect critically and constructively on their own ethical views, to better understand the contrasting positions others may take on these questions, and be better equipped to enter into a meaningful dialogue with others about ethical issues related to wildlife management and conservation.

References

Baker, S.E., Cain, R., Van Kesteren, F. et al. (2013). Rough trade: animal welfare in the global wildlife trade. *BioScience* 63 (12): 928–938.

Beauchamp, T. and DeGrazia, D. (2019). *Principles of Animal Research Ethics*. New York, USA: Oxford University Press.

Clark, J.A. and May, R.M. (2002). Taxonomic bias in conservation research. *Science* 297 (5579): 191–193.

Cooke, S.J. and Cowx, I.G. (2004). The role of recreational fishing in global fish crises. *BioScience* 54 (9): 857–859.

D'Cruze, N., Galarza, F.E.R., Broche, O. et al. (2021). Characterizing trade at the largest wildlife market of Amazonian Peru. *Global Ecology and Conservation* 28: e01631.

Fox, H.E., Mous, P.J., Pet, J.S. et al. (2005). Experimental assessment of coral reef rehabilitation following blast fishing. *Conservation Biology* 19 (1): 98–107.

Gamborg, C., Jensen, F.S., and Sandøe, P. (2016). A dividing issue: attitudes to the shooting of rear and release birds among landowners, hunters and the general public in Denmark. *Land Use Policy* 57: 296–304.

Gastañaga, M., MacLeod, R., Hennessey, B. et al. (2011). A study of the parrot trade in Peru and the potential importance of internal trade for threatened species. *Bird Conservation International* 21 (1): 76–85.

Giles, R.H. (1978). *Wildlife Management*. New York, USA: W.H. Freeman.

Kellert, S. (1986). Social and perceptual factors in the protection of animal species. In: *The Preservation of Species* (ed. B. Norton), 50–76. Princeton, USA: Princeton University Press.

Knight, S. and Barnett, L. (2008). Justifying attitudes toward animal use: a qualitative study of people's views and beliefs. *Anthrozoös* 21 (1): 31–42.
Lacalli, T. (2022, 1844). An evolutionary perspective on chordate brain organization and function: insights from amphioxus, and the problem of sentience. *Philosophical Transactions of the Royal Society B* 377: 20200520.
Manfredo, M.J., Teel, T.L., and Dietsch, A.M. (2016). Implications of human value shift and persistence for biodiversity conservation. *Conservation Biology* 30 (2): 287–296.
Newman, J., Varner, G., and Linquist, S. (2017). *Defending Biodiversity*. Cambridge, UK: Cambridge University Press.
Oxford English Dictionary (2021). https://www.oed.com
Prokop, P. and Randler, C. (2018). Biological predispositions and individual differences in human attitudes toward animals. In: *Ethnozoology* (ed. R.R.N. Alves and U.P. Albuquerque), 447–466. London, UK: Academic Press.
Redpath, S., Gutiérrez, R., Wood, K., and Young, J. (2015). *Conflicts in Conservation*. Cambridge, UK: Cambridge University Press.
Ribeiro, J., Reino, L., Schindler, S. et al. (2019). Trends in legal and illegal trade of wild birds: a global assessment based on expert knowledge. *Biodiversity and Conservation* 28 (12): 3343–3369.
Sandøe, P., Corr, S., and Palmer, C. (2015). *Companion Animal Ethics*. Oxford, UK: Wiley.
Schlottmann, C. and Sebo, J. (2018). *Food, Animals and the Environment: An Ethical Approach*. New York, USA: Routledge.
Schmitz, O.J., Wilmers, C.C., Leroux, S.J. et al. (2018). Animals and the zoogeochemistry of the carbon cycle. *Science* 362 (6419): eaar3213.
Soulé, M. (1985). What is conservation biology? *Bioscience* 35 (11): 727–734.
Woodroffe, R., Thirgood, S., and Rabinowitz, A. (eds) (2005). *People and Wildlife: Conflict or Co-Existence?* Cambridge, UK: Cambridge University Press.

2 Valuing Wildlife

2.1 The Value of Tigers

Fewer than 5000 individuals of the two main subspecies of tigers, the Continental tiger and the Sunda Island (Sumatran) tiger, remain in the wild, and the majority of them are found in India. Tigers no longer live in an estimated 96% of their historic range and three subspecies have already become extinct: the Caspian tiger from western Asia, and the Javan and Balinese tigers that once lived in Indonesia (Yamaguchi et al. 2013). Because they are so rare, tigers are classified as endangered by the International Union for the Conservation of Nature, and trade in tigers or their body parts is internationally banned under the Convention on International Trade in Endangered Species. In many countries where wild tiger populations remain, tigers are expensively (and expansively) protected in reserves, sometimes involving the relocation of human populations. Owing to such protective measures, some wild tiger populations are slowly increasing, especially in India where they are also used to attract tourists (Figure 2.1), but others, including the critically endangered Malaysian populations, are nonetheless declining towards extinction (Jhala et al. 2021).

In contrast to wild populations of tigers, however, captive populations are thriving. There are around 5000 captive tigers in the United States alone (World Wildlife Fund 2014)

Wildlife Ethics: The Ethics of Wildlife Management and Conservation, First Edition. Clare Palmer, Bob Fischer, Christian Gamborg, Jordan Hampton, and Peter Sandøe.

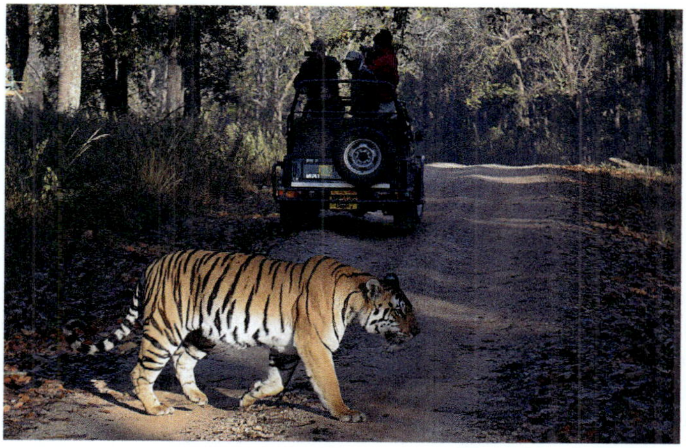

Figure 2.1 A tourist jeep closely approaching a wild tiger in an Indian national park. *Source:* MaxPixel.net/CC0 1.0.

and perhaps 8000 captive tigers in Asia, the majority in China (Abbott and Van Kooten 2011). Far more tigers exist in captivity than in the wild. In the USA, while a small number of tigers are on display in zoos accredited by the American Zoological Association (AZA) (for more discussion of the role of zoos in conservation, see Chapter 14), the rest are kept in roadside zoos or as exotic pets in private households. In East and Southeast Asia, many captive tigers are kept in what are widely labeled tiger farms, sometimes for entertainment but also contributing to markets in tiger parts (Dinerstein et al. 2007).

That humans hunt, keep, display, trade, breed, and protect tigers, both in and from the wild and in captivity, suggests that they are seen as extremely valuable to us, in a variety of ways. Many – although not all – of these values are what are called *instrumental values*: they are values derived from the *uses* humans have for tigers (Latombe et al. 2022). These use values explain some tiger declines in the wild as well as why tigers are kept in captivity. But their decline in the wild is also due to other factors, including loss of habitat and reduced availability of prey owing to human expansion into tiger territory.

Another reason for the decline of tigers is what we might call an instrumental *disvalue*: tigers are not only resources, they are also threats – they kill people or prey on livestock on which people depend for their livelihood. Often, this results in long-standing, negative human–wildlife relationships, sometimes called human–wildlife conflicts, where tigers may be killed to protect humans from, or to avenge, tiger attacks. The latter phenomenon is known as retaliatory killing targeted on large carnivore species globally (Inskip et al. 2014), as well as other wildlife species associated with significant disvalues (e.g., infectious disease; see Chapter 16).

Finally, alongside these instrumental values and disvalues, it's also sometimes claimed that tigers have *intrinsic value* or *moral status*; that what matters about tigers isn't just whether they are useful or threatening to humans, but also that they have some kind of independent value in themselves (Latombe et al. 2022). Such claims, though, raise another crucial distinction in the ways people may value wild animals – either as *individuals* or as valued *species*. So, when someone maintains that tigers have intrinsic value, they may mean that each individual tiger, because it is a living, feeling being, has intrinsic value. Alternatively, however, they may mean that the tiger species *as a whole* has such value, and individuals have value because they are members of that valuable species. As we'll see throughout this book, concern about killing or harming *individual animals* is often very different from worrying about threats of extinction to a *whole population* or *species*. A species might, after all, go extinct without any individual species member being harmed or killed by humans; and harming individual species members could, in some cases, help a species to survive (for instance, by confining individual species members for the purpose of captive breeding, as discussed in Chapter 14).

Understanding the ways in which tigers (or any other wild animals) are valued is central to wildlife ethics. Numerous attempts to categorize such values exist. Many such categorizations have been proposed by economists, who understand these values mainly in terms of different kinds of preference satisfaction, measured in terms of people's willingness to pay or to accept compensation to access, promote, or protect such values. These economic categorizations are very useful and we'll draw on these ideas and economic terminology below. However, we'll also talk about related *ethical* ideas, which often reflect rather different commitments, commitments not reliant on preference satisfaction and willingness to pay.

2.2 Instrumental or Use Value of Wildlife

Let's begin by thinking about use value or instrumental value, most naturally illustrated by money. Suppose that someone has a \$100 bill. That's valuable to the person who owns it, but it probably isn't *any particular bill* that the person values. If the person had the opportunity to exchange the \$100 bill for five \$20 bills, they would probably be indifferent to the trade. In other words, the person doesn't care about the \$100 bill itself at all; they care about what the bill can do for them in terms of the goods and services it can secure. Something that's of instrumental value is useful because it can get someone what they want. If they can get that same thing some other way, then that's just as good.

Wild animals have this kind of instrumental or use value to humans in multiple ways; this usefulness is captured in the term "wildlife resources." Following a standard economists' distinction, in the following we've divided such use values into direct use and indirect use, and further subdivided direct values into consumptive and nonconsumptive values. Starting with direct consumptive values, we'll talk about these different categories in turn.

2.2.1 Consumptive Use Value

The most obvious benefits humans gain from wild animals are in terms of direct consumptive use, where wild animals are killed and their bodies consumed or used in other ways. Tigers are an obvious example here (rhinos are another; see Chapter 10). One of the reasons for the decline in tiger populations has been the demand for tiger body parts in traditional Chinese medicine; this demand has driven tiger poaching and an extensive illegal traffic in tiger parts (Abbott and Van Kooten 2011). While tiger hunting is outlawed almost everywhere due to the scarcity of tigers, the hunting of other wild animals for meat, hide and fur, horns, and tusks is commonplace across the world. Among high-latitude human communities, such as Indigenous communities in Siberia and Alaska, fur and hides are valued for their warmth, water resistance, and durability. And there are many communities where meat from wild animals is an important protein source. One study surveyed nearly 8000 households across the Global South and found that 39% of them (extrapolated to ~150 million households) eat wild meat (Nielsen et al. 2018). It's worth noting that while the term "bushmeat" is sometimes used as a catchall phrase for the meat of wild animals, it's nearly always used with negative connotations to refer to practices in the forests and savannas of sub-Saharan Africa. By contrast, when supermarkets in Australian cities sell kangaroo meat (see Chapter 5), no one calls it bushmeat, though the product fits the definition.

2.2.2 Nonconsumptive Use Value

However, not all direct uses of wild animals are consumptive in the sense that the animals are used up – literally, consumed – in the pursuit of the activity. Wild animals can also be valued for *nonconsumptive use*. An obvious example is where wild animals are a spectacle; humans enjoy *watching* them. Looking at, photographing, and filming wild animals in their native habitat is a key element of many vacations and other recreational pursuits – for instance, safaris to seek wild-living tigers in reserves in India (Figure 2.1) – and also day-to day wildlife walks or birdwatching. Wildlife documentaries are another form of nonconsumptive use. Looking at wildlife, of course, applies to captive as well as wild-living animals. Wherever tigers are on display, for example, they attract an interested and excited human audience – whether that's a tiger farm in Southeast Asia or a US roadside zoo. Opportunities to be fascinated and entertained by wild animals are part of their enduring, nonconsumptive instrumental value.

Wild animals also attract interest as educational devices and as the subjects of scientific research, both in captivity and in the field. Sometimes, wild animals are used consumptively in research (for instance, when killed as part of an educational or research project); more commonly, animals are captured, trapped, tracked, watched, filmed, or followed. In parts of India, for instance, remote wildlife cameras are used in tiger-based citizen science projects both to help local people learn about the tigers and to gather data about the number and behaviors of local tigers.

Wild animal species can also carry various different kinds of *cultural and symbolic* value. Some of these values seem to fit fairly comfortably into nonconsumptive use values. For instance, the tiger has high cultural value in China, where every 12th year is the auspicious Year of the Tiger and where tigers are understood to symbolize power and strength (Abbott and Van Kooten 2011). The bald eagle is the national symbol of the United States owing to its majestic appearance and because it was believed, through its sweeping flight, to embody freedom.

It's worth noting, though, that being a culturally important symbol as a *whole* species doesn't necessarily bestow protection on *individual* species members; it's because of the symbolic power and strength tigers carry, after all, that the parts of individual tigers have become so important in Chinese medicine. However, some cultural and spiritual values don't seem to be instrumental or resource based, even in the nonconsumptive sense. We'll consider these cultural values together with *esthetic* value below.

The idea of resources can be interpreted more broadly than just being available to deliver well-defined products and services. It's possible to care about large herbivores such as elephants or moose, for instance, not (or not only) because they can be directly used as game, where they are subsequently turned into food or ornamental products. People may also value wild animals because they have more indirect, but extremely important, ecological functions.

2.2.3 Indirect Ecological Instrumental Values

Wild animals may be of more *indirect* instrumental value to humans via the roles they play in ecosystems. The most straightforward example might be the members of what are termed keystone species – species thought to be critical to particular ecosystems taking the form they do (Mills et al. 1993). Keystone species include apex (top) predators such as gray wolves. It's been claimed that their reintroduction to Yellowstone National Park significantly altered the entire ecosystem (Ripple and Larsen 2000). Keystone species also include animals referred to as ecosystem engineers, such as Eurasian beavers (reintroduced to Scotland and Denmark in order to help restore lost habitats for other species and so to increase ecosystem diversity [Gamborg and Sandøe 2004]). Wild animals that are not members of keystone species may still have important roles in ecosystems, even though those roles are not fully understood. Ecosystems are themselves instrumentally valuable, insofar as they provide humans with "ecosystem services" such as water filtration, watershed protection, and carbon sequestration (see Chapter 7). (Economists sometimes call these nonmarketable values.) Wild animals, then, are of indirect instrumental value as partial constituents of such valuable ecosystem processes.

2.3 Nonuse Values of Wildlife

Alongside use or instrumental values, economists have also identified a category of nonuse values, sometimes also called 'passive use values' (although there's some disagreement between models as to what falls under nonconsumptive use values and nonuse values). The kinds of values identified here are also helpful for thinking about the ways in which wildlife can be valued ethically.

2.3.1 Option Value

Option value is sometimes described as a *passive* use value because it doesn't abandon the idea of use (even consumptive use) altogether. Rather, option value refers to the value of not using something *now*, but instead keeping it as an option for possible use in the future. In economics, option value is primarily understood in terms of willingness to pay – that is, willingness to pay to withhold the use of some resource now to ensure there's an option to use it in the future. So, for instance, people may be willing to pay to protect tigers now and not to drive them to extinction, so that it's possible to access their instrumental value (e.g., being able to photograph them in a wildlife reserve; Figure 2.1) in the future. This kind of option value can be interpreted in terms of human wellbeing on a relatively short time scale. That is, even though it might improve the wellbeing of some individuals to hunt tigers to extinction now, it's rational *for those same individuals* to maintain tiger populations in case they want to use them later on.

In general, option value appears to be closely related to sustainable wildlife management (see Chapter 7) where hunting is restricted in the present to ensure that there's a sufficiently large wild animal population for continued use down the line.

2.3.2 Bequest Value

Like option value, bequest value doesn't reject all use in the future, whether consumptive or nonconsumptive. Here, though, the users are *future* people. The idea is that it's valuable to ensure that future generations are bequeathed access to a resource but doing so requires restraint in the present. This idea can be found (though the phrasing here could be taking both option and bequest value into account) in US legislation, where wildernesses:

> shall be administered for the use and enjoyment of the American people in such manner as will leave them unimpaired for future use and enjoyment as wilderness.
>
> (US Wilderness Act 1964, p. 1)

Again, in economics, bequest value is measured in terms of willingness to pay – for instance, in terms of the satisfaction that present generations gain from paying to protect wildernesses for the use of future generations. Many ethicists, however, maintain that in making this argument, economists are putting the cart before the horse. That is, wildlife ought to be preserved for future generations not just on account of the satisfaction that it would bring *present* generations to benefit future generations, but because of the positive impact that such preservation would have on the wellbeing of future people themselves. Our willingness to pay for the wellbeing of future generations may, therefore, be seen as a reflection of what we owe to them.

The philosopher John Nolt (2015), for instance, argues that just as distance is irrelevant to the value of individual human beings (people are not of greater moral significance because they are born in London rather than Lahore), so time is also irrelevant. Thus, someone born in 2000 has the same moral significance as someone born in 2100. So, if access to wildlife resources, wilderness experiences, and seeing charismatic species such as tigers are regarded as important to *present* human beings, then present generations have a moral responsibility to ensure that these opportunities are also available for *future* generations to experience.

2.3.3 Existence Value

In economics, existence value is measured by what people are willing to pay for the feeling of satisfaction of knowing that some being, place or thing continues to exist, even if they will never visit it or experience it for themselves. In the context of wild animals, this means something like a person's willingness to pay for the satisfaction gained from the continued existence of the Sumatran tiger species, even if the individual does not have the possibility or lacks any intention of ever going to Sumatra or visiting a Sumatran tiger in a zoo (Latombe et al. 2022). (This could be understood as the limit case of nonconsumptive use, where the use is simply the benefit of knowing that the animals are there, but we'll follow the economists in separating the ideas.)

Such feelings of satisfaction do count for something in ethics (since they would constitute satisfied preferences, or boost happiness, either of which can be argued to be important for welfare; see Chapter 5). However, it could also be argued here that economists, in putting forward this notion of existence value, are in fact grasping at a distinct yet related idea that ethicists call *intrinsic* value. According to this idea, the continued existence of a wild animal species (like the Sumatran tiger) matters in its *own right* and not because it is instrumental to creating human satisfaction or pleasure. We'll return to this idea shortly. First, we'll consider both esthetic value and the ways in which wildlife may bring instrumental *disvalues* – that is, the *negative* impacts of wildlife on human societies.

2.3.4 Esthetic and Related Values

Esthetic value is an important component of the way wildlife is valued. One thing that's important about tigers is how they appear – the controlled savagery of their faces, their glossy fur with its intricate patterning. The esthetics of the tiger was the inspiration for a famous poem, William Blake's *The Tyger*, from the Romantic period (1794):

> Tyger Tyger, burning bright, / In the forests of the night, / What immortal hand or eye, / Could frame thy fearful symmetry?

Esthetic values may be so important that changing the way a species appears – such as dehorning rhinos to protect them from poachers – could change their value for tourism (see Chapter 10). Esthetic values associated with wildlife may not only be about the value of individual species members or the appearance of an animal; whole landscapes in which wild animals play a part – the herds of caribou on snowy North American plains, the African Serengeti teeming with large ungulates, or brightly colored tropical fish surrounding a Pacific Ocean coral atoll – may be esthetically valued. And people don't only esthetically value what they *see*; smells, textures, and sounds, such as the melodies of the dawn chorus in spring, may also be important. (Reduced birdsong, for instance, has been one of the losses associated with native bird species extinctions in New Zealand; see Chapter 12.)

Economists frequently place esthetic, cultural, and spiritual values in the category of nonconsumptive use values. Here, wildlife satisfies human preferences in important cultural, spiritual, and esthetic ways. Without denying that *some* esthetic value may be like this, most environmental estheticians argue that esthetic judgments arise from more complex relationships between object and subject. If that's so, then esthetic value seems to be more than just about satisfying our preferences, which is why we're suggesting here that it falls into a separate category. On some recent accounts, esthetic value can best be understood as a form of *relational* value, inasmuch as part of what it means for us to flourish as humans is to esthetically experience and appreciate entities in our environment (Muraca 2016). It may even be that esthetic qualities can be valued intrinsically (see section 2.5). In addition, as Emily Brady (2003) argues, the intensity and multisensory nature of esthetic experience may underpin or stimulate ethical responses to protect what is valued esthetically, leading us to think about what Holmes Rolston III (2002) calls the relation between beauty and duty.

The argument that esthetic values can't easily be pigeon-holed into nonconsumptive use values also applies to some cultural, symbolic, and spiritual values. Cultures can be understood as systems of meaning, the ways in which people make sense of and find patterns in the world around them. In this way, cultural and spiritual belief systems about our relations with nature are formed (Goodin 1992). On some cultural and spiritual views, nonhuman nature, not least some wild animals, can be thought of as sacred or totemic. This idea is found in many Indigenous and tribal cultures where local communities set aside areas and protect animals for spiritual reasons (Milton 1999). These kinds of values can move far beyond both direct and indirect use, and may take relational or even intrinsic forms of valuation.

2.4 Wildlife and Instrumental Disvalue

So far, this chapter has discussed the multiple ways in which wild animals are of instrumental or relational value to us. However, when thinking about wildlife management and conservation, we also need to think about the ways in which wildlife is of *negative* value – where it has what we might call instrumental *disvalue*. These disvalues can be so serious that they threaten human lives or are of major economic or ecological significance; or they may alternatively be more of a nuisance. Many of these disvalues will be considered in much more detail in later chapters (see Chapters 11, 12, and 16). For instance, Jones et al. (2008) estimate that between 1940 and 2004, zoonoses from wildlife accounted for approximately 43% of emerging infectious human diseases. Since these diseases can severely affect the welfare of humans, causing suffering, death, and economic and social turmoil, they obviously constitute a major disvalue.

While less concerning than zoonotic transmission in terms of scale, wild animals may also pose threats of attack to humans and domesticated animals. The most common threat is of snakebite (Figure 2.2); an estimated 5.4 million venomous snakebites are received by people each year (World Health Organization 2021), of which between 20 000 and 94 000 are deadly. Less common are attacks by big cats such as tigers, other large mammals including moose, hippos and elephants, large crocodilian reptiles, and sharks (although it's worth noting that domestic dogs kill far more people, approximately 25 000 each year). Although wild animal attacks can be sensationalized, they do present significant threats to human safety and, as mentioned above, can also lead to retaliatory killings of particular "guilty" individual wild animals (Inskip et al. 2014).

Other instrumental disvalues or threats posed by wild animals are economic. Wild animals, including mammalian herbivores and frugivorous (fruit-eating) birds, may damage and consume crops and grazing intended for humans and domesticated animals. Wild pigs and elephants can move *en masse* over land, trampling and destroying crops. In some countries, this kind of threat can significantly undermine the subsistence abilities of rural populations, posing real concerns for human welfare (Mackenzie and Ahabyona 2012).

Threats to human safety and to human structures and crops from animals such as tigers and elephants are not just material and visible; they are also psychological and emotional. Living around predators and animal crop-raiders can generate feelings of

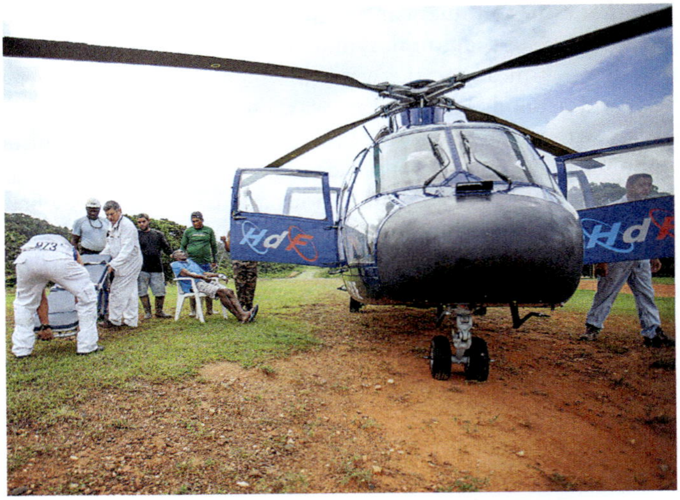

Figure 2.2 A human victim of venomous snake bite is evacuated to a hospital via helicopter in French Guiana. *Source:* Courtesy of Laszlo Kupi.

stress, fear, and anger and negatively shape the ways in which people live their lives, even if such attacks never actually materialize.

Finally, where wild animals have nowhere else to go, or where human-created environments are attractive to them, they may end up living alongside humans and behaving in ways that humans regard as a nuisance. Macaques and seagulls may steal and pester for food; coyotes in suburban areas may prey on companion animals; the creation of lightly treed suburban lots with ornamental planting and tree-edge habitat attracts and sustains "overabundant" deer populations (see Chapter 11). This kind of wild animal nuisance, while not threatening to human welfare or economies on the scale of other threats, is still a significant instrumental disvalue posed by wild animals.

So far, then, we've looked at many ways in which wildlife can be instrumentally valuable to us or instrumentally disvalued by us, essentially taking a human-centered or *anthropocentric* ethical worldview (see more in section 2.4). However, some of the most important ways in which wildlife is valued, especially in relation to wildlife management and conservation, are not instrumental at all.

2.5 Wildlife and Intrinsic Value

The idea of wild nature, including wildlife, having *intrinsic* value has always been at the heart of debates about conservation. It appears in some of the classic texts of conservation biology, such as Michael Soulé's landmark paper *What is conservation biology?* (1985) and the article *Principles of Conservation Biology* published by the Education Committee of the Society for Conservation Biology (Trombulak et al. 2004). (See also Chapter 7.)

But what's meant by the term "intrinsic value"? In order to think about different possible meanings, let's go back to tigers, and consider the case of Nadia. Nadia is one of the tigers in the Bronx Zoo in New York City. She became well known in 2020 as one of the big cats in the zoo that contracted COVID-19.

Let's suppose that someone is a frequent visitor to the Bronx Zoo and is very fond of Nadia in particular. When this person hears that Nadia has contracted SARS-CoV-2 (the virus causing COVID-19), they are deeply worried about Nadia's wellbeing. We could say that this person cares about Nadia because they regard her as having intrinsic value. What might be meant by saying this?

One possible meaning is that the person values Nadia as an *individual* in a certain way – intrinsically. Nadia is being valued as an end in herself, not because of her instrumental value to the person doing the valuing, or to the zoo, or to people in general. Intrinsic value in nature is often described like this: "Intrinsic values are those values of nature itself, independent of any usefulness to humans" (Trombulak et al. 2004, p. 1182). So, if this person says they value Nadia intrinsically in this sense, they aren't valuing her, for instance, because they find Nadia entertaining or because it excites them to see Nadia roaring in her enclosure. The person values her intrinsically, in herself – as Nadia. If something happened to her, replacing her with another tiger wouldn't make up for the loss. No other tiger – nor any other animal – could substitute for her.

But another possible meaning is that the person values Nadia as a *member of the tiger species*. So understood, the tiger *species* is being valued intrinsically, independently of any usefulness the continued existence of the species might have. This might be, for instance, because a world with tigers is believed to be better than a world without tigers and that nothing could substitute for tigers were they to become extinct. In that case, what matters is not the continued existence of Nadia as an individual but the continued existence of generations of tigers, of which Nadia is just a transient part.

Another question here concerns the *origin* or *basis* of intrinsic value. That is, *why* do things have intrinsic value? So far, we've discussed intrinsic *valuing* as something a human being does: it's a certain expression of someone's evaluative attitudes and judgments (Sandler 2012). This subjective idea of intrinsic value is similar but not identical to the economist's idea of existence value; unlike existence value, intrinsic value isn't about the valuer's *experience* of satisfaction from the protection of the value. The idea of intrinsic value is sometimes associated with the view that what has intrinsic value is outside the market and cannot and should not be priced (see the discussion of markets for rhino horn in Chapter 10). In any case, the crucial issue we're interested in here is whether subjective valuing is all there is to intrinsic value.

Suppose it is. Then, it follows that if no one were to value some thing or being intrinsically, it would have no intrinsic value. However, many conservationists and some ethicists argue that certain individuals (including human individuals) and/or species and ecosystems are valuable in themselves, valuable *objectively*, even if their value is not acknowledged. For instance, it has been claimed that "Species have value in themselves, a value neither conferred nor revocable, but springing from a species' long evolutionary heritage and potential" (Soulé 1985, p. 731). On this view, species have *objective* intrinsic value even if no human actually recognizes or confers this value; so, for instance, on

Soulé's view, the tiger species would have intrinsic value, even if no one cared about tigers. This view has an obvious attraction for conservationists; it gives a straightforward justification for maintaining that someone is just mistaken if they don't value, say, species, or ecosystems, or whatever's at issue.

This view, which Ronald Sandler (2012) calls the "natural historical view" of intrinsic value, has had some influence in environmental ethics, especially in the work of Rolston (1988; 2002). In a criticism of the view that intrinsic value is *merely* subjective, Rolston (1988) argued that it's strained and inadequate to treat value in nature like the light in a fridge – when humans are looking, the value lights up, and when they shut the door, the value disappears. He rejects the view that "[v]alues in flora and nonsentient fauna are only 'on' when humans are perceiving them, and otherwise 'off'" (Rolston 1988, p. 116). For Rolston, value in nature and in evolutionary processes is objective, not dependent on human perceptions; humans recognize value, rather than constituting its source.

However, Rolston's position is contested within environmental ethics. Many find the idea mysterious, raising questions about what exactly objective intrinsic value *is* and how to discover it if it's out there. Fortunately, we do not need to pursue this theoretical discussion about the origins of intrinsic value in detail here. In most cases, it works well just to take intrinsic value as referring to something that matters in itself, irrespective of where this value is thought to originate.

2.6 Moral Status and Moral Significance

Sandler (2012) also identifies yet another account of intrinsic value, which he calls the inherent worth view. In this view, things or beings have intrinsic value if they can be argued to have a good of their own, if things can go better or worse for them (again, independently of whether someone actually values them in this way). So, for instance, as we'll see in Chapter 5, some people argue that wild animals as individuals have intrinsic value because they can have positive or negative welfare, which is to say that things can go better or worse for them – even if no human actually values their welfare (perhaps because they are regarded as pests).

A number of philosophers argue in response that just because some being has a good of its own does not mean that it should be protected. For instance:

> The gardener knows what it is for greenfly to flourish, recognizes they have their own goods, and has a practical knowledge of what is good for them. No moral injunction follows. She can quite consistently believe they ought to be done harm.
>
> (O'Neill 1992, p. 131)

By John O'Neill's argument, a further reason is needed beyond just *having* a good to explain why that particular good should be protected or promoted – or, otherwise put, why that being should be given *moral status*.

Moral status (or alternatively, moral considerability or moral standing; these terms mean essentially the same thing) is an expression used to refer to things, systems, or beings that are thought to matter in their own right, normally because they have interests, and because it can be argued that there's reason to think that these interests matter. As Mary Anne Warren puts it:

> If an entity has moral status, we may not treat it in just any way we please; we are morally obliged in our deliberations to give weight to its needs, interests or wellbeing. Furthermore, we are morally obliged to do this not merely because protecting it may benefit ourselves or other persons, but because its needs have moral importance in their own right.
>
> (Warren 1997, p. 3)

In the context of environmental values, a number of different kinds of things or beings have been taken to have moral status. Aside from individual animals (which we'll discuss more in Chapter 5), some philosophers – called *biocentrists* – argue that all individual living things have moral status; others – *ecocentrists* – contend that whole ecosystems or species have moral status (for more, see Chapters 3 and 4). In almost all these discussions of moral status, what's at stake are beings or things that can in some sense have a good of their own and can be made worse or better off – not necessarily in terms of conscious experience, but in terms of flourishing, meeting (even unconscious) goals, or being healthy.

The relationship between intrinsic value and moral status is potentially confusing because, as we've seen, the term "intrinsic value" is used in different ways. If intrinsic value is used in the inherent worth sense of Sandler (2012), where something has a good of its own, it's relatively close to moral status. But if intrinsic value is taken to mean subjective, noninstrumental value, then the two do not necessarily overlap – something can be valued intrinsically without thinking that it has moral status. So, for instance, it might be argued that Vermeer's painting from 1665, *Girl with a Pearl Earring*, has noninstrumental intrinsic value; it has value in itself – nothing could substitute for it if it were lost or destroyed. However, this doesn't imply that the painting has moral status, since a painting doesn't have a good of its own and can't be made better or worse off. (It would be odd to say of a restored painting that its *welfare* had been improved, for instance.) This also seems to be true, in the environmental context, of biodiversity or states of affairs like wildness. Such items can certainly be valued intrinsically, but if moral status requires having a good of one's own, it's going to be very difficult to argue that either has moral status (see Chapters 3 and 4).

That something or some being has moral status doesn't, in itself, tell us how *much* it matters in comparison with other things or beings. But it can be argued that some things or beings with moral status matter more or have greater *moral significance* than others. The most common justification for attributing more or less moral significance has to do with the kinds of *capacities* that a being has. Some people argue that in the case of animals at least, possessing more complex cognitive capacities provides a reason for greater moral significance. On this view, while both a lion and a human have moral status, the human's moral significance is greater because of her more complex cognitive capacities. If there is a conflict of interests between a human and a lion (and those interests are equally significant from the point of view of the beings concerned, and nothing else of moral importance is at stake), then fulfilling the human's interests should take priority over fulfilling the lion's interests since the human has greater moral significance.

It's worth noting, though – as we'll discuss below – that if we were to base differences in moral significance on individuals' complex cognitive capacities alone, then some *humans* would appear to be much more morally significant than others. Babies, for instance, would appear to be worth less than adults. What's more, entities such as individual plants or ecosystems, even if they were attributed moral status, couldn't have much moral significance at all, since they lack complex cognitive capacities.

This discussion of moral considerability and significance brings us to views in which either only human individuals matter in their own right or humans matter much more than everything else. These views form part of a group of positions that fall under the heading of *anthropocentrism*.

2.7 Anthropocentrism

If wildlife and other elements of the nonhuman world are valued only in an instrumental sense, that is, solely according to their use value for humans, this seems to correspond to what's called a human-centered or *anthropocentric* worldview. The majority of environmental ethicists are critical of this position; indeed, it's often argued that this kind of anthropocentrism is "the ethical attitude the field [of environmental ethics] was created to overcome" (Minteer 2008, p. 58). One example of a prominent rejection of anthropocentrism can be found in an article published by Eileen Crist in *Science* in 2018. Here, she maintains that an anthropocentric worldview "forms the tacit postulate from which people source meaning and justification to disregard virtually any limitation of action or way of life in the ecosphere and toward nonhumans" (Crist 2018, p. 1242). Crist, like many environmental ethicists, sees anthropocentrism as the ethical part of a broader position of human exceptionalism on which humans are regarded as being unique among organisms, and divided from other animals by their exceptional capacities and abilities (Srinivasan and Kasturirangan 2016).

However, some clarifications are necessary here. Anthropocentrism can be understood in different ways and comes in different degrees. Here, we've been taking it to mean an ethical position within which wildlife and other elements of the nonhuman world either matter only inasmuch as they are useful to humans and affect human interests (a *strong* form of anthropocentrism, although in practice it may be ameliorated by the various nonuse values of nature described above). However, it can also be interpreted to mean the view that while humans matter more than anything else, some other beings do have a lesser degree of intrinsic value or moral status (a *weaker* form of anthropocentrism).

On a strongly anthropocentric view, causing the extinction of species and the loss of wildlife habitat would be ethically unproblematic if doing so served human interests. On a weakly anthropocentric view, human interests are always more important than wild animal interests or the value carried by species, but there could be occasions when some highly significant wild animal interest or species value could trump a trivial human interest. So, for instance, killing endangered but beautifully plumaged birds in order to put feathers on fashionable ladies' hats, as was common in the US in the nineteenth century, could be justified on strong anthropocentric arguments (unless killing the endangered birds seemed overall to be against human interests). However, it's unlikely to be justifiable on weaker anthropocentric accounts, where the continuance of the species, together with the birds' serious interests in going on living, might together outweigh human interests in attractive hats.

Someone who is *nonanthropocentric*, in contrast, maintains that the nonhuman world or some aspects of it, including wild animals, do matter ethically and that their significance can be high – and according to some, as high as the significance of human beings. However, different forms of nonanthropocentrism are also possible. After all, the term "nonanthropocentrism" just tells us that humans are not the only beings of moral importance; it does not tell us what the other things are. There are a number of possible nonanthropocentric candidates, e.g., that all sentient beings, all individual living organisms, or all species and ecosystems are of moral importance (the latter two positions are biocentrism and ecocentrism, respectively).

Before concluding this chapter, we should also note a significant debate about the importance or usefulness of the distinction between anthropocentrism and nonanthropocentrism, at least in a policy context. Some argue that views like that of Crist (2018), in which anthropocentrism is seen as the root of all environmental evils, are profoundly mistaken and, that if anthropocentrism were to be developed in a sufficiently wide-ranging way, including all the values discussed earlier in this chapter, it would result in very similar policy prescriptions to nonanthropocentrism, but without adopting nonanthropocentrism's controversial commitments.

To explain this a bit more, let's consider the influential *convergence hypothesis* of philosopher Bryan Norton (1991). Norton argues that the reason environmentally destructive policies are implemented is not because anthropocentrism is the dominant ethical view. Instead, it's because our ideas of anthropocentrism – in terms of what really matters for humans – are far too limited and shortsighted. If the indirect use and nonuse instrumental values discussed earlier in this chapter were taken more seriously – including the significance and range of the ecosystem services on which human beings rely, as well as the option and bequest value of various dimensions of the natural world – then radically different policies would be adopted. And, Norton (1991) argues, those long-view anthropocentric policies would be very similar to the ones that someone who defended a nonanthropocentric view would also adopt. So, there should be convergence – at least at the policy level – between suitably wide-ranging anthropocentric policies and those flowing from nonanthropocentrism. If that's the case (he suggests), why bring more controversial, nonanthropocentric views into a policy-making arena dominated by anthropocentric economists, social scientists, and so on, since doing so causes unnecessary disagreement? On this argument, the chances of environmental collaborations leading to successful policy changes would be improved if everyone worked with anthropocentric approaches.

Unsurprisingly, this kind of view has been rejected by many nonanthropocentrists on both empirical and theoretical grounds. *Empirically*, it's been argued that even rich and extended anthropocentric views would diverge from nonanthropocentric views in some policy cases – for instance, that some kinds of climate engineering might benefit humans overall but be very harmful to some wildlife (Nolt 2011). Second, it's also been argued that Norton's claim that nonanthropocentric views are more controversial and less popular is false. There's certainly some empirical evidence of unease among conservationists, at least, about a move toward anthropocentric justifications for conservation (Fisher and Brown 2014). Moreover, the rise in "wildlife mutualism" – where the coexistence of humans and wild animals in a kind of community is fundamental (see Chapter 8) – suggests that there's a growing popular movement away from regarding wildlife in purely anthropocentric terms.

Third, there have been several *theoretical objections* to anthropocentrism on the grounds that valuing the natural world intrinsically is in itself important. After all, in the case of humans, even if the same policy outcomes from an approach that instrumentalizes others could be achieved, it could nevertheless be maintained that this would be the wrong way to treat people. In another version of this objection, Katie McShane (2007) argues that nonanthropocentrism is important in terms of our attitudes and feelings toward the nonhuman world; she makes the case that love, respect, and awe, for instance, are not compatible with regarding the nonhuman world in the terms of anthropocentrism. A possible rejoinder from a weakly anthropocentric view could be that heeding values such as respect and awe for wild animals is essential to achieving long-term human wellbeing. They are relational values, part of what makes us flourish as humans. But this debate is far from settled.

2.8 Conclusion

This chapter has introduced some key ideas about valuing wildlife, focusing on different kinds of instrumental and intrinsic value. It has also explored the concepts of anthropocentrism and nonanthropocentrism. In the next two chapters, we'll look in more depth at specific ideas regarding wildlife and conservation values: the value of wildness, biodiversity, ecosystems, and species.

References

Abbott, B. and Van Kooten, G.C. (2011). Can domestication of wildlife lead to conservation? The economics of tiger farming in China. *Ecological Economics* 70 (4): 721–728.

Blake, W. (1794). The Tyger. In: Songs of Experience.

Brady, E. (2003). *Aesthetics of the Natural Environment*. Edinburgh, UK: Edinburgh University Press.

Crist, E. (2018). Reimagining the human. *Science* 362 (6420): 1242–1244.

Dinerstein, E., Loucks, C., Wikramanayake, E. et al. (2007). The fate of wild tigers. *BioScience* 57 (6): 508–514.

Fisher, J. and Brown, K. (2014). Ecosystem services concepts and approaches in conservation: just a rhetorical tool? *Ecological Economics* 108: 257–265.

Gamborg, C. and Sandøe, P. (2004). Beavers and biodiversity: the ethics of ecological restoration. In: *Philosophy and Biodiversity* (ed. M. Oksanen), 217–236. New York, USA: Cambridge University Press.

Goodin, R.E. (1992). *Green Political Theory*. Cambridge, UK: Polity Press.

Inskip, C., Fahad, Z., Tully, R. et al. (2014). Understanding carnivore killing behaviour: exploring the motivations for tiger killing in the Sundarbans, Bangladesh. *Biological Conservation* 180: 42–50.

Jhala, Y., Gopal, R., Mathur, V. et al. (2021). Recovery of tigers in India: critical introspection and potential lessons. *People and Nature* 3 (2): 281–293.

Jones, K.E., Patel, N.G., Levy, M.A. et al. (2008). Global trends in emerging infectious diseases. *Nature* 451 (7181): 990–993.

Latombe, G., Lenzner, B., Schertler, A. et al. (2022). What is valued in conservation? A framework to compare ethical perspectives. *NeoBiota* 72: 45–80.

Mackenzie, C.A. and Ahabyona, P. (2012). Elephants in the garden: financial and social costs of crop raiding. *Ecological Economics* 75: 72–82.

McShane, K. (2007). Anthropocentrism vs. nonanthropocentrism: why should we care? *Environmental Values* 16 (2): 169–186.

Mills, L.S., Soulé, M.E., and Doak, D.F. (1993). The keystone-species concept in ecology and conservation. *BioScience* 43 (4): 219–224.

Milton, K. (1999). Nature is already sacred. *Environmental Values* 8 (4): 437–449.

Minteer, B.A. (2008). Anthropocentrism. In: *Encyclopedia of Environmental Ethics and Philosophy* (ed. J.B. Callicott and R. Frodeman), 58–62. Farmington Hills, USA: Gale.

Muraca, B. (2016). Relational values: a Whiteheadian alternative for environmental philosophy and global environmental justice. *Balkan Journal of Philosophy* 8 (1): 19–38.

Nielsen, M.R., Meilby, H., Smith-Hall, C. et al. (2018). The importance of wild meat in the global south. *Ecological Economics* 146: 696–705.

Nolt, J. (2011). Nonanthropocentric climate ethics. *WIREs Climate Change* 2: 701–711.

Nolt, J. (2015). *Environmental Ethics for the Long Term: An Introduction*. New York, USA: Routledge.

Norton, B. (1991). *Towards Unity amongst Environmentalists*. Oxford, UK: Oxford University Press.

O'Neill, J. (1992). The varieties of intrinsic value. *Monist* 75 (2): 119–137.

Ripple, W.J. and Larsen, E.J. (2000). Historic aspen recruitment, elk, and wolves in northern Yellowstone National Park, USA. *Biological Conservation* 95 (3): 361–370.

Rolston, H. (1988). *Environmental Ethics*. Philadelphia, USA: Temple University Press.

Rolston, H. (2002). From beauty to duty: aesthetics of nature and environmental ethics. In: *Environment and the Arts: Perspectives on Environmental Aesthetics* (ed. A. Berleant), 127–141. New York, USA: Routledge.

Sandler, R. (2012). Intrinsic value, ecology, and conservation. *Nature Education Knowledge* 3 (10): 4.

Soulé, M. (1985). What is conservation biology? *BioScience* 35 (11): 727–734.

Srinivasan, K. and Kasturirangan, R. (2016). Political ecology, development, and human exceptionalism. *Geoforum* 75: 125–128.

Trombulak, S.C., Omland, K.S., Robinson, J.A. et al. (2004). Principles of conservation biology: recommended guidelines for conservation literacy from the education committee of the society for conservation biology. *Conservation Biology* 18 (5): 1180–1190.

US Government (1964). *US Wilderness Act*. Washington, D.C., USA: US Government.

Warren, M.-A. (1997). *Moral Status: Obligations to Persons and Other Living Things*. Oxford, UK: Oxford University Press.

World Health Organization (2021). Snakebite envenoming. www.who.int/news-room/fact-sheets/detail/snakebite-envenoming

World Wildlife Fund (2014). More tigers in American backyards than in the wild. www.worldwildlife.org/stories/more-tigers-in-american-backyards-than-in-the-wild

Yamaguchi, N., Driscoll, C.A., Werdelin, L. et al. (2013). Locating specimens of extinct tiger (*Panthera tigris*) subspecies: Javan tiger (*P. t. sondaica*), Balinese tiger (*P. t. balica*), and Caspian tiger (*P. t. virgata*), including previously unpublished specimens. *Mammal Study* 38 (3): 187–198.

The Value of Wildness and Ecosystems

3

3.1 Why Are Wild Animals Valued?

In Chapter 2, we looked at different possible ways of valuing wildlife, in particular the framework ideas of *instrumental* and *intrinsic* value. In Chapters 3–5, we're going to flesh out these ideas, examining how wild animal management and conservation might be justified. Such justifications are diverse – they concern animals as part of ecosystems, as populations, as species, and as individuals – and these different levels of concern can come into conflict with one another, forcing people to make difficult choices.

In this chapter, we'll first consider the value of wild animals just inasmuch as they are *wild*. Wildness, in other words, can itself be one reason why they are important. Next, we'll think about the role of wild animals as contributors to, and members of, ecosystems, something we briefly touched upon in Chapter 2, which we termed indirect ecological instrumental value. Since the flourishing of ecosystems has been a longstanding environmental concern, the role of wild animals as contributors to ecosystems is also highly significant. In Chapter 4, we'll look at two further, closely related ways of valuing wild animals: either they are valuable due to their contribution to biodiversity, or because of their embodiment, or membership, of a particular

Wildlife Ethics: The Ethics of Wildlife Management and Conservation, First Edition. Clare Palmer, Bob Fischer, Christian Gamborg, Jordan Hampton, and Peter Sandøe.

species. Finally, in Chapter 5, we'll consider the importance of animals as *individuals*. Here value is located in the *welfare* of wild animals and the significance that can be ascribed to their lives.

Thinking about wild animals in all these ways requires bringing scientific debates in biology, ecology, and animal cognition into conversation with value theory and ethics. Differences in interpretations of the relevant science (for instance, about the relevant dependencies within ecosystems), as well as different prioritizations of the various values at stake, underpin many of the ethical conflicts around the management and conservation of wild animals. Nevertheless, these values also provide reasons as to why people should want to conserve them at all.

We'll start with a controversial case in conservation ecology, that of a nature restoration (or perhaps rewilding) experiment – the Oostvaardersplassen in the Netherlands. Disagreement over how to manage this area brings all these values into play – as well as the conflicts between them.

3.2 The Case of Oostvaardersplassen

Formed from a polder – land reclaimed from the sea – in the Netherlands, and originally intended for an industrial scheme, Oostvaardersplassen was repurposed as a habitat for waterfowl in the 1970s. After some years, concerns grew that a dense tree canopy would make the land no longer suitable for waterfowl. The most obvious way to prevent a forest growing was by introducing large herbivores (Figure 3.1). However, the introduction of domesticated herbivores, such as regular cattle, seemed inappropriate in an area that was supposed to be "wild." And, with the exception of red deer, the relevant native wild herbivores – that is, aurochs (a kind of wild cattle) and tarpan (a kind of wild horse) – are now extinct.

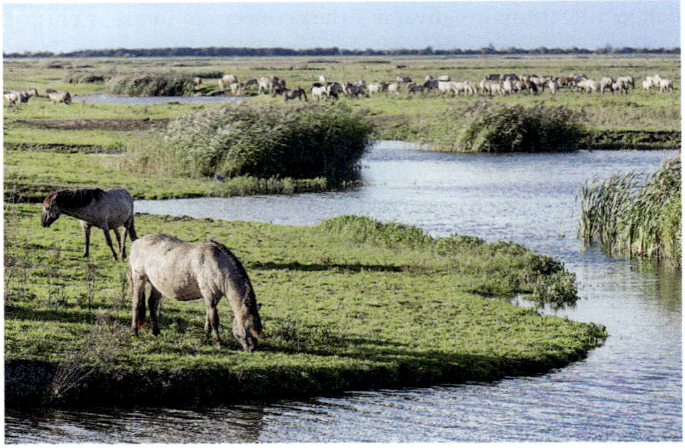

Figure 3.1 "Wild" horses in the Dutch national park, Oostvaardersplassen. *Source:* T.W. Van Urk/Dreamstime LLC, reproduced with permission.

To prevent the forest from growing while keeping Oostvaardersplassen wild, conservation managers decided to introduce nonnative herbivores alongside red deer that could perform a functionally similar role to extinct wild herbivores, without needing constant human intervention and supervision. To this end, Heck cattle and Konik ponies were introduced to Oostvaardersplassen (Lorimer and Driessen 2014). Heck cattle are varieties "back-bred" from domestic cattle to look more like the extinct aurochs, based on the belief that aurochs' genes are still present in existing domestic cattle. (That said, despite being very hardy, they do not closely resemble aurochs.) Konik ponies are small, tough horses from Poland, once believed to be genetically descended from the likewise extinct tarpan (though recent genetic evidence now suggests otherwise [Lovász et al. 2021]).

After being introduced to Oostvaardersplassen, these herbivores successfully performed the intended ecological functions: they prevented formation of a closed forest canopy and ensured the continuation of the wildfowl habitat. But they also reproduced, creating larger herbivore populations. Oostvaardersplassen is not very large: about 22 mile^2 (57 km^2), with fencing preventing herbivores from dispersing elsewhere (Kopnina et al. 2019) and no large predators. Consequently, the populations of Heck cattle, Konik ponies, and red deer increased even though the resources to feed them did not. Without human management or natural predators, winter resources ran low and in cold winters some of the herbivores died.

A reactive management approach was adopted – that is, reacting to changes after they happen (e.g., killing deer once they were very sick or starving). The most notable incident occurred during the hard winter of 2017–2018, when an estimated 3300 animals (more than 60% of the herbivores there) starved and were ultimately shot (Theunissen 2019). Since Oostvaardersplassen is located near roads and railways, these starving animals attracted public attention – and outcry. The response (in 2018) was to increase active management of the reserve, which involved culling and keeping herbivore numbers down to a fixed number of 1500. However, the policy was, and unsurprisingly still is, also controversial – especially among the general public and various animal welfare and animal rights organizations (Sandøe et al. 2022).

3.3 Key Ethical Questions: Wildness and Ecosystems

The Oostvaardersplassen rewilding case, while important in itself, raises deeper questions about wildlife management and conservation. Some of these questions are about definitions: What counts as a "wild animal"? Can de-domesticated animals like Heck cattle be called wild? If animals are fed, culled, or relocated – that is, actively managed – are they, and is Oostvaardersplassen as a whole, really wild?

Some questions are more ethical in nature. For instance: why, and to what extent, does wildness matter? Should wildlife be managed to sustain certain ecosystem states, or to increase or maintain biodiversity? Is one state of an ecosystem (say, a closed forest canopy) "worse" than another state (say, an open grassland)? How should decisions be made about what's "good" for an ecosystem (and why does *that* matter)? Should the welfare of individual Konik ponies or Heck cattle be taken into account alongside conservation values? Generally, starving wild animals aren't offered assistance; what's more, they have traditionally been managed in terms of whole populations, not as individuals. Is there any reason the Oostvaardersplassen should be regarded as an exception?

These kinds of questions will recur through this chapter and the next two chapters. Here, we want to use Oostvaardersplassen to provide an overview of conceptual and ethical issues that the ideas of "wildness" and "ecosystems" raise for wildlife management and conservation.

The meaning and value of wildness matter for wildlife ethics. First, some debates (about wild animals and wild places and ecosystems) have at their root disagreements about what's actually meant by "wild" (and this may indeed be one element of what makes the Oostvaardersplassen case so difficult). Second, it's sometimes argued that moral responsibilities toward wild animals are different from those owed to domesticated animals (e.g., Donaldson and Kymlicka 2011; Palmer 2010). For instance, while people generally agree that farmers and equestrians should get veterinary treatment for sick cattle and horses (and this, indeed, may be legally mandated in some places), it's not usually argued that vets should be assigned to wild areas to treat sick wildlife. This is not only because of the strain this would place on resources, but more importantly because it's widely thought that there are no obligations to intervene when wild animals are sick or dying (or at least not when humans have no responsibility for the situation). And third, in the case of land and ecosystems in particular, wildness, or naturalness, is frequently believed to carry some special value that should be protected.

When thinking about why wildlife matters, it's also important to consider the ecosystems or ecological communities (we won't distinguish between these terms for now) in which they are located. We'll focus on less managed, or "wilder" ecosystems rather than agricultural or urban ecosystems. Wild animals partly constitute such systems, and they have important ecological functions in them. On some accounts, as we'll see below, the reason why wild animals matter is because they are crucial to ecosystem flourishing.

We'll begin by exploring the idea of wildness and why it might matter ethically. Then we'll consider the value of wilder ecosystems or ecological communities, drawing throughout on the work of one of the leading historical thinkers in this area, Aldo Leopold.

3.4 Wildness

The term "wildness" can be used in many ways and applied to different beings, states, and places – which, not surprisingly, can lead to confusion. What's more, it rarely makes sense to think of wildness as a binary property – for instance, that a place is either wild or it's not. In most of its uses, wildness can be thought of as falling along a scale of "more" or "less," though how this scale is measured depends on what wildness is thought to be.

3.4.1 Wild Animals

Let's start by thinking about what might be meant by "wild" when we talk about "wild animals" or "wildlife," elaborating on our discussion in Chapter 1. In common parlance, "wildness" is often seen as standing in opposition to "tameness." According to this usage, a "wild" animal keeps a distance from humans or is afraid, uncomfortable, or aggressive in response to human interaction. A second sense of "wild" (perhaps more useful to our discussion) is wild as "not domesticated." Animals that are wild in this sense make their own reproductive choices and are genetically adapted to their wild environments – unlike domesticated animals, which are bred by humans and have become adapted genetically to a life close to humans. So, for instance, in the Oostvaardersplassen case, the extinct aurochs in their original context could be understood as wild in the sense of being undomesticated, while current cattle breeds, by contrast, are domesticated rather than wild.

This does, though, raise questions about where to place the Heck cattle. Are they wild or domesticated? They have been bred by humans, but the goal is to place them in environments where they would be largely unmanaged. Sometimes this is called "de-domestication," the term for an intentional process, undertaken over many generations, of trying to turn animals that are domesticated in terms of human breeding into animals that can live independently, without human support (Gamborg et al. 2010). Similarly, "feral" animals are domesticated animals that now live independently of human provision and make their own reproductive choices, though not generally because humans intended them to do so (Hill et al. 2022). These animals seem to fall along a wildness–domestication spectrum.

Finally, there exists a set of interpretations of animal wildness that centers on the idea of autonomy, where animals are relatively free from human constraints and are able to do what they want – to the extent possible. So, in this sense wild animals are simply animals that are free to express or fulfill essential capacities and behaviors and, in species where this applies, purposes and desires, without being inhibited by humans. Human constraints here could be intentional (for instance, by caging animals) or much more indirect (for instance, where the presence of humans or domesticated animals leads to animals foraging in the dark rather than the daytime due to hunting pressure or disturbance) (Lewis et al. 2021). On this interpretation, centered on autonomy, any animal, whether domesticated, de-domesticated or feral, if they are living reasonably free from human constraints, is wild.

All these senses of "wild animal" are useful, but one thing that emerges from considering them together is that an animal can be wild in one sense while not being wild in another. An animal could be simultaneously tame, undomesticated, and able to make autonomous choices. Think, for example, of a friendly free-roaming squirrel that has chosen (in some sense at least) to feed on hand-fed nuts from local householders. This multiplicity of meanings points to the importance of sorting out what's being valued in any particular case, especially since wildness in all these senses is scalar (so, an animal can be more or less wild in several senses simultaneously). To clarify this further, we'll look at the Oostvaardersplassen case again in more detail below.

Before doing that, though, we need also to think about what's meant by wildness in *places*, what we could think of as ecosystems or "wild nature."

3.4.2 Wild Places, Wild Nature

Understanding what's meant by the wildness of places, or "wild nature," is tricky because, as with wild animals, there are different senses of wildness at play here. Almost all these different understandings agree that wildness is best interpreted as being relational: the *absence* of some kind of relationship between human beings and other parts of the world (e.g., a relationship of creation, control, influence, or impact).

Perhaps the best known account of wild nature is found – as the concept of wilderness – in the text of the US Wilderness Act of 1964:

> A wilderness, in contrast with those areas where man and his works dominate the landscape, is hereby recognized as an area where the earth and its community of life are untrammeled by man, where man himself is a visitor who does not remain ... an area retaining its primeval character and influence ... which is protected and managed so as to preserve its natural conditions ... with the imprint of man's work substantially unnoticeable.
>
> (US Wilderness Act 1964, p. 2)

Here a wilderness, understood as the wildest kind of place, is interpreted as being apart from humans, not controlled, changed, shared with, influenced, or even touched by people (though, interestingly, according to the definition, a place with these characteristics can still be *managed* to preserve "natural conditions").

This sense of wildness as being "apart from humans" is very common, and used much more generally than just in referring to areas designated as wildernesses. However, it has also given rise to significant objections. One set of objections rejects the dualism implicit in this idea of wildness; because it is defined in terms of the *absence* of certain relations with humans, the suggestion seems to be that humans are not part of nature at all. Other objections concern the application of this human-exclusive idea of wildness to particular places, where it may both deny the influence and management of past generations of humans and lead to the exclusion of present humans who live or use the land. It's argued that wildness in this sense ignores the presence and effects of traditional or Indigenous hunter-gatherers and agriculturalists (Fletcher et al. 2021) and hardly applies at all in other human-dominated landscapes, such as much of Europe (Callicott and Nelson 1998).

William Cronon (1995) suggests, in a much taught and reproduced paper *The Trouble with Wilderness*, that (rather as discussed in the context of wild animals) wildness in nature more broadly could be understood as a kind of "otherness," the autonomy and independent existence of the nonhuman world. In this sense, wildness can be found anywhere; it's about elements of the nonhuman world "doing their own thing," perhaps unpredictably, and outside human intentional management or control (see also Birch 1990). This would apply regardless of whether the place concerned is an urban, suburban, rural, or other landscape.

One further issue here makes a practical difference for wildlife management and conservation: namely, whether the wildness being aimed at is thought of as *historical*, concerning the degree of human involvement in how things or states originated, or *compositional*, where what matters is achieving a particular desired "natural" end-state, irrespective of human involvement in getting there. In the context of ecological restoration, for instance, wildness value is understood as present in the "end-state" or compositional sense when restoration has put back what would have been there had humans not carried out some earlier destruction in the first place (Gamborg and Sandøe 2004). Historical wildness, on the other hand, is where wildness is understood as an absence of human influence on the origin/making of an ecosystem. So, an ecological restoration, even if deliberately designed to be identical to what was present before some destruction, would not be wild in terms of *origin*, just because it was designed by humans (Elliot 1982). However, inasmuch as it closely resembles what would have been there without human intervention, it could be seen as wild in terms of *composition*.

What emerges from this discussion is that depending on how wildness is defined, what it means to *protect* wildness can vary dramatically.

3.4.3 Wildness Value

People may also *value* wildness in different ways, as we saw in Chapter 2. Some ways can be thought of as falling into the category of nonconsumptive use value (such as the emotional and spiritual experience of being able to visit places and seek or see animals that pursue their own, independent lives). Others may be nonuse values, such as the bequest value of knowing that future generations will also be able to have similar experiences, or the existence value of knowing that such wild places and beings exist even if one is never going to see them. Many people also deeply value wild places and animals intrinsically – they judge that such places are important in themselves, independently of any experiences or satisfactions that visiting them, or knowing that they exist, could bring.

That many people have a deep, strong, and stable subjective value for something such as wildness (Sandler 2012) may itself provide a reason for protecting it. However, this isn't necessarily an overriding reason. (After all, people can be very deeply attached to all sorts of trivial things, such as reality TV shows.) The reason most commonly given for protecting wildness is that doing so is a form of human humility and restraint, where humans "acknowledge that limits to human mastery and domination of the world are imperative" (Hettinger and Throop 1999, p. 13). In a related argument, Ned Hettinger (2005) has also taken up the idea of wildness as nature's autonomy, arguing that it's arrogant and hubristic to try to dominate and manage the purposeful and self-driven living world around us. Of course, these arguments too are controversial. For instance, it isn't clear what might be meant by the "autonomy" of nature, nor why this autonomy ought to be respected. Letting nature take its course, after all, produces significant human and nonhuman suffering through infectious diseases, disasters, and so on.

This discussion seems to have taken us quite far from Oostvaardersplassen. But we're now in a better place to analyze some of the value concerns underlying that case.

3.5 Back to Oostvaardersplassen

Oostvaardersplassen is often described as a rewilding project (Kopnina et al. 2019). Given that the land was claimed by people from the sea, however, its wildness is not, strictly speaking, either historical or compositional; it has a human origin, and no former composition of plants or animals to recapture. However, in a looser sense, wildness of both kinds seems to have been important in how the project was conceived: the goal was to create habitat for wildfowl resembling other habitat lost in the region (a weaker kind of compositional wildness) and once the wildfowl were established, to step back and allow human influence to wash out and natural processes to take back over (an idea of historical wildness that could strengthen over time). Difficulties arose, however, when the natural processes pushed toward a forest, meaning that the habitat for important wildfowl species began to vanish. Without intervention into natural processes, these wildfowl species would disappear.

This worry about species loss underpinned the decision to introduce herbivores to contain forest growth. But bringing in domestic cattle or horses – domestic both in the sense of having been selectively bred, as well as adapted to live alongside and be supported by humans – would mean a loss of compositional wildness and, since they would need ongoing care, make it difficult to step back later and just let natural processes take over (Gordon et al. 2021). This would imply a loss of potential historical wildness too. But wild herbivores, such as aurochs and tarpan, being extinct, weren't an option. Introducing Heck cattle and Konik horses was the compromise. Even though they wouldn't be there without human introduction, they had been bred to resemble the tarpan and aurochs, were able to perform similar ecosystem functions, and were relatively hardy.

How wild are these animals? To the extent that Heck cattle, for instance, are left to roam in Oostvaardersplassen, they are wild in the sense of being reasonably autonomous (though not entirely so, since they are prevented from migrating by fences); and they are what we've called "de-domesticated" in that they were intentionally and selectively bred to live independently of human intervention and to be as similar as possible to the undomesticated aurochs. But the autonomy and independence of the Heck cattle and Konik horses did not spare them from high mortality over hard winters due to insufficient food resources. It's worth noting, though, that these losses were primarily due to the small size of Oostvaardersplassen and the lack of predators; had the animals been able to roam freely, their survival rates might have been better. After all, enclosed in a small enough space, many tarpan and aurochs may not have survived the winter either.

But with the deaths of so many animals, arguments about intervention began. Those against intervention maintained that such a death rate would be expected also in wild, unrestricted populations in a hard winter, and that the value of natural processes – historical wildness value – should be prioritized. Those in favor of intervention pointed out that the Heck cattle and Konik horses were not really wild animals in any important sense of the word. Using the definitions above, after all, these animals were bred by people; people were responsible for putting the animals in the reserve; their autonomous movement was constrained by fences; and their ecosystem lacked predators (Sandøe et al. 2022). Since they weren't really "wild" animals, they should be assisted in one way or another, or at least euthanized rather than left to protracted deaths from starvation.

This analysis highlights another important idea: some believe that what's owed to an animal differs depending on whether or not it's thought to be wild. Although there are cases where people feed wild animals during a hard winter (usually either those valued as game animals or wild birds), there's not thought to be any general *duty* to do so. However, if a farmer were to allow her horses to starve to death in a hard winter, she would be thought to have done something wrong (and in many countries, there would be legal ramifications). De-domestication, though, muddies the waters here; it's unclear whether these animals should be treated according to the norms of agriculture or those of wildlife management. The former generally takes care of individuals; the latter has historically operated at the level of populations.

We can't resolve all the issues around the management of Oostvaardersplassen here, of course; much more could be said about this case. But perhaps we've moved a little closer to an answer to the question posed at the beginning of the chapter: Is Oostvaardersplassen really wild? As we've seen, the answer depends on what dimensions of wildness are under consideration. Oostvaardersplassen was created by humans and the herbivores placed there were bred by humans. In this historical sense, it doesn't seem very wild. On the other hand, the animals there are free to make their own autonomous choices (though constrained by fences) and, within the context of a human-created environment, nonhuman nature is largely free to "do its own thing." So, in this sense Oostvaardersplassen and its inhabitants are fairly wild.

Of course, we should not forget that the purpose of introducing herbivores to Oostvaardersplassen was for them to serve as "proxy animals" performing the role of members of other, now extinct, wild animal populations, in order to create something like a wild *ecosystem*. Wild ecosystems are not only important in terms of their *wildness* value, but also because the flourishing of ecological systems and communities is also frequently argued to be valuable. We'll turn to this in the next section.

3.6 The Value of Wildlife in Ecosystems

While many people now take it for granted that ecosystems are valuable – and that wild animals are valuable, at least in large part, because of their roles in ecosystems – these ideas are relatively recent. The term "ecosystem" was coined by the ecologist Arthur Tansley (1935), and became increasingly popular in the late twentieth century. Indeed, the ecosystem idea gave rise to a branch of ecology – ecosystem ecology – with an emphasis on ecological analysis at the level of ecosystems (rather than, say, at the level of species populations or specific habitats). At this time, the idea of managing wildlife for ecosystems also became increasingly important; for instance, a wildlife manager might control or encourage the expansion of particular species populations depending on the impact these populations were believed to have on the ecosystem in which they were located.

This brief description, however, glosses over significant controversies and difficulties. If people are going to manage wildlife for the sake of ecosystems, they need to be able to specify both the ecosystem that's supposed to benefit and the value of the relevant state of an ecosystem that management is supposed to promote. However, there still isn't any widely agreed definition of what an ecosystem is, nor how one ecosystem should be distinguished from another. Moreover, there's little agreement about how coherent an ecosystem is. Thus, it's an open question whether an ecosystem is an individual thing that could be described as having persistent or resilient or "healthy" states. (The alternative view is that it's something much more inchoate – or even chaotic.)

To look at these questions a little more closely, we need to introduce the work of Aldo Leopold, whose influence has been fundamentally important in the development of ecosystem-centered wildlife management and conservation. Leopold's work will give us a further handle for tackling the values at stake in the Oostvaardersplassen case.

3.6.1 Aldo Leopold's Land Ethic

Aldo Leopold is a key figure in environmental ethics and wildlife management; more specifically, he was the founder of the science of game management (see Chapter 7). However, he's most widely known for his posthumously published collection of essays, *A Sand County Almanac* (1949), and for his role in creating the Gila Wilderness Area, the first official wilderness in the USA, in 1924. Leopold's work brought wildness and ecosystems together; he maintained that wildernesses were the healthiest kind of ecosystems known. What's more, he argued, such healthy ecosystems are *morally* important, and our priority in terms of managing wildlife should be to support and protect such ecosystems. So, for Leopold, the focus of moral concern for wildlife management and conservation should be at the level of populations and systems, not at the level of the individual animal. As his support for game management indicates, on Leopold's view, there's no problem in thinking of individual wild animals as "game" for hunting; what matters is that if hunted, then animals are hunted at levels that permit the thriving of wildlife populations and the healthiness of the ecosystems to which they contribute.

The best-known statement of Leopold's view is found in his essay "The Land Ethic" in *A Sand County Almanac*. This book wasn't intended to be a rigorous scientific or philosophical work; it's aimed at a popular audience. Nonetheless, the ideas in "The Land Ethic" are both striking and radical. Most famously, Leopold claimed toward the end of this essay:

> A thing is right as it tends to preserve the integrity, stability and beauty of the biotic community. It is wrong as it tends otherwise.
>
> (Leopold 1949, p. 242)

The meaning of these sentences isn't straightforward and immediately raises some tricky questions. Let's start by thinking about the object of Leopold's concern: the "biotic community." Elsewhere in his essay, Leopold says that the biotic community includes "soils, waters, plants and animals, or collectively, the land." It isn't completely clear whether Leopold is referring here to what we would now call an ecosystem (he was writing soon after the term was first coined and it wasn't widely adopted until the 1950s and 1960s). It does, however, seem that Leopold is interested in all the organisms – including humans – in a specified area of landscape. While there's room for debate about precisely how Leopold's idea relates to modern ecology (see Millstein 2018), in terms of wildlife management, it may not matter exactly what he had in mind. What does matter is whether there's something here – a biotic or ecological community, an ecosystem, or some combination – that's of *ethical* importance.

If the focus is on *instrumental* values, broadly construed – that is, what is now commonly thought of as ecosystem services (more on these in Chapter 7), taken to include noneconomic, nonuse values – then there are no obvious difficulties here. These values are fairly uncontroversial, and there's generally no need to carefully delineate any particular ecological community or system to recognize that these values are provided to humans by the natural world. Thought of in this way, wildlife is valuable because it contributes to ecosystem services that all humans rely on and need. On this view, putting the herbivores into Oostvaardersplassen, for the sake of a flourishing system, is valuable to *humans*.

Nevertheless, on a straightforward reading of "The Land Ethic," Leopold seems to be claiming something further: that a biotic community has *moral status*. It matters directly, in itself; it can be harmed and benefited; it has particular states (e.g., integrity, stability) that should be preserved for ethical reasons; and helping to preserve those ecological states should at least be a goal, or possibly *the* goal, of wildlife management. One possible interpretation of what Leopold means when he discusses the "integrity" of the biotic community is that it contains the full range of native species. In Oostvaardersplassen, some species (the tarpan and aurochs) that would have been native to areas like this have gone extinct. If what matters are the ecological *functions* of species, then the substitution of so-called proxy species – here the Heck cattle and Konik horses – would certainly seem to be "right." Or, at least, it would be "right" if they contributed to the maintenance of the biotic community as a whole.

There are two main debates concerning Leopold's claim that ecosystems or ecological communities have moral status – a claim that's since been developed and defended by others, notably J. Baird Callicott (1989). One of the debates is about how best to describe the subject of the claim. Are there real ecological "things" that actually can be picked out here, ecological *individuals* in some sense, with both identifiable boundaries and at least some degree of internal coherence? This seems to be needed as a foundation for Leopold's Land Ethic. The second debate is about the moral claim. Even if there are such ecological "individuals," do they have *interests?* Can they be better or worse off? And if they can, does this imply that they matter ethically? Do they have moral status?

The debates are linked. Roberta Millstein (2018), for instance, argues that so-called ecosystem-communities can indeed be identified as ecological individuals, bounded in space and time, continuous through time despite changes, and integrated in terms of causal interactions between their parts. This, she maintains, gives the parts a shared fate, such that it could make sense to say that such "individuals" have a collective welfare and that they have interests.

However, this view is widely contested. One alternative position is that ecosystems are not bounded individuals, but rather that *people* identify particular causal connections or relationships at the scale on which they want to work, and then draw corresponding ecosystem boundaries. Further, referring to what's sometimes called a shift of paradigm in ecology, emphasis has moved to a focus on dynamic *change* and disturbance (Pickett and Ostfeld 1995). But if ecological systems or communities are in a state of flux, doesn't this raise questions about Leopold's idea of the "integrity and stability" of the biotic community? And what of the idea that ecological communities can have interests? Suppose, after all, that ecological communities have limited inner coherence; they are constantly changing without an inbuilt direction (based largely on the chanciness of what happens around them, such as nonnative species moving in, human activity, a changing climate, and so on) and any boundaries they have are those humans arbitrarily choose. In that case, it isn't clear what *could* be in the "interests" of ecosystems (short of avoiding total destruction). There may be changes, but it will be hard to say what constitutes a change to a better or worse state.

These questions bring us back to Oostvaardersplassen. Here, herbivores were introduced in order to produce a particular state of the ecosystem: one with wildfowl habitat. Does this mean that the Oostvaardersplassen with herbivores, wildfowl, and no forest was in a "better" state than an Oostvaardersplassen with a forest but no herbivores or wildfowl (which is where it was headed without intervention?) Was it "in the interests" of the polder ecosystem to have herbivores introduced – just as, it's sometimes argued, it was in the interests of the Greater Yellowstone ecosystem discussed in Chapter 2 to have wolves reintroduced? Or was the real motive at Oostvaardersplassen simply to prioritize the species that people valued the most – namely, waterfowl?

Ethicists often argue that the attribution of interests to ecosystems or ecological communities is key to their having moral status (since it means that they have, in some sense, their own good, and that's what the attribution of moral status serves to highlight). But as we've seen, whether ecosystems or ecological communities are sufficiently defined or coherent to have interests is itself contested. Even if they *do* have interests, it may be argued that these are not of the right kind for moral status. On some moral views, for instance, only the interests of *conscious* beings matter (see Chapter 5). At the very least, ecosystem interests would be rather different, since they can't enjoy their own flourishing or suffer if (for instance) a hurricane devastates them.

Whatever we conclude about these questions, it's nevertheless the case that preserving ecological communities *in* certain states, or restoring ecosystems *to* certain states, is a significant part of current wildlife conservation and management. If people value ecosystems intrinsically, wanting them to flourish independent of any potential usefulness, these activities might be defended, regardless of whether or not ecosystems can be said to have moral status. What's more, ecosystems also have high instrumental value in terms of providing ecosystem services; Oostvaardersplassen, for instance, has the function of reducing flood risks, providing recreational opportunities, and so on.

In any event, managing wildlife seems to be essential to creating, sustaining, and protecting valuable ecosystems and these ecosystems, in turn, make the existence of populations of wild animals possible. We'll explore this a little further in section 3.8, at the end of this chapter.

3.7 Managing Wildlife for the Ecosystem

"Thinking like a Mountain" is another of Leopold's most famous essays (Leopold 1949, p. 137). It's also a useful place to start in thinking about managing wildlife for an ecosystem. At the time Leopold wrote this essay, part of his job was to carry out predator control in the American Southwest for the Forest Service. One day, when he and his colleagues saw an older wolf and grown wolf pups in a stream below their lunch spot, their immediate response was to shoot the animals. Clambering down to the stream, after the firing, Leopold reached the older wolf just in time to watch a "fierce green fire dying in her eyes" (Leopold 1949, p. 138). He reflects: "I was young then, and full of trigger-itch; I thought that because fewer wolves meant more deer, that no wolves would mean hunter's paradise. But after seeing the green fire die, I sensed that neither the wolf nor the mountain agreed with such a view" (Leopold 1949, p. 139).

Leopold uses this "fierce green fire" to develop a telling reflection on predator elimination policies. Without predators (like wolves), the population of prey animals (like deer) would expand to the point that the deer exhaust the available resources. And then what? "In the end, the starved bones of the hoped-for deer herd, dead of its own too-much, bleach with the bones of the dead sage, or molder under the high-lined junipers"

(Leopold 1949, p. 140). Here, Leopold is arguing that removing predators leads both to the death of the prey and the destruction of the community in which both predator and prey operated. "Thinking like a Mountain," for Leopold, is taking the perspective of the whole land community: in this case the relationship between the deer, the wolves, and the resources on which the deer live.

From the perspective of the biotic community, the job of the wolf is to trim the deer herd to fit the resources the land provides; to kill all the wolves is to undermine the integrity and stability of the entire system. And, he notes, if wolves are cleared to run cattle on a range, then the cowman has, essentially, to perform the role of the wolf and trim cattle numbers to fit that range – the alternative is the devastation of the ecosystem through overgrazing. From this, we can infer what Leopold might have said about the human role in Oostvaardersplassen: if predators could not be reintroduced, then the population of Heck cattle and Konik ponies should be reduced by people in order to allow the ecological community to flourish; so here humans should "play wolf." Interestingly, in the initial breeding program at Oostvaardersplassen, animals were meant to be selected by (what was called) "looking through the eyes of a wolf," a method designed to counter the risk that the selection would be (too) anthropocentric (Gamborg et al. 2010).

We should also note that, as mentioned above, Leopold's message in "Thinking like a Mountain" was not that there's anything wrong with hunting (in fact, he remained a keen hunter all his life; Figure 3.2). Nor did he think that the lives of *individual* wolves should be protected because they are, as individuals, of any special value. Rather, hunting that doesn't disturb the land community is perfectly permissible; hunting that promotes its integrity and stability is even ethically desirable. Hunting is only a problem when it has negative impacts on the "healthy" functioning of the whole land community, and the elimination of predators is likely to have just such a negative impact.

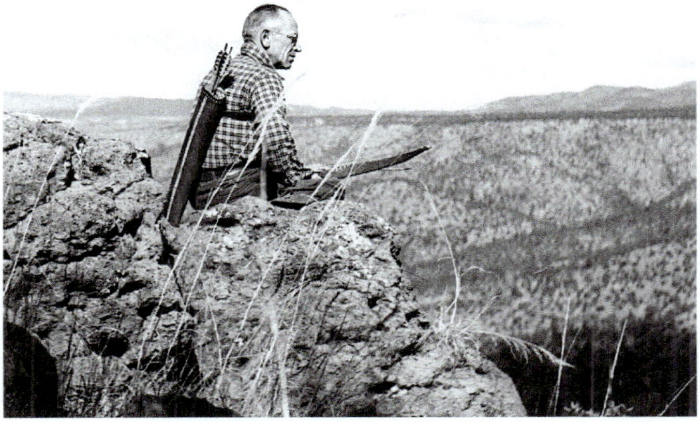

Figure 3.2 Aldo Leopold bow hunting in Mexico in 1938. *Source:* U.S. Department of Agriculture/flickr/CC BY 2.0.

This emphasis on the integrity of the whole land community, and in particular the idea that native community members (like wolves and deer) have become adapted to one another, also informed Leopold's increasing wariness toward nonnative species. In his essay "The Land Ethic," he notes, for instance, that "native plants and animals kept the energy circuit open; others may or may not" (Leopold 1949, p. 218). Leopold was not in principle opposed to nonnative species (though he does seem to have thought that native species in place had esthetic virtues that nonnative ones lacked). However, since they didn't evolve "in place" as part of particular ecological communities, there's no reason to assume that nonnative species will have useful functions in them – and a chance they will be damaging. As Daniel Simberloff (2012, p. 496) argues, Leopold fundamentally "stresses coevolution as the reason why nonnative species are so likely to become runaways that destabilize native ecosystems and why it is difficult if not impossible to construct stable, 'healthy' ecosystems out of them."

In recent years, the worry about nonnative species has become a central concern of wildlife management (where the issue may be damage to human interests such as crops) and wildlife conservation (where human introductions of wild animals from elsewhere may impact whole ecological communities); we'll discuss this further in Chapter 12 in the context of the "Predator-Free New Zealand" policy. In any case, it seems likely that Leopold would have found policies to control nonnative species when they have negative impacts on ecological communities desirable; such policies line up well with the principal concerns of the Land Ethic.

3.8 Some Concluding Thoughts

In this chapter we've considered the value of wildness and of ecosystems, and how these values relate to wildlife conservation and management. These values can be in tension; active wildlife management itself may conflict with protecting wildness value, since (on at least some interpretations of wildness) the less management, the more wildness. However, there are also ways in which wildlife management can protect or help to restore wildness. The removal of destructive nonnative species introduced by humans may not only improve the functioning of an ecosystem, but could also return it to a state with less human influence, making it compositionally wilder. (That doesn't, of course, mean that other values, such as animal welfare, would not be at stake in such a removal.)

Oostvaardersplassen is a "rewilding" project to create a functioning wild ecosystem. However, this very idea presents multiple difficulties. First, Oostvaardersplassen is of human origin – the land was created from the sea – and so is not historically wild. Second, the wildlife there doesn't closely resemble what would have been there without human intervention so it isn't strongly compositionally wild. Third, given its small size, fencing, and the absence of predators, it doesn't function as a self-contained ecosystem in a Leopoldian sense; humans are needed to cull the herbivores as it doesn't contain native predators. At the same time, though, Oostvaardersplassen isn't entirely without wildness value; in particular, the herbivores and other animals live autonomous lives relative to most domestic animals (Sandøe et al. 2022). It's also important in terms of having a flourishing, valued ecological community that provides habitat for rare species, and significant increases in biodiversity in comparison to the pre-project state.

Overall, Oostvaardersplassen seems to fit the bill of what has been called "new nature" – nature that becomes a relatively independent entity, having been designed and re-created (Doevendans et al. 2007) with the particular goal of biodiversity conservation. This takes us to the topic of our next chapter: the value of species and biodiversity.

References

Birch, T. (1990). The incarceration of wildness: wildernesses as prisons. *Environmental Ethics* 12 (1): 3–26.

Callicott, J.B. (1989). *In Defense of the Land Ethic: Essays in Environmental Philosophy*. New York, USA: State University of New York Press.

Callicott, J.B. and Nelson, M. (1998). *The Great New Wilderness Debate*. Athens, USA: University of Georgia Press.

Cronon, W. (1995). The trouble with wilderness. In: *Uncommon Ground: Rethinking the Human Place in Nature* (ed. W. Cronon), 69–90. New York, USA: W.W. Norton.

Doevendans, K., Lörzing, H., and Schram, A. (2007). From modernist landscapes to new nature: planning of rural utopias in the Netherlands. *Landscape Research* 32 (3): 333–354.

Donaldson, S. and Kymlicka, W. (2011). *Zoopolis: A Political Theory of Animal Rights*. New York, USA: Oxford University Press.

Elliot, R. (1982). Faking Nature. *Inquiry* 25 (1): 85–93.

Fletcher, M.-S., Hamilton, R., Dressler, W., and Palmer, L. (2021). Indigenous knowledge and the shackles of wilderness. *Proceedings of the National Academy of Sciences* 118 (40): e2022218118.

Gamborg, C. and Sandøe, P. (2004). Beavers and biodiversity: the ethics of ecological restoration. In: *Philosophy and Biodiversity* (ed. M. Oksanen), 217–236. New York, USA: Cambridge University Press.

Gamborg, C., Gremmen, B., and Sandøe, P. (2010). De-domestication: ethics at the intersection of landscape restoration and animal welfare. *Environmental Values* 19 (1): 57–78.

Gordon, I.J., Manning, A.D., Navarro, L.M., and Rouet-Leduc, J. (2021). Domestic livestock and rewilding: are they mutually exclusive? *Frontiers in Sustainable Food Systems* 5: 68.

Hettinger, N. (2005). Respecting Nature's autonomy in relationship to humanity. In: *Recognizing the Autonomy of Nature* (ed. T. Heyd), 86–98. New York, USA: Columbia University Press.

Hettinger, N. and Throop, B. (1999). Refocusing ecocentrism: de-emphasizing stability and defending wildness. *Environmental Ethics* 21 (1): 3–21.

Hill, K., Szydlowski, M., Heaney, S.O., and Busby, D. (2022). Uncivilized behaviors: how humans wield "feral" to assert power (and control) over other species. *Society & Animals* (published online ahead of print 2022). doi: https://doi.org/10.1163/15685306-bja10088.

Kopnina, H., Leadbetter, S., and Cryer, P. (2019). Learning to rewild: the failed case of the Dutch "new wilderness" Oostvaardersplassen. *International Journal of Wilderness* 25 (3): 72–89.

Leopold, A. (1949). *A Sand County Almanac*. Oxford, UK: Oxford University Press.

Lewis, J.S., Spaulding, S., Swanson, H. et al. (2021). Human activity influences wildlife populations and activity patterns: implications for spatial and temporal refuges. *Ecosphere* 12 (5): e03487.

Lorimer, J. and Driessen, C. (2014). Wild experiments at the Oostvaardersplassen: rethinking environmentalism in the Anthropocene. *Transactions of the Institute of British Geographers* 39 (2): 169–181.

Lovász, L., Fages, A., and Amrhein, V. (2021). Konik, tarpan, European wild horse: an origin story with conservation implications. *Global Ecology and Conservation* 32: e01911.

Millstein, R. (2018). Is Aldo Leopold's 'land community' an individual? In: *Individuation, Process, and Scientific Practices* (ed. O. Bueno, R. Chen, and M.B. Fagan), 279–302. Oxford, UK: Oxford University Press.

Palmer, C. (2010). *Animal Ethics in Context*. New York, USA: Columbia University Press.

Pickett, S. and Ostfeld, R. (1995). The shifting paradigm in ecology. In: *A New Century for Natural Resources Management* (ed. R.L. Knight and S.F. Bates), 261–278. Washington, D.C., USA: Island Press.

Sandler, R. (2012). Intrinsic value, ecology, and conservation. *Nature Education Knowledge* 3 (10): 4.

Sandøe, P., Gamborg, C., and Palmer, C. (2022). Will the use of domesticated animals in rewilding projects compromise animal welfare? In: *Transforming Food Systems: Ethics, Innovation and Responsibility* (ed. D. Bruce and A. Bruce), 159–164. Wageningen, Netherlands: Wageningen Academic Publishers.

Simberloff, D. (2012). Integrity, stability and beauty: Aldo Leopold's evolving view of non native species. *Environmental History* 17 (3): 487–511.

Tansley, A.G. (1935). The use and abuse of vegetational concepts and terms. *Ecology* 16 (3): 284–307.

Theunissen, B. (2019). The Oostvaardersplassen fiasco. *Isis* 110 (2): 341–345.

US Government (1964). *US Wilderness Act*. Washington, D.C., USA: US Government.

The Value of Species and Biodiversity

4

4.1 The Scottish Wildcat

The European wildcat (*Felis silvestris silvestris*) – or as it's called in Scotland, the Highland tiger (Figure 4.1) – was once widely distributed across the United Kingdom. But by the late nineteenth century, largely due to habitat loss and to being trapped and shot as pests, wildcat populations became confined to remoter parts of Scotland. Hunting pressures subsequently eased, especially as gamekeepers (professionals employed to protect game) were called up in the First World War, allowing wildcat numbers to expand again. Later in the twentieth century, though, a new apparent threat appeared: the spread of domesticated cats (*Felis catus*) introduced to England by the Romans and originating from the African wildcat. Domesticated cats can introduce infectious diseases into wildcat populations, but strikingly they can also readily interbreed with them, producing fertile wildcat/domesticated cat hybrids. Now it's thought that fewer than 100 genetically nonhybrid Scottish wildcats persist in the wild (among thousands of domestic cats), with the majority of "wildcats" in Scotland being genetic hybrids, leading to the conclusion, in a 2019 report, that Scottish wildcats are on the brink of extinction (Breitenmoser et al. 2019).

Wildlife Ethics: The Ethics of Wildlife Management and Conservation, First Edition. Clare Palmer, Bob Fischer, Christian Gamborg, Jordan Hampton, and Peter Sandøe.

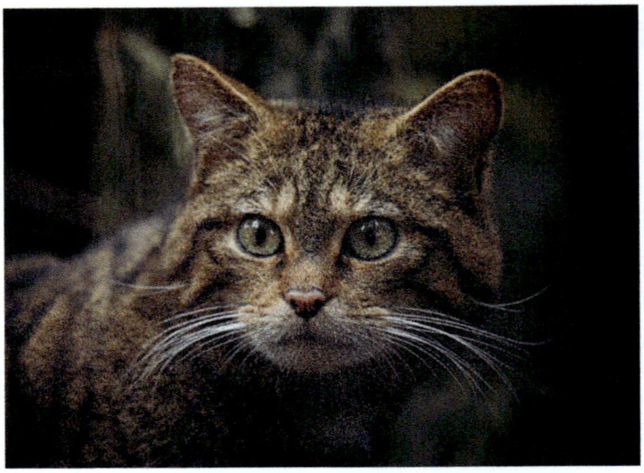

Figure 4.1 A Scottish wildcat in Edinburgh Zoo. *Source:* Courtesy of the Royal Zoological Society of Scotland.

Since any remaining genetically "pure" wildcats are scattered over a relatively large area, hope of increasing their numbers will require a plan to create protected areas with buffer zones – that is, zones where privately owned or feral domesticated cats are either excluded or vaccinated and neutered to prevent further hybridization and disease transmission (Kitchener et al. 2005). Conservationists have recommended that Scottish wildcats from existing less hybridized captive populations should be used in captive breeding and reintroduction projects and that wildcats from continental European populations, whose genes are relatively close to those of Scottish wildcats, should also be introduced to the area (Breitenmoser et al. 2019). Combined, these strategies have the goal of creating a sufficiently large population of relatively pure Scottish wildcats to increase, or at least stabilize, the population.

This hybridization issue isn't unique to Scottish wildcats. Interbreeding between wild and domesticated animals presents a conundrum for wildlife managers globally. For example, an almost identical concern exists in contemporary Australia, involving the dingo (often termed *Canis dingo*, although this nomenclature is controversial) and domestic dogs (*C. familiaris*) (Daniels and Corbett 2003). And all this conservation activity raises a difficult question: Why? Why should anyone care about the loss of Scottish wildcats – or any other species? Why does it matter whether the cats roaming in the Scottish Highlands and Islands are "pure" European wildcats or hybrids between wildcats and domesticated or feral cats?

In this chapter, we look more closely at the value of preserving species and the closely related idea of protecting biodiversity. We'll consider why species or biodiversity might be of value, and in what sense it might be claimed that *all* species are valuable. We'll also try to identify some of the ways in which these values might feed into wildlife management and conservation decisions, which we'll explore in more detail in the second part of the book.

We'll start with some conceptual questions. What, exactly, is a species? What is biodiversity? As the case of the European wildcats in Scotland suggests, the answers to these questions aren't straightforward. Then, revisiting many of the concepts from Chapter 2, we'll consider some key issues about the value and ethical significance of species and biodiversity.

4.2 What is a Species?

Species are the "fundamental taxonomic units of biological classification" (Ereshefsky 2017). However, what's *meant* by "a species" isn't at all straightforward. There's ongoing debate about how to define species, what kind of things they are, and even whether they are a "real" category found in nature, or rather are a way in which humans impose structure onto the natural world. Not all these debates need to be considered here, but we do need to look a little more closely at "species concepts," of which there are many (dozens, in fact). Here we'll discuss just two important concepts that highlight why the idea of a species is so complex and why this complexity might matter for conservation.

Most people, if asked for their definition of a species, would give a version of what's called the *biological* species concept, formulated by Ernst Mayr. This takes species to be "groups of actually or potentially interbreeding populations which are reproductively isolated from other such groups" (Mayr 1940, p. 256). To be a member of the same species, on this definition, organisms should be able to interbreed and to produce fertile offspring. This concept of species is widely used and often unproblematic. However, it fits awkwardly with some conservation concerns – including those being expressed in the case of the Scottish wildcats.

The biggest threat to these wildcats, according to the 2019 report, is not so much habitat loss or being killed on the road; it's domesticated and feral cats. This isn't primarily because feral and domesticated cats pass diseases to wildcats but because they *mate* with them, producing fertile offspring that are hybrids of domesticated cats and wildcats. The worry is that all these hybrid cats – the "hybrid swarm" as the 2019 report calls them – mean that Scottish wildcats will be completely lost (Breitenmoser et al. 2019). And yet, on the biological species concept, this seems impossible; after all, these cats are interbreeding to produce fertile offspring.

This takes us to the *evolutionary* species concept, which emphasizes ancestry rather than interbreeding: "a species is a lineage of ancestral descendant populations which maintains its identity from other such lineages and which has its own evolutionary tendencies and historical fate" (Wiley 1978, p. 18). Being a member of a species is like being a family member, related by descent; if you don't have the right ancestry, you're not part of the family – however similar you may look and even if you can breed successfully. It is this genetic, ancestry-related understanding of a species that lies behind the claim that Scottish wildcats are at the brink of extinction. Scottish wildcats are genetically distant from domesticated cats, which as mentioned descend from African, not European wildcats, and are regarded as being members of a different species (domesticated cats are the species *F. catus*, not *F. silvestris*). However, Scottish wildcats are genetically close to other European wildcat populations (also *F. silvestris*). So, on this account of species, while breeding with captive Scottish wildcats and other European wildcats could allow Scottish wildcats to continue in something relatively similar to their current form, breeding with domesticated cats risks losing what's distinctive about the Scottish populations.

In discussing these two species concepts, we are not trying to suggest that one species concept is better than another (indeed, pluralism about species concepts in different contexts is very common). Neither are we commenting here on ethical arguments for or against valuing and protecting "pure" species such as the Scottish wildcat while reducing or removing hybrids. The main goal here is just to show that talking about species and species extinction is not completely straightforward; the species concept adopted will, in some cases, affect whether a species is thought to be threatened. Let's now turn to the equally complex notion of *biodiversity*.

4.3 What is Biodiversity?

Perhaps the best known definition of biodiversity comes from the *Convention on Biodiversity* (1992):

> Biological diversity means the variability among living organisms from all sources including, inter alia, terrestrial, marine and other aquatic ecosystems and the ecological complexes of which they are a part; this includes diversity within species, between species, and of ecosystems
>
> (Secretariat of the Convention on Biological Diversity 2012)

As this definition makes clear, biological diversity comes in many forms. Diversity *within* species refers to genetic and phenotypic variation both between individual members of a species and between species populations. Worry about this kind of biodiversity is playing a significant role in the drive to conserve Scottish wildcats. Although they are very similar genetically to other European wildcats, there's still enough that's genetically distinct to argue that the Scottish wildcats contribute significantly to the diversity of the European wildcat gene pool. If they do, then there's a case to be made that they should be protected.

Diversity *between* species is measured as the number of different species (species richness) plus the number of individuals of each species present. *Ecosystem biodiversity* refers to diversity between ecosystems. This can be understood in different ways, but the focus is usually on the variation between ecosystems in a region, nation, or globally (e.g., diversity of ecosystems such as oak savanna, desert grassland, short-grass prairie).

This means, then, that biodiversity can be measured in different ways, both in terms of different units (by genes, species, ecosystem types, etc.) and different kinds of divergence. So, suppose someone were measuring biodiversity in some particular location. They could measure simply by number of species present (species richness), which is probably the most common measurement. But they might also want to consider diversity *between* species – on this measure, they'd add species evenness to species richness. Hence, if there were 99 oak trees and one gray squirrel, there would be less biodiversity than if there were 50 oak trees and 50 gray squirrels, even though in both cases, species richness would be the same (two species).

In addition, the level at which biodiversity is measured matters, in particular the difference between local and global levels. Working only at *local* levels, adding a non-native species into an area would actually increase biodiversity (Wallach et al. 2020). But at a *global* level, of course, moving a species from one place to another doesn't increase biodiversity. Indeed, if the effect of the movement is that biodiversity is lost in the new location, as when an introduced species negatively impacts a native species, then we could simultaneously (until and unless the local species goes extinct) see a rise in local biodiversity and a loss in global biodiversity. (For more discussion of nativeness, see Chapter 12.)

These multiple levels of biodiversity (within and between species and ecosystems), along with complexity within each level, make measuring biodiversity difficult. Indeed, there are profound scientific disagreements about whether *any* simple proxy is adequate to measure biodiversity. The most common proxy is species richness but this alone, for instance, wouldn't catch evenness of distribution or stability over time. In this book, we won't adopt one kind of definition in preference to others, but we'll try to be clear when we use the term "biodiversity" what interpretation and level we have in mind.

Now that we've outlined what "species" and "biodiversity" might be taken to mean, we'll consider why they might be thought of as *valuable*.

4.4 Values of Species and Biodiversity

A first point to make here is that to value species or biodiversity is not the same as valuing *individual* wild animals. Where *species* are the focus of value, individual species members don't matter so much in themselves; instead, they matter because they manifest the valued characteristics of the species as a whole (genetically and/or in terms of reproductive capacity, esthetics, ecological function, and so on). If the focus of value is *biodiversity*, then individuals again matter not so much in themselves, but because of what their genes or their species membership (and so on) contribute to valued biodiversity.

This distinction between species and individuals is important because there can be conflicts between the welfare of individual species members and the goal of protecting or promoting the value of the whole species. It may be, for instance, that if people move wildcats from other parts of Europe to Scotland to promote a breeding program, then those individual wildcats could have much worse lives, as individual animals, after the move than they would have had if left alone. While the translocation may mean that genetic biodiversity within the Scottish wildcat species improves, which is good in terms of the persistence of the species, at least some translocated wildcats may have difficulty adjusting to hunting in new territory, be vulnerable to unexpected threats, or end up in conflicts with resident wildcats (Harrington et al. 2013), all of which may negatively affect their welfare. The interests of individual species members may not, therefore, be best served by policies to conserve the whole species to which these individuals belong, nor by policies to protect biodiversity.

4.4.1 Direct Instrumental, Option, and Bequest Values

In Chapter 2, we looked at different categories of instrumental value. Species and biodiversity clearly offer a good deal of instrumental value. Some of this instrumental value is *direct* – for instance, the genetic diversity of certain wild species may be exploited to introduce traits such as disease resistance into domesticated animals. These direct instrumental values clearly provide reasons for protecting some wildlife species/biodiversity from overexploitation and extinction. However, the number of species with direct, proved usefulness, whether of a consumptive or nonconsumptive variety, is likely to be relatively small. Scottish wildcats, for instance, are not obviously of direct instrumental value in this sense (though were there to be a chance of actually spotting them, they might offer economic potential for attracting tourists, akin to tiger tourism; see Chapter 2).

One way of responding to this is to say that while there are many wild animal species that do not appear to be useful to humans, current appearances may be deceiving. In the *future*, some particular species or forms of biodiversity may in fact turn out to be very useful (although this isn't known now, as it is difficult to anticipate future needs). To be on the safe side, then, every species had better be preserved – a response that moves toward the idea of universal *option* value. This, we should note, is a so-called *precautionary* argument for protecting species and biodiversity. It may not be possible to establish the direct instrumental value of a particular species here and now, but because it might have instrumental value in the future, it's important to err on the side of safety by preserving it as a *possible* future resource.

One difficulty with this argument is that it may not take into account the opportunity costs of preserving species – the loss of things that, in all likelihood, would have been gained by letting the species go. Moreover, given the precautionary nature of this argument, those things are lost in favor of highly uncertain future benefits.

Let's take a case from the US to illustrate this point: that of the snail darter. This is a species of small freshwater fish declared endangered under the US Endangered Species Act in 1975. It became an early test case for the Act when the completion of a massive dam project was temporarily stopped because the dam threatened to destroy the snail darter's only known migratory route (Plater 2013). The fish species had no known current use value. Of course, it could have been maintained that the continuance of snail darters had option or bequest value. Perhaps at some point in the future, snail darters might become useful, maybe even to create a medicine to cure a rare disease. On the other hand, the dam project offered some *immediate* benefits, including many jobs and downstream flood regulation. Given this, if what matters is use value, then there's clearly a question about whether it makes sense to prioritize possible future benefits (option value), which after all may never materialize or be insubstantial, over the immediate, significant, and known benefits. From a (direct) use value point of view, "[e]ven if we can show that some bit of biodiversity is, in fact, useful to us, we need to show that it is more useful than whatever we want to do that might endanger it" (Newman et al. 2017, p. 43).

This particular case has a happy ending: the dam was ultimately completed, a population of snail darters was relocated to a river in Tennessee, and some years later, the species was reclassified as recovered (Plater 2013). However, since the instrumental value of developing a species' habitat now often feels more salient than distant possible benefits in cases where a species is threatened, there is what Lovejoy (1986) calls "the incremental problem" of species loss. When cases are taken one by one, and the values at stake are all directly instrumental, current use tends to outweigh uncertain option and bequest values, with species paying the price.

4.4.2 Indirect Instrumental Value: Ecological Value

Other arguments for the protection of species and biodiversity take a broader approach, focusing on the more *indirect* instrumental value species and biodiversity have in ecosystems and in providing – as the Millennium Ecosystem Assessment in 2005 puts it – "regulating" and "supporting" ecosystem services (Millennium Ecosystem Assessment Board 2005). These include functions such as storing carbon, filtering water, forming soils, and creating ecosystems (see also Chapter 7). Indeed, there wouldn't *be* any ecosystems without species and biodiversity; the latter are part of what constitute the former. So, however ecosystems are valued – whether intrinsically or instrumentally – species and biodiversity are vital ecologically. But this says nothing about *which* species matter in a given ecosystem or the *kind* and *amount* of biodiversity that's important. Answering these questions is difficult and much contested; in particular, there's a long and unresolved debate about the importance of biodiversity for ecosystems. Largely, the debate concerns the claim that a relationship exists between higher biodiversity and increased stability; this, in turn, is complicated by disagreements about what's meant by ecosystem stability (an issue that emerged in Chapter 3).

Sometimes it's claimed that *species* are of ecological value because every species occupies a unique and equally vital niche in its ecosystem. However, the evidence doesn't seem to support so strong a view. Not all species are equally important in ecosystems, partly because there's often "species redundancy," meaning that multiple species can perform similar functions, allowing other species to take over the function if one species is lost. Having said this, there isn't species redundancy for *every* function and there's often poor understanding of how much redundancy any particular ecosystem includes. Some keystone species, for instance, could cause major changes in an ecosystem if lost.

One well-known way of thinking about the relationship between species and ecosystems is what's called the "rivet popping" analogy. The analogy likens an ecosystem to an airplane and species to rivets that hold the plane's wings together (Ehrlich and Ehrlich 1981). The argument acknowledges that not all the rivets (species) are essential to the plane's wings staying attached (ecosystem functioning). In principle, it's possible to pull out *some* rivets (species) without thereby compromising the integrity of the plane (ecosystem) as a whole. However, some rivets nevertheless *are* essential; it's just that it might not be possible to know in advance *which* ones. What's more, even in the case where species redundancy allows other species to move in when one species is lost, as species numbers decline, available redundancy is reduced. Additionally, if new pressures emerge – for instance, the climate shifts – then, as there are fewer species remaining in an ecosystem, the ecosystem has fewer resources with which to adapt and could become less resilient. So, as species disappear, the chance of system breakdown increases, all else being equal. Thus, the loss of wild animal species *can* be highly ecologically significant; however, the significance of the loss varies by species, with the added difficulty that it may not be known which species really matter in advance. This would suggest that ecological security is best achieved by maintaining species richness.

Relatedly, Bryan Norton (1988) developed the idea of the *contributory* value of species and biodiversity to ecosystems. He argues that species can contribute new adaptations, new relationships, and new niches to ecosystems, as well as being key to speciation – all of which allow for an increasing spiral of biodiversity. However, when species are lost, then these ecological relationships start to weaken and unravel as other species that were wholly or partially dependent on the lost species become somewhat more vulnerable. So, losing species leads to a spiraling decline in biodiversity, ultimately making future extinctions more likely.

Combined, these arguments suggest that, in a general sense, retaining species and biodiversity supports ecosystems and that losing them undermines ecosystems, with impacts that affect humans and other animals who depend on the services ecosystems provide. However, such arguments also suggest that *particular* species are of variable importance to ecosystems and that the loss of some species may well make little or no difference to ecosystem functioning.

For this reason, it's worth noting that if what's important is just the ecological role of a species, hybridization may not be a problem, provided that the hybrid performs the same function as the "pure" original. Daniels and Corbett describe this approach:

> Protecting animals for where and how they live, and for their cultural or ecosystem function value rather than focusing on their appearance, offers the best solution for maintaining their conservation status.
>
> (Daniels and Corbett 2003, p. 213)

So, *if* Scottish wildcat hybrids carried out the same ecological function as "pure" Scottish wildcats *and* the main reason for valuing them was this function, then their hybridization would not affect their value (a discussion is ongoing about whether at least some hybrid wildcats can be "functional wildcats"). All this suggests, then, that excepting the case of keystone species, such ecological arguments may not be particularly helpful to campaigns to protect *individual* species.

There's one further issue to consider here, namely that not all species and biodiversity in any particular place may have originated there or migrated without human intervention; they may be *introduced* or "invasive" species (see Chapter 12). This leads us to consider something we noted above, what Newman et al. (2017) call the "scale" problem. According to a 2019 Assessment Report from the Intergovernmental Science-Policy Platform on Biodiversity and Ecosystem Services (IPBES), roughly one million animal and plant species are at risk of extinction, the average abundance of native land-based species is down over 20% in the last 150 years, and more than 680 vertebrate species have gone extinct due to human action since the sixteenth century (Brondizio et al. 2019). Still, at local or regional level, not only may there be no overall loss of biodiversity, but there may be an *increase* in biodiversity due to introduced species (Newman et al. 2017). So, it would be an oversimplification to think that, in terms of ecological value, the goal is to try to ensure the highest level of biodiversity or the greatest species richness. That would seem to imply that introduced species are desirable or even that *more* species should be introduced or artificially created.

So, while maintaining a high number of species and high biodiversity makes sense at a *global* level, at local or regional levels, maintaining or increasing species richness and high biodiversity may not necessarily be the most important goal. But other things are also at stake in the way species are valued – such as animals' geographic origins and the appearance of species' members.

4.4.3 Esthetic and Cultural Values

The beauty of Amazonian parrots. The fearsome roaring of lions. The fascinating strangeness of the long-nosed giant anteaters. As we noted in Chapter 2, one of the principal ways in which people value species is *esthetic*: how members of species look, sound, smell, feel, and in some cases, taste. Elliott Sober (1986) argued that the main way people value species is very like the way in which works of art are valued. In particular, *rarity* is important in the valuation of works of art; he notes: "a work of art may have enhanced value just because there are very few other works by the same artist, or from the same historical period, or in the same style" (Sober 1986, p. 190). Similarly, in the case of wildlife species, a species that has few living members, or is from a clade with only a few surviving species, may be especially valued. Of course, for rarity to enhance value in this way, a species would have to be valued in the first place; rarity doesn't by itself provide value. There are, after all, plenty of rare things that people would prefer to be even rarer, especially those species involved in transmitting infectious diseases to humans (see Chapter 16), like the tsetse fly of central Africa that transmits trypanosomiasis or "sleeping sickness" (Bouyer et al. 2019).

A more complex version of this esthetic approach to wildlife can be attributed to Lilly-Marlene Russow (1981). She argues, rather like Sober (1986), that the main value species have is esthetic. In fact, she maintains that to value a species esthetically is not really to value the *species*, but the esthetic qualities of individual species members that are encountered: "What we value, then, is the existence of that individual and the existence (present or future) of individuals like that" (Russow 1981, p. 111). In the case of Scottish wildcats, for instance, she might say that what is valued is the distinctive appearance or "pelage," especially the characteristic thick and blunt tail, with black rings and a black tip, as well as the wildcat's elusive and untamable nature, which sets it apart from domesticated cats. This raises questions, though, about the value of hybrid wildcats, which can be difficult to distinguish from "pure" wildcats – at least to the less experienced eye.

Rarity plays an important role for Russow (1981), as it did for Sober (1986); she maintains that people find the unusual experience of seeing members of rare species much more exciting than seeing everyday species, and that this creates a motivation to protect these rarer species in the hope of having such encounters again. Though Russow (1981) doesn't mention it, this view also may have the unfortunate implication that it would be good to make species rare in order to gain heightened excitement from encountering their members! To put the point another way, if rarity makes a species more valuable, then is there a loss in value when conservationists succeed in making a species' members more abundant?

Esthetic value is also important in thinking about *biodiversity*. In addition to the specific way an individual animal *looks*, humans also seem to appreciate *variety*: the contrasts of colors, shapes, smells, and textures between different species. So, it's not just that the pink of the lesser flamingo is of value in an east African savanna landscape; the vivid pink of the flamingo contrasts with the black and white of the zebra or the yellow and brown of the giraffe. In some cases, it's the actual juxtaposition of members of different wildlife species in their ecosystem context that's judged esthetically important, not just the individual species members in abstraction from their context. In this way, differences might be valued as they are encountered alongside each other.

Broadly, esthetic responses such as awe, disgust, admiration, excitement, and attraction in the context of species and biodiversity can have both positive and negative implications for wildlife conservation and management. While cuteness or charisma brings some wild animal species a high degree of attention and protection, lack of appeal can mean others are neglected. For instance, zoos may prioritize species that they think visitors want to see (see Chapter 14), especially mammals, while other more endangered but less charismatic or endearing animal species – such as reptiles or amphibians – are less well represented (Brereton and Brereton 2020). And attracting esthetic attention can also have negative implications for conservation: beauty can be regarded as collectable, as in the case of some butterfly species, and deliciousness can be bad for both species and biodiversity – not to mention for individual animals.

In addition, members of some wildlife species won't be regarded as esthetically valuable by many people; they might be dull, drab, or too small to attract much notice. This might mean, as some estheticians have argued, that there's a need to rethink how wild animals are valued esthetically. So, for instance, Glenn Parsons (2007) argues that our esthetic focus should not be on factors such as cuteness or sleekness, but on looking fit for function. So, when looking at an animal, we should think about how its bodily form fits its form of life – how the narrow shoulders of the cheetah fit it for running, the wide snout of the hog fits it for rooting; these elements are "perfectly shaped and positioned to carry out the actions [the animal] must perform" (Parsons 2007, p. 168). This would give a much broader scope for esthetic value. In practice, though, it seems unlikely that this view of wild animal esthetics will be widely adopted (even though there are some people who do admire the hooks on the mouth parts of intestinal worms) and so some species just won't do well measured in esthetic terms.

Let's move now to *cultural* values, which are often of huge importance in efforts to protect particular species in particular places. (Although this has only played a minor role in arguments for their protection, Scottish wildcats have a long history of featuring on the heraldry of Scottish clans.) Take, for instance, the Monkey Forest in Ubud on the island of Bali in Indonesia. This is a site managed by the local community to protect Balinese long-tailed macaques and other local biodiversity. The site is marketed to, and succeeds in attracting, tourists (Figure 4.2). But it's also much more than this. The long-tailed macaques have important cultural and spiritual values connected to Hanuman, the monkey god, and the "old men of the village" tell stories about the sacred nature of the macaques (Wheatley and Harya Putra 1994). The sacredness of members of this species, and the ways in which it's appropriate for the community to respond to them, suggest that there are deep *relational* values at stake here; ensuring the right relationship with the macaques is understood as part of what it is for the local community and culture to flourish. For instance, although the community perceived that there were too many macaques, relocation or fertility control was rejected because "the monkeys were sacred and cannot be interfered with" (Wheatley and Harya Putra 1994, p. 252).

While many species and much biodiversity have value in one or more of the senses discussed above, these arguments don't provide a strong reason to protect *all* species. But claims that *all* species should be protected (at least from human threats), even where they lack obvious usefulness, are not unusual. Justifying this view is likely to require an argument based on species having value *in themselves* (rather than on

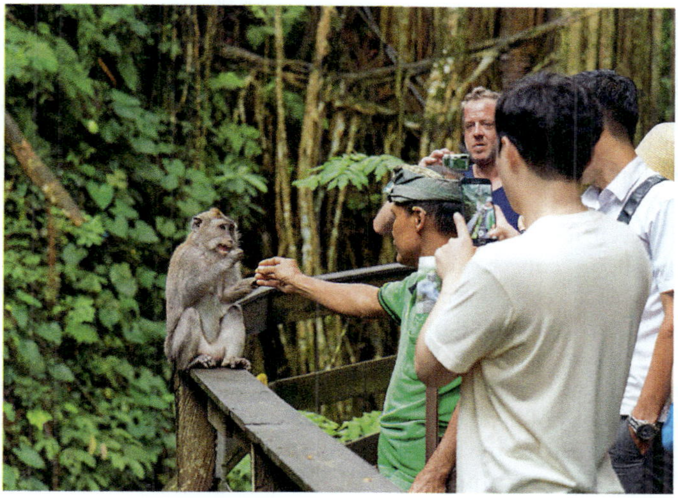

Figure 4.2 Tourists viewing a habituated and hand-fed long-tailed macaque on the Indonesian island of Bali. *Source:* Constantin Stanciu/Dreamstime.com, reproduced with permission.

variable characteristics such as their use, beauty, function, and so on), which brings us to the ideas of species' and biodiversity's intrinsic value or moral status.

4.4.4 Intrinsic Value of Species and Biodiversity

Claims that all species have *intrinsic* value, or that biodiversity has intrinsic value, are frequently made by conservationists. The very first sentence of the preamble to the Convention on Biological Diversity, for instance, begins: "Conscious of the intrinsic value of biodiversity ..." (Secretariat of the Convention on Biological Diversity 2012).

However, as we saw in Chapter 2, "intrinsic value" can mean rather different things. In this context, the most likely meaning for the claim is that species and biodiversity are being valued *noninstrumentally* – that is, valued in and for themselves, independently of any use value they may have for us. This idea of intrinsic value is often contrasted with the framework of "ecosystem services" and the focus on "nature's contributions to people," which is central, for instance, to the IPBES (Brondizio et al. 2019). Claims that species and/or biodiversity have intrinsic value are usually seen as important to moving away from an *anthropocentric* toward a more *ecocentric* valuation of species and biodiversity.

This claim needn't imply, however, that *all* species and *all* biodiversity are necessarily valuable. Not many people, for instance, would argue that the creation of new strains of lab rat would add valuable biodiversity to the world. In this context, naturalness, and often nativeness, is what ties particular species and biodiversity to intrinsic value. This takes us back to the "natural historical" sense of the intrinsic value of biodiversity (see Chapter 2) which Soulé claims is based on "species" long evolutionary heritage and potential (Soulé 1985).

This, though, raises its own questions (though we don't have room to explore these in depth here). For example, why would having "long evolutionary heritage" bestow intrinsic value? In the case of species, does this mean that species that evolved more recently should be valued less? But why should the *age* of a species be relevant to its value?

While consistent with the idea that intrinsic value here refers to noninstrumental value, something more specific may be meant when intrinsic value is attributed to species: that they have *interests* and can be harmed and benefited. The idea of interests can't easily be applied to biodiversity, which can't obviously be "harmed" and "benefited"; indeed, even the idea that species have interests is highly contested. But still, at least in casual speech, it's possible to make sense of the idea that extinction (for instance) is "bad for" the species concerned.

Ian Smith (2016) developed a more rigorous account of this idea, arguing that species can have interests and a good of their own, and that this good consists in reproducing successfully and remaining safe from extinction. And while, as we noted in Chapter 2, this doesn't necessarily require us to *preserve* that value, Smith argues that it would nevertheless be *virtuous* of us to do so, at least in cases where we are the ones threatening the species. Returning to the Scottish wildcats, on this view it would be in the interests of the wildcat *species* to be protected from hunting and habitat loss and for wildcats to mate successfully with other wildcats to produce wildcat offspring – and not to mate with domesticated cats. And because humans are the main reason for the decline of Scottish wildcats (through hunting, habitat reduction, and introducing domesticated cats), on Smith's argument, it would be virtuous for humans now to develop policies that protect and support Scottish wildcats.

4.5 The Moral Status of Species

Smith's (2016) argument about the intrinsic value of species gets very close to making the case that certain species have *moral status*. Indeed, some attempts have been made to make this case more directly. These generally draw on versions of the evolutionary species concept discussed earlier in the chapter – that species are more like individuals or families than like classes of things; they are continuous lineages restricted over time and space, with a relationship of genetic inheritance. Based on this model of what a species is, Lawrence E. Johnson (2003, p. 479), for instance, argues that a species is a *living entity* and has interests in "coherent and effective functioning as the particular ongoing life process which it is." Possessing such interests, he argues, give species moral status and, therefore, humans have duties to try to protect species from extinction.

This kind of argument is both complex and controversial, depending as it does on contested ideas about what a species is and whether, even if a species does have interests, those interests matter morally. After all, a species as a whole (as opposed to its members) can't *feel* anything, experience anything, or care about anything so why should there be any duties toward it? It's not as though (for instance) the wildcat *species* minds about hybridization. (And for that matter, it's not as though individual Scottish wildcats mind either; they are, after all, actively engaging in the mating process.) It's also difficult, on some occasions, to work out what exactly the interests of a species would be and how this interest relates to the interests of its individual members. For instance, would the interest of a species really be promoted if all its members had miserable lives? Or would it then rather be in the interest of the species to become extinct?

Given all these concerns, the jury is still out on whether whole species (as opposed to individual species members) can and do have moral status. However, it's likely that this is an area where ethical debate will develop further in the near future.

4.6 Conclusion

This chapter has considered different ways in which species and biodiversity might be argued to be valuable and so worthy of protection. Many species and much biodiversity are clearly of instrumental value, both directly and indirectly. Some species and much biodiversity are of high cultural and aesthetic value; and these values together give present generations good reason to protect these species and biodiversity for future generations. These values, though, won't necessarily include all wildlife species; a few may fall through the cracks because they aren't obviously valuable on any of these grounds. Arguments about species' moral status, if they could be made to stick, would provide an ethical foundation to protect *all* wildlife species.

However, having grounds for protection doesn't necessarily help in dealing with some of the tough questions in conservation: what to do when values are in tension and choices have to be made between them. For instance, it may be necessary to choose between animal welfare and species protection (an issue we discuss in Chapter 12 in the context of introduced species in New Zealand). And if interventionist policies are adopted to protect species and biodiversity, this may mean that wildness value is lost. So, for instance, Wildcat Haven, one of the organizations trying to protect Scottish wildcats, comments: "Scottish wildcats epitomise the solitary, independent superpredator and the mysterious and wild spirit of the Highlands in a way that no other animal can" (Wildcat Haven n.d.). But can that "mysterious and wild spirit" persist through captive breeding and the translocation of wildcats from elsewhere in Europe?

Choices may even need to be made between different forms of biodiversity. For example, the Evolutionary Distinctive and Globally Endangered (EDGE) Program at the Zoological Society of London emphasizes EDGE species – species that have a long evolutionary history and few close relatives, such as the echidnas (Isaac and Pearse 2018). This program, then, focuses conservation funding on species with high phylogenetic distinctiveness, rather than on species just as endangered but less evolutionarily distinctive. This raises questions about how to value different forms of biodiversity in relation to one another, and how to make choices between them, in terms of scarce conservation funding. The case studies in the second part of the book will look more closely at wildlife management and conservation dilemmas like these.

References

Bouyer, J., Carter, N.H., Batavia, C., and Nelson, M.P. (2019). The ethics of eliminating harmful species: the case of the tsetse fly. *Bioscience* 69 (2): 125–135.

Breitenmoser, U., Lanz, T. and Breitenmoser-Würsten, C. (2019). Wildcat in Scotland: review of conservation status and activities. www.nature.scot/doc/wildcat-scotland-review-conservation-status-and-activities

Brereton, S.R. and Brereton, J.E. (2020). Sixty years of collection planning: what species do zoos and aquariums keep? *International Zoo Yearbook* 54 (1): 131–145.
Brondizio, E.S., Settele, J., Díaz, S. and Ngo, H.T. (eds) (2019). Global assessment report on biodiversity and ecosystem services of the Intergovernmental Science-Policy Platform on Biodiversity and Ecosystem Services. https://ipbes.net/global-assessment
Daniels, M.J. and Corbett, L. (2003). Redefining introgressed protected mammals: when is a wildcat a wild cat and a dingo a wild dog? *Wildlife Research* 30 (3): 213–218.
Ehrlich, P. and Ehrlich, A. (1981). *Extinction*. New York, USA: Random House.
Ereshefsky, M. (2017). Species. In: Edward N.Z. (ed.) The Stanford Encyclopedia of Philosophy (Fall 2017 edition). https://plato.stanford.edu/entries/species
Harrington, L.A., Moehrenschlager, A., Gelling, M. et al. (2013). Conflicting and complementary ethics of animal welfare considerations in reintroductions. *Conservation Biology* 27 (3): 486–500.
Isaac, N.J. and Pearse, W.D. (2018). The use of EDGE (evolutionary distinct globally endangered) and EDGE-like metrics to evaluate taxa for conservation. In: *Phylogenetic Diversity* (ed. R.A. Scherson and D.P. Faith), 27–39. Cham, Switzerland: Springer.
Johnson, L. (2003). Future generations and contemporary ethics. *Environmental Values* 12 (4): 471–487.
Kitchener, A.C., Yamaguchi, N., Ward, J.M., and Macdonald, D.W. (2005). A diagnosis for the Scottish wildcat (*Felis silvestris*): a tool for conservation action for a critically-endangered felid. *Animal Conservation Forum* 8 (3): 223–237.
Mayr, E. (1940). Speciation phenomena in birds. *American Naturalist* 74 (752): 249–278.
Millennium Ecosystem Assessment Board (2005). *The Millennium Ecosystem Assessment*. Washington, D.C., USA: Island Press www.millenniumassessment.org/en/index.html.
Newman, J., Varner, G., and Linquist, J. (2017). *Defending Biodiversity: Environmental Science and Ethics*. Cambridge, UK: Cambridge University Press.
Norton, B. (1988). *Why Preserve Natural Variety?* Princeton, USA: Princeton University Press.
Parsons, G. (2007). The aesthetic value of animals. *Environmental Ethics* 29 (2): 151–169.
Plater, Z.J.B. (2013). *The Snail Darter and the Dam*. New Haven, USA: Yale University Press.
Russow, L.M. (1981). Why do species matter? *Environmental Ethics* 3: 101–112.
Secretariat of the Convention on Biological Diversity (2012) *The Convention on Biological Diversity*. www.cbd.int/intro
Smith, I. (2016). *The Intrinsic Value of Endangered Species*. New York, USA: Routledge.
Sober, E. (1986). Philosophical problems for environmentalism. In: *The Preservation of Species: The Value of Biological Diversity* (ed. B.G. Norton), 173–194. Princeton, USA: Princeton University Press.
Soulé, M. (1985). What is conservation biology? *Bioscience* 35: 727–734.
Wallach, A.D., Lundgren, E., Batavia, C. et al. (2020). When all life counts in conservation. *Conservation Biology* 34 (4): 997–1007.
Wheatley, B.P. and Harya Putra, D.K. (1994). The effects of tourism on conservation at the monkey forest in Ubud, Bali. *La Revue d'Écologie* 49 (3): 245–257.
Wildcat Haven (n.d.). The Scottish wildcat. www.wildcathaven.com/scottish-wildcat
Wiley, E.O. (1978). The evolutionary species concept reconsidered. *Systematic Biology* 27 (1): 17–26.

Valuing Wild Animals as Individuals

5

5.1 Introduction

Modern-day Australians face challenges knowing what to do with the continent's iconic kangaroos. These challenges don't primarily relate to the concepts of biodiversity we explored in Chapter 4 as, with the exception of tree kangaroos, no kangaroo species in Australia is threatened with extinction. On the contrary, kangaroos have become so abundant in the past two centuries that their populations number in the millions. In fact, kangaroos can become so populous that their very abundance regularly leads to their death via starvation (Figure 5.1). Because many Australians don't like to see kangaroos suffer, much discussion about kangaroos has centered on a relative newcomer into debates about values in wildlife management: *animal welfare*.

Unfortunately, there are many threats to kangaroo welfare, both nonhuman and human in origin (Wilson and Edwards 2019). On the nonhuman side, kangaroos undergo heavy parasitic infestations and face mass mortality events during the irregular droughts that characterize Australia's climate. They can also suffer due to both the presence and absence of predators. Dingoes chase and kill kangaroos when the two species live in the same area, which is stressful for the individual kangaroos being chased (Allen et al. 2019). At the same time, one of the factors that explains the explosion in kangaroo

Wildlife Ethics: The Ethics of Wildlife Management and Conservation, First Edition. Clare Palmer, Bob Fischer, Christian Gamborg, Jordan Hampton, and Peter Sandøe.

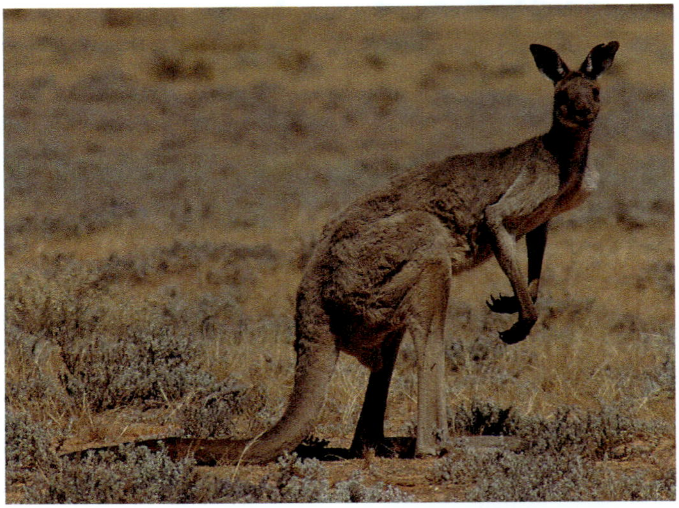

Figure 5.1 An emaciated kangaroo facing starvation during drought in semi-arid inland Australia. *Source:* Courtesy of Graeme Coulson.

populations is a lack of natural predators in many areas. High populations can result in kangaroos starving partly due to intraspecific competition for resources.

On the human side, kangaroos are frequently struck by vehicles on Australia's highways and in cities (Descovich et al. 2015). Additionally, they are the target of a large-scale commercial harvesting industry for their meat and leather. There are also potential welfare impacts of nonlethal population management strategies. In cities, for instance, kangaroos are captured and subjected to fertility control to avoid killing them (a modern approach to managing hyperabundant urban animals; see Chapter 11). Depending on how we understand the notion of welfare, the loss of the ability to make mating decisions could be a welfare impact, as could the loss of positive experiences associated with reproduction.

Additionally, there are difficult questions about welfare across a kangaroo's lifespan. Some deaths for adult kangaroos may be relatively quick, for instance when shot or struck by cars. Still, there's the question of whether it's bad for those animals to have shorter lives than they would have had otherwise. Additionally, there are questions about differences between juveniles and adults. Some of the kangaroos struck by cars are females carrying juvenile kangaroos (joeys) in their pouches. As young marsupials, some of these younger joeys may lack the neurological development widely thought to be necessary for sentience, but older joeys are generally recognized as sentient, and may die slow deaths from starvation or lack of maternal care if their mother dies (Sharp and McLeod 2016). So, how should those nuances factor into our assessment of the overall welfare impact?

These questions force us to consider how we define welfare and raise the possibility that there might be different conceptions of what welfare is. In this chapter, we discuss the development of the concept of animal welfare as it emerged out of intensive farm animal production. We present what might be thought of as the mainstream view of wildlife welfare, the so-called Five Domains model, and consider how wildlife welfare might be assessed based on this approach. Finally, we present and discuss challenges to the mainstream view of wildlife welfare, including alternative interpretations of what welfare should be understood to be.

5.2 The Idea of Wild Animal Welfare

In previous chapters, we focused on the value of wild animals to humans and as members of valuable species and ecosystems. Our concern here is what's important from the point of view of the wild animals themselves. Or, to put the question more generally: What is animal welfare?

The concept of "animal welfare" is typically applied to *individual* animals. When doing so, it's assumed that things can go better or worse for them and that what is done or happens to them can be good or bad for them. Nonliving things, like cars or stones, don't have states of welfare; while cars can break down or fall apart, there aren't states that are better or worse for *them*. Humans, of course, might prefer that cars *not* break down or that certain rock formations not crumble – but not for the sake of the cars or rock formations themselves.

What about plants? While it's true that things can be said to go better or worse for them, there remains an important difference between plants and sentient animals. In this book, as we noted in Chapter 1, we're concerned about wildlife as beings that have *interests*, understood as being aware of, and caring about, what happens to them and having the capacity for both positive and negative mental experiences (Beausoleil et al. 2018). Concern for animal welfare, then, is a concern for what is done or happens to sentient nonhuman animals for their *own* good, rather than for the good of humans, species, ecosystems, or anything else.

Historically, questions about *wild* animal welfare have most often been raised in situations where humans keep or manage wild animals and make decisions that affect their welfare, such as zoos. Considerable efforts have been made to measure and improve the welfare of captive wild animals, especially for large mammalian species such as elephants (Mason and Veasey 2010). Less attention has been devoted to the welfare of wild and free-roaming animals with which humans interfere, such as the animals that people hunt for food or leather (like Australian kangaroos), though research efforts in these areas are ramping up. Still, it remains the case that the main conversation about animal welfare has not been, first and foremost, about wild animals but about *domesticated* ones. To understand debates about wild animal welfare, then, we need to understand their roots in the study of animal welfare as it emerged in farm animal production.

5.3 Animal Welfare: From Avoiding Suffering to Positive Welfare

The modern discussion of animal welfare dates back to the 1960s. At that time, there were increasing public misgivings about conditions in intensive farm animal production (Sandøe and Jensen 2011). This led the United Kingdom government to form the

Brambell Committee to investigate and report on welfare conditions in British livestock farming. In 1965, the Committee produced a document called *Report of the Technical Committee to Enquire into the Welfare of Animals Kept under Intensive Livestock Husbandry Systems* (Brambell 1965). The Brambell Report, as it became known, was theoretically important for the way it conceptualized animal welfare. It was also practically important because its recommendations formed the basis of subsequent British and European animal welfare legislation.

While previous animal protection legislation had focused on preventing "pointless" suffering – suffering that brought with it no economic or other human benefits – a major conceptual shift took place in the Brambell Report and the animal welfare legislation that followed it. This new approach involved protecting animals against the adverse consequences of practices genuinely useful to efficient food production. The Brambell Report understood animals' needs as requirements that, if not met, would cause them to suffer. This interpretation also came with a new and wider understanding of suffering, which had previously been conceptualized only in terms of persistent and significant pain. The Brambell Report introduced the idea that suffering could also follow from the frustration of "behavioral urges" in the form of discomfort, stress, and other negative mental states. This sense of suffering made it possible to criticize the confinement of sows and calves, not based on the claim that confinement causes pain but rather that animals were prevented from engaging in behaviors they were highly motivated to perform (Kilgour 2012).

Following the Brambell Report, the influential "Five Freedoms" notion of animal welfare was subsequently formulated in the United Kingdom by the Farm Animal Welfare Council (1979). The Five Freedoms also reflected the idea that suffering includes mental states other than the feeling of undergoing physical pain: freedoms from (i) thirst and hunger, (ii) discomfort, (iii) pain, injury or disease, (iv) behavioral frustration, and (v) fear and distress. However, there's one important limitation about both Brambell and the Five Freedoms: namely, the focus on the absence of suffering. Important though that is, it ignores *positive* welfare – that is, the presence of positive states like satisfaction and pleasure.

A more recent development in the idea of welfare, then, includes such *positive* welfare states alongside avoiding *negative* welfare states (harms or suffering) when thinking about what makes for good welfare (Mellor and Beausoleil 2015). These include opportunities for pleasurable experiences such as social play, courtship or parenting. These states are valuable in themselves, but can also be valuable instrumentally; for instance, positive social engagement may also help animals to cope with injuries or illnesses.

This brings us to the "Five Domains" model of animal welfare, which has had various manifestations since its first conceptualization in 1994. The model from 2015, represented in Figure 5.2, builds on the foundations of the Brambell Report and the Five Freedoms model and includes positive welfare states alongside the negative ones (Mellor and Beausoleil 2015). The basic idea of the model is that the welfare status of an animal is a direct function of the feelings of the animal, the so-called mental domain. The more that positive experiences prevail over negative experiences, the better the overall welfare state. This experience-based position is called "hedonism" in the philosophical literature (Robbins et al. 2018) and has, to date, been the mainstream view of animal welfare,

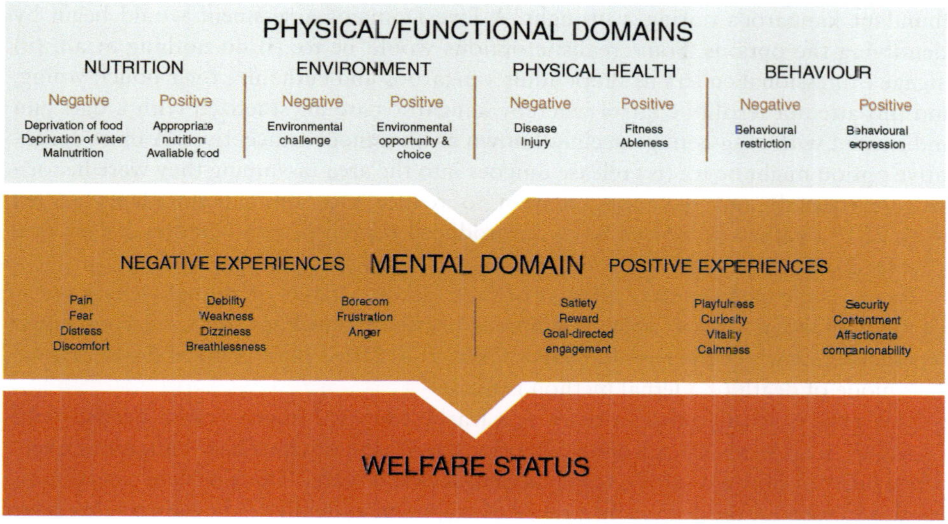

Figure 5.2 The 2015 version of the Five Domains model of animal welfare. *Source:* Adapted from Mellor and Beausoleil (2015).

where it is generally called the "affective state approach" (Fraser and Duncan 1998). We'll look at some alternative understandings of welfare later in the chapter.

However, there's no direct way to measure the experiences or feelings of animals. Therefore, even if animals' welfare is determined by the overall quality of their experience, the study of their welfare has to be focused on detectable *indicators* of their experiences. This is why the Five Domains model interprets the experiences of animals as the function of four other aspects or "domains" of animals' lives: their nutritional state, the environment in which they live, their physical health, and their behavioral opportunities. In short, then, the model says that animals' welfare is determined by the quality of their experiences *and* that our best evidence regarding the quality of their experiences comes from the four domains at the top of Figure 5.2. The assessment of animal welfare, using such welfare indicators, is the task of animal welfare science, an empirical discipline concerned with documenting and measuring impacts of different ways of housing, managing, and using animals (Fraser 2008). In the following section, we give some examples of how such assessments can be carried out in the context of wildlife.

5.4 Using the Five Domains Model to Assess Wild Animal Welfare

The Five Domains model is often used to assess the welfare impact of wildlife management practices such as the control of unwanted nonnative animals and overabundant native species (Baker et al. 2016).

Let's go back to the example of overabundant kangaroos presented at the start of the chapter and suppose that the aim is to try to decide whether – and if so, how – to manage abundant kangaroos during a drought. A Five Domains assessment would begin by identifying the options. Some realistic options would be to: (i) do nothing at all, (ii) engage professional cullers to shoot adult kangaroos and euthanize their pouch young, and (iii) attempt fertility control whereby kangaroos are anesthetized with a dart gun and treated with long-acting vaccines known as immunocontraceptives. A more speculative option might be to: (iv) release dingoes into the area (assuming they were historically extirpated) and rely on predation to reduce prey animal abundance (Allen et al. 2019), rather as wolves were reintroduced to Yellowstone National Park (see Chapter 2).

To assess the likely welfare impacts of each option, a panel of animal welfare scientists would assign scores to the magnitudes of negative feelings the kangaroos might experience in each of the five domains (Baker et al. 2016) both prior to death and via their mode of death (if a lethal method is used).

This task is hardly straightforward. Clearly, educated guesswork is needed with respect to the relevant background conditions, as it isn't obvious how kangaroos experience thirst or how stressful it is for them to seek out water. This problem can be mitigated, at least to some degree, by a range of empirical animal-based measures that have been developed with the goal of objectively assessing aspects of an animal's physiology or behavior.

However, interpreting these measures can be problematic. For example, an animal's blood cortisol level is often taken to be evidence of stress (not just as a physiological phenomenon, but as a marker of a particular negative subjective experience; Gentsch et al. 2018). This is because cortisol tends to increase when animals are in situations associated with protracted pain or physiological exertion, such as having recently experienced a severe injury or having recently escaped from a predator. However, cortisol levels can also be high during play and can be very low in some animals who exhibit depressive behavior. So, cortisol is really a measure of *excitement* or *arousal*, which bears a more complex relationship to stress (Dawkins 2021). Additionally, very short-term cortisol responses are particularly difficult to interpret. For instance, a short-term cortisol response could tell us little about the intensity of stress a kangaroo experiences in the few seconds it takes to die from a bullet. The use of this type of physiological marker is therefore challenging when studying stress (whether in kangaroos or other animals).

Of course, simple metrics, such as the duration of a procedure, can also be used to get some idea of the duration of suffering. However, such estimates are often based on optimal conditions, where plans go exactly as expected. Suppose, for instance, that someone uses the amount of time it takes for a bullet to kill an animal to estimate the welfare impact of that death. They might assume that there's almost no impact as death (or more accurately, "insensibility") is practically immediate after a head shot. But how often does death happen this way under typical conditions? So, it's more accurate when animal welfare studies report the frequency of "adverse animal welfare events" (see Chapter 15 on the use of this metric in research) – which here means cases of protracted death – to allow more nuanced interpretation of the welfare consequences.

So far, we've focused on trying to account for what kangaroos might experience in each hypothetical scenario. But kangaroos, of course, are not the whole picture. There are many other wild animals in the same ecosystems that will be affected by any kangaroo management decision made. After all, most of the ways in which humans harm animals are not intentional or even direct (Fraser and MacRae 2011). In fact, most are derived from processes of which scientists may not be fully aware, such as small mammals being killed during land clearing, fish being killed by toxic blue-green algae blooms arising from nutrient-rich run-off from cropping land, or bats perishing during extreme heat waves due to climate change. A holistic assessment of the animal welfare effects of kangaroo management would need to include consideration of *indirect* and *unintentional* animal welfare impacts. These would include native reptiles that may die from loss of grass tuft habitat if inflated kangaroo populations are not reduced (Howland et al. 2014). It may also include eagles that are poisoned via lead bullet fragments if kangaroos are shot *en masse* (Hampton et al. 2022). Finally, there will be welfare effects on kangaroo predators and scavengers whatever management decisions are taken.

These points are not necessarily challenges to the Five Domains model as such; they can be taken as reasons to be careful when applying the model. There are, however, also some conceptual challenges to the model that deserve attention.

5.5 Two Challenges to the Mainstream View of Animal Welfare

In what follows, we'll consider two influential challenges to the mainstream view of animal welfare. The first questions the affective state approach that stands behind the Five Domains model. The second challenges the assumption that death isn't a welfare issue.

5.5.1 Beyond Feelings: The Importance of Natural Behavior

So far in this chapter, we've focused on the mainstream idea that welfare is determined solely by animals' positive and negative subjective experiences. However, that view has some challenging implications when applied to wild animals. Let's take our kangaroos as an example here. In good times, kangaroos may have positive experiences from eating, drinking, moving freely, and engaging with other kangaroos. But as we saw at the beginning of this chapter, living in the wild also poses a host of welfare challenges in terms of parasites, disease, drought, fires, and predation.

Indeed, evolutionary biologists from Charles Darwin to Richard Dawkins have pointed out that the mechanisms of natural selection will generally result in extensive animal suffering in nature, since insofar as natural selection maximizes anything, it's *fitness*, not positive experiences. Building on this, others have argued that suffering is particularly common among the members of *r*-selected species – that is, species that produce many offspring, each of which has a relatively low probability of surviving to adulthood, as opposed to *k*-selected species, which produce fewer offspring and invest more in each one (see Horta 2017). Kangaroos are *k*-selected species and even their lives can be difficult. Compared to kangaroos, though, most *r*-selected animals have relatively short lives, many of which end painfully. So, assessing the welfare of wild animals based on their subjective experiences may lead to the conclusion that many or most wild animals have relatively *low* welfare, and some may not even have lives worth living.

These issues need not be taken as an objection to the affective state approach behind the Five Domains model. It could simply be concluded that many animals have worse lives than predicted based on the romanticized portraits found in some nature documentaries.

Indeed, as we'll see in Chapter 6, on some ethical views, poor wild animal welfare *in itself* is a reason to intervene to attempt to improve the lives of wild animals. If their welfare is really so bad, it might be concluded that there are more extensive reasons to intervene than might have been guessed.

However, this may also raise the question whether welfare really is only about animals' subjective experiences. After all, the welfare challenges of freedom of movement and association in intensive production from which the dominant animal welfare model arose are very different from the welfare challenges of free-roaming wild animals. One historically influential alternative to the affective state approach maintains that welfare is determined by living "naturally," what is sometimes called a "species-typical life." The idea here is that animals have, to some degree at least, species-specific "natures" that determine what's good for members of their kind. To be clear, the view here is *not* that if animals live according to their natures, then they are likely to have good experiences – essentially staying wholly within the affective state framework. Instead, the view is that animals living according to their natures constitutes good welfare *independently* of the resulting experiences. This view is rooted in parallel discussions about human wellbeing, where a long-standing and influential contender to the affective state approach has been a view called "perfectionism." According to that view, a good human life is one where important human potentials are realized (Appleby and Sandøe 2002).

Of course, someone who holds a "naturalness" view of animal welfare doesn't have to reject the importance of an animal's subjective states altogether. It's generally argued that *both* what an animal experiences *and* the ability to perform natural behaviors matter for an animal's welfare. The main thought here is that what an animal experiences doesn't capture *all* that we should take into account when considering welfare. So, for instance, many amphibians and reptiles seem to do well in terms of affective states in well-managed zoos. However, someone might worry that they are not exhibiting the full range of behaviors that they would exhibit in the wild and take this fact alone to imply that welfare is compromised (Robbins et al. 2018) (see also Chapter 14).

On a "naturalness" view of animal welfare, then, being able to realize natural, species-specific potentials is a constituent of a good life (Musschenga 2002). It makes sense that it's good for animals to be able to do the things that come naturally to them – control territory, find mates, search for food, and so on. Moreover, animals may be worse off insofar as they are denied these opportunities. So, for instance, even if a gray wolf born in a zoo has never hunted with a pack and isn't in any conscious sense aware of missing anything, nonetheless (on this view) something *is* lacking. The animal has been denied the opportunity to fulfill his or her species-specific nature (Clubb and Mason 2007) – which is taken to be of value in its own right.

The naturalness view of welfare can also be controversial when natural behavior creates negative subjective feelings. For instance, while fighting between male members of a species may be natural, it's also stressful; can cause injury; and gives rise to pain, fear, and other negative experiences. If welfare is measured in terms of subjective experiences, fighting that results in injury seems to bring about poor welfare, especially for the loser. But from a natural behavior account of welfare, both animals will have good welfare, as they are free to do what comes naturally. This suggests that when someone accepts a naturalness account of welfare that includes a place for subjective experiences, they will need to explain how the two welfare determinants trade off against one another when they conflict.

Going back to the kangaroos, what would an exclusive focus on naturalness imply about kangaroo welfare, when kangaroos are so abundant that they are low on resources? If natural behavior alone is our guide, perhaps dying of predation, thirst or starvation is not welfare negative; after all, it's a natural occurrence that kangaroos have undergone for millions of years. If welfare was assessed based on natural behavior, that might also suggest that fertility control has undesirable welfare outcomes. After all, this type of intervention works by denying kangaroos the opportunity to reproduce, which means they often won't experience the full range of behaviors associated with reproduction, including courting and copulation (Hampton et al. 2015). A hybrid, "naturalness + subjective experiences" view would, of course, deliver different results, though it isn't clear what they are, since it's unclear how two independent determinants of welfare would interact.

However one interprets welfare, it's clear that for any particular wild animal species, making judgments about the base rate of welfare *independent* of human management is important for assessing the welfare impacts of human activities and management. Assessing a welfare base rate may cast the welfare impacts of different forms of management, including lethal management, in a different light. On an affective state view of welfare, for instance, we might think that lethal management is bad for individual animals for two possible reasons: first, because the process of dying may be painful; second, because death deprives them of a future of good experiences. If, however, it's likely that most members of a particular population would live unpleasant lives and die painfully as a result of predation, starvation, or disease, then on an affective state view, painless lethal management may actually be a welfare benefit rather than a welfare harm; death at human hands may mean that those animals may have been spared from worse fates in the wild. This kind of calculation has been used, for instance, more generally in considering the management of hyperabundant native animals (see Chapter 11).

These observations, however, raise a further question. We just suggested that someone could take the view that lethal management is bad for animals insofar as death deprives them of good experiences in the future. But this assumes that killing itself is a welfare issue, even if done painlessly. This is the second challenge we'll consider to the mainstream view of animal welfare.

5.5.2 Is Killing a Welfare Issue?

So far, our discussion of animal welfare has ignored one important issue: namely, the significance of death. Is death, and any act of killing that brings it about, a welfare issue?

Clearly, the process leading to death can be bad for animals: dying can be painful, whether due to injury, disease, or another cause. Of course, dying isn't always painful, or at least not very painful. When veterinarians euthanize animals, they aim to cause no more pain than a needle prick. Some forms of predation may also be so quick that the prey animal is barely aware of what's happening. However, we need to separate questions about dying, which can involve suffering that is bad for animals, from death itself. So, leaving the process of dying aside, is death itself bad for animals? Is it bad for an animal not to continue living? Do we harm animals when we kill them?

There are views – most famously the view held by the Greek philosopher Epicurus – on which death doesn't harm *anyone*, human or nonhuman. Epicurus maintained that you can only be harmed by having negative experiences. A dead person has no experiences and so, obviously, no negative experiences. Of course, both in the human case and in the case of some nonhumans, Epicurus would grant that the death of an individual matters to other individuals who are still alive. But that doesn't make it bad for the one who died. On this view, then, lethal management of animals would only harm them insofar as it causes them pain. If it can be done painlessly, it causes no harm at all.

However, hardly anyone actually holds this view about humans. The standard objection to Epicurus is simple: while a person who dies won't have any negative experiences after their death, they are nonetheless missing out on all the positive experiences they would otherwise have had – positive experiences that, on balance, may outweigh any negative experiences. And if they would have had mostly positive experiences, then it seems that death *is* bad for them, as they're losing a good future.

While this issue might seem abstract, it has enormous practical relevance. Let's suppose that death itself is *not* bad for animals. Then, a wildlife manager who culls animals painlessly hasn't harmed those animals at all, even though they are now dead. Of course, if the manager had caused pain, that would have been bad on most theories of welfare. But if death isn't bad for animals, then that pain would have been the only harm. By contrast, if death is bad for animals, then even if the wildlife manager kills the animals painlessly, they've been harmed. And if the animals had long, positive lives ahead of them, then it could be that they were harmed enormously. So, when we try to quantify the impact that an action has on wildlife, it matters a great deal both whether death is a harm and, if it is, then how great that harm is.

The objection to Epicurus says that death harms humans insofar as it deprives them of a future that would have been good for them (Kasperbauer and Sandøe 2016). This is a *comparative* account of the badness of death. What makes death bad – when it is bad – is the contrast with how things would have gone for the individual had she survived. If we extend that view to animals, then it implies that if an animal is suffering intensely with no hope of improvement – for instance, with an unbearably painful parasitic infection or having been severely wounded with no chance of survival – then death is not bad, because it doesn't deprive the animal of anything good. Indeed, death is good insofar as it ends suffering – this is the foundation for the euthanasia of sick animals by veterinarians. But in other cases, death would be a welfare loss. Consider, for instance, a young female kangaroo basking in the sun with her healthy offspring, full after grazing on abundant green grass in an optimal habitat. That kangaroo appears to have pleasant experiences ahead. So, if a harvester were to shoot her, the kangaroo would be harmed: she would lose those future positive experiences.

By contrast, noncomparative accounts say that what makes death bad is not just explained in terms of the potential welfare lost for the animal in question. Some argue, for instance, that death is bad for an individual simply because death destroys something inherently valuable – namely, the individual herself. On such a view, lethal animal management also involves harming animals, even if done painlessly, at least on the assumption that each individual animal is a valuable being.

A different sort of noncomparative account follows from an alternative theory of welfare, both to the hedonistic and the naturalness account: the desire-satisfaction account, one that has been widely discussed in the case of human beings. This account forms another challenge to the hedonism of the Five Domains model. Like hedonism, the desire-satisfaction account focuses on animals' subjective states. But what matters here is not happiness or misery but getting or doing what one wants – satisfying one's desires – and avoiding what one doesn't want – not having desires frustrated (Dawkins 2021). Of course, satisfying one's desires may make one feel happy but on this account, it's the *satisfaction of the desire*, not the happy feelings, that count for welfare. On this view, death harms insofar as it frustrates a being's most fundamental desire: to go on living, even though the frustration is never actually experienced, of course, because the being is dead.

It's clear how this works in the case of humans, where people have forward-looking desires for how their lives will go, premised on the desire to go on living. For this to work in the case of animals, it would need to be established whether an animal either actually has a desire to live (which would mean having some kind of understanding of self, life, and death) or, at least, that the animal has desires about the future that imply or depend on a desire to go on living. So, the implications of the desire-satisfaction view seem to depend on the cognitive capacities of particular species. It's more likely that elephants and chimpanzees have such desires, for instance, than crocodilians and chickadees. See Palmer (2010) for a more extensive discussion of the issues here.

To give just one example of the practical relevance of all this to assessing wild animal welfare, Baker et al. (2016) offer a model of the welfare impact of a management intervention. This particular model has two parts. The first scores the welfare impacts of both lethal and nonlethal management interventions using a version of the above-mentioned Five Domains model. The second part focuses on lethal intervention specifically and scores interventions based on (i) time to loss of consciousness and (ii) level of suffering. Two scoring matrices determine where the intervention falls on a graph. Figure 5.3 shows a graph representing the welfare impact of three methods of crow management:

- shooting crows in the chest with a shotgun
- trapping crows and then killing them by cervical dislocation
- scaring crows using gas guns.

The striking result here is that, according to the model, the welfare impact of scaring crows with gas guns is greater than the welfare impact of shooting crows. This is because death itself has no place in the analysis: the model assumes that welfare is exhausted by what happens *before* animals die. So, if wildlife managers are committed to minimizing welfare impacts and use this model to assess those impacts, then they will reach the conclusion that a lethal option is better than a nonlethal one.

The authors of this study are aware of the limits of this model, writing that "an ideal welfare assessment model would allow direct comparison of the total impact of any management interventions, whether lethal or non-lethal" though they worry that "such a model might be impossible to achieve" (Baker et al. 2016, p.14). Whether that's so depends on one's philosophical commitments. If, for instance, hedonism and a comparative account of the badness of death are endorsed, then it's clearly possible to offer a unified account of such welfare impacts. To assess the total impacts on a particular

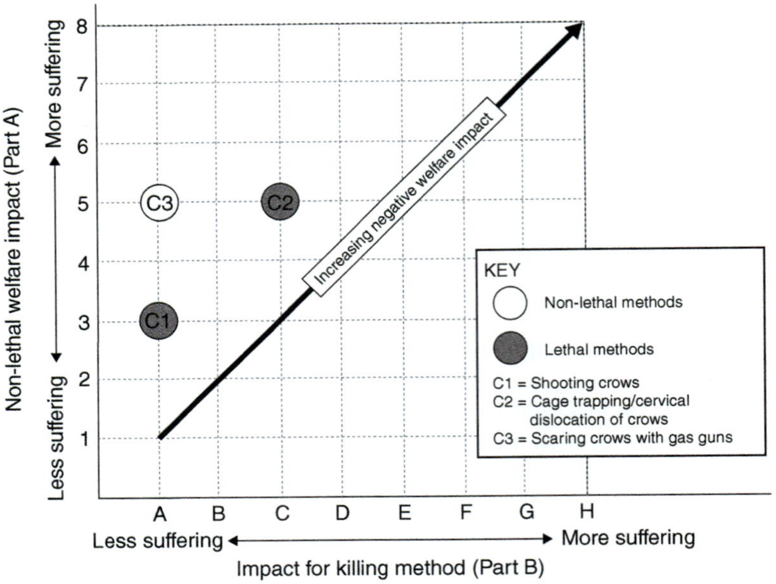

Figure 5.3 A Five Domains assessment of animal welfare outcomes for management intervention applied to crows in the United Kingdom that compares lethal and nonlethal methods. *Source:* Baker SE, Sharp TM, Macdonald DW (2016) Assessing animal welfare impacts in the management of European rabbits (*Oryctolagus cuniculus*), European moles (*Talpa europaea*) and carrion crows (*Corvus corone*). PLoS ONE 11(1): e0146298. CC BY 4.0.

crow, the balance of pleasures and pains that the crow would experience without the intervention – that is, the balance of pleasures and pains across the rest of its natural lifespan – should be compared to the balance of pleasures and pains that the crow experiences with the intervention. Of course, getting the relevant data would be difficult. In principle, though, it would be possible for experts to make reasonable estimates, drawing on the average life expectancy for crows, the quality of the lives of crows in the wild, plus the same sort of information that informed the model that Baker et al. (2016) employed. The point is that theories of welfare and death's relationship to welfare either permit or prohibit more comprehensive welfare assessment tools.

5.6 Conclusion

This book isn't the place to defend particular accounts of welfare or death's relationship to it. What matters here is just that we recognize that such accounts represent significant theoretical choice points in thinking about what's important for animals. That being said, there is an asymmetry here, because most accounts of welfare agree that positive and negative subjective experiences matter for welfare, even if they disagree about how much these experiences matter and whether other factors (such as natural behavior and desire-satisfaction) matter too.

In the rest of the book, when we talk about "animal welfare," we will generally be referring to the mainstream hedonist view represented by the Five Domains model. However, where it's interesting or important to give a broader account, we'll include discussion of welfare in terms of natural behavior and/or the desire-satisfaction account and will include discussion of the welfare consequences of death.

We should make one final point. A theory of welfare – or a commitment to the other values we've discussed in earlier chapters, such as species, ecosystems, wildness, and so on – doesn't itself determine what ought to be done in a particular situation. People have very different ideas about what should be *done* with values – whether, for instance, the goal is to try to protect them and prevent them from being violated or, on the other hand, to maximize them, such that more is always better. So, even if two people agree about all the welfare facts in a given case, they may think that very different practices are best. To understand those disagreements, we turn to ethical theory – how those values are handled – which is the subject of the next chapter.

References

Allen, B.L., Allen, L.R., Ballard, G. et al. (2019). Animal welfare considerations for using large carnivores and guardian dogs as vertebrate biocontrol tools against other animals. *Biological Conservation* 232: 258–270.

Appleby, M.C. and Sandøe, P. (2002). Philosophical debate on the nature of well-being: implications for animal welfare. *Animal Welfare* 11 (3): 283–294.

Baker, S.E., Sharp, T.M., and Macdonald, D.W. (2016). Assessing animal welfare impacts in the management of European rabbits (*Oryctolagus cuniculus*), European moles (*Talpa europaea*) and Carrion crows (*Corvus corone*). *PLoS ONE* 11 (1): e0146298.

Beausoleil, N.J., Mellor, D.J., Baker, L. et al. (2018). "Feelings and fitness" not "feelings or fitness" – the raison d'être of conservation welfare, which aligns conservation and animal welfare objectives. *Frontiers in Veterinary Science* 5: 296.

Brambell, F.W.R. (1965). *Report of the Technical Committee to Enquire into the Welfare of Animals Kept under Intensive Livestock Husbandry Systems*. London, UK: Her Majesty's Stationery Office.

Clubb, R. and Mason, G.J. (2007). Natural behavioural biology as a risk factor in carnivore welfare: how analysing species differences could help zoos improve enclosures. *Applied Animal Behaviour Science* 102 (3–4): 303–328.

Dawkins, M.S. (2021). *The Science of Animal Welfare: Understanding What Animals Want*. New York, USA: Oxford University Press.

Descovich, K., McDonald, I., Tribe, A., and Phillips, C. (2015). A welfare assessment of methods used for harvesting, hunting and population control of kangaroos and wallabies. *Animal Welfare* 24 (3): 255–265.

Farm Animal Welfare Committee (1979). *Five Freedoms*. London, UK: Farm Animal Welfare Council.

Fraser, D. (2008). Understanding animal welfare. *Acta Veterinaria Scandinavica* 50 (1): S1.

Fraser, D. and Duncan, I.J. (1998). 'Pleasures', 'pains' and animal welfare: toward a natural history of affect. *Animal Welfare* 7 (4): 383–396.

Fraser, D. and MacRae, A.M. (2011). Four types of activities that affect animals: implications for animal welfare science and animal ethics philosophy. *Animal Welfare* 20 (4): 581–590.

Gentsch, R.P., Kjellander, P., and Röken, B.O. (2018). Cortisol response of wild ungulates to trauma situations: hunting is not necessarily the worst stressor. *European Journal of Wildlife Research* 64: 11.

Hampton, J.O., Hyndman, T.H., Barnes, A., and Collins, T. (2015). Is wildlife fertility control always humane? *Animals* 5 (4): 1047–1071.

Hampton, J.O., Pay, J.M., Katzner, T.E. et al. (2022). Managing macropods without poisoning ecosystems. *Ecological Management and Restoration* 23 (2): 153–157.

Horta, O. (2017). Animal suffering in nature: the case for intervention. *Environmental Ethics* 39 (3): 261–279.

Howland, B., Stojanovic, D., Gordon, I.J. et al. (2014). Eaten out of house and home: impacts of grazing on ground-dwelling reptiles in Australian grasslands and grassy woodlands. *PLoS ONE* 9 (12): e105966.

Kasperbauer, T.J. and Sandøe, P. (2016). Killing as a welfare issue. In: *The Ethics of Killing Animals* (ed. T. Višak and R. Garner), 17–31. Oxford, UK: Oxford University Press.

Kilgour, R.J. (2012). In pursuit of "normal": a review of the behaviour of cattle at pasture. *Applied Animal Behaviour Science* 138 (1–2): 1–11.

Mason, G.J. and Veasey, J.S. (2010). What do population-level welfare indices suggest about the well-being of zoo elephants? *Zoo Biology* 29 (2): 256–273.

Mellor, D. and Beausoleil, N. (2015). Extending the 'Five Domains' model for animal welfare assessment to incorporate positive welfare states. *Animal Welfare* 24 (3): 241–253.

Musschenga, A.W. (2002). Naturalness: beyond animal welfare. *Journal of Agricultural and Environmental Ethics* 15 (2): 171–186.

Palmer, C. (2010). *Animal Ethics in Context*. New York, USA: Columbia University Press.

Robbins, J., Franks, B., and von Keyserlingk, M.A. (2018). 'More than a feeling': an empirical investigation of hedonistic accounts of animal welfare. *PLoS ONE* 13 (3): e0193864.

Sandøe, P. and Jensen, K.K. (2011). The idea of animal welfare developments and tensions. In: *ICVAE First International Conference on Veterinary and Animal Ethics* (ed. C. Wathes, S. May, S. McCulloch, et al.), 11–17. University of London: Royal Veterinary College.

Sharp, T.M. and McLeod, S.R. (2016). Kangaroo harvesters and the euthanasia of orphaned young-at-foot: applying the theory of planned behaviour to an animal welfare issue. *Animal Welfare* 25 (1): 39–54.

Wilson, G.R. and Edwards, M. (2019). Professional kangaroo population control leads to better animal welfare, conservation outcomes and avoids waste. *Australian Zoologist* 40 (1): 181–202.

The Role of Ethical Theories

6

6.1 Introduction

The last few chapters have focused on *values*. Our values, however, don't tell us how to act; they only tell us what should be taken into account when deliberating. *Ethical theories* include values, but they also provide guidance about what to *do* with these values. As we'll see in this chapter, that guidance can be quite different from theory to theory.

We can find examples of this guidance in existing policies in wildlife management and conservation. Some policies are constructed with the aim of maximizing a threatened population's size; others are designed to ensure that rights aren't violated in pursuit of a conservation goal. But while these ideas are often present, their relationship to ethical theories is often *implicit* rather than explicitly and systematically formulated. This chapter aims to explain leading ethical theories in a structured way, how they differ from one another, and their respective implications for wildlife management and conservation.

To get started, we'll consider a case. In 1987, the US Fish and Wildlife Service (USFWS) listed the black-capped vireo (*Vireo atricapilla*) – a small songbird – as endangered under the Endangered Species Act of 1973. As of 2018, the USFWS

Wildlife Ethics: The Ethics of Wildlife Management and Conservation, First Edition. Clare Palmer, Bob Fischer, Christian Gamborg, Jordan Hampton, and Peter Sandøe.

considers this species "recovered" but it's generally accepted that the vireo is a conservation-reliant species: it won't survive without intervention (Wilsey et al. 2014). This is, in part, because it occupies a limited range, extending from Oklahoma through central and west Texas into Mexico. Black-capped vireos breed in early successional shrublands and, historically, wildfires were the disruptions that created these habitats, clearing out the Ashe juniper, a native tree in these regions, and making room for the shrubby cover that the vireos need for their nests. But disturbance-dependent habitats are in sharp decline across the US; fires are frequently suppressed, and shrublands are either eliminated for agriculture or are allowed to grow out of the early successional stage. This has meant dramatic loss of breeding habitat for the black-capped vireo.

Additionally, the vireo is threatened by the brown-headed cowbird, a native brood parasite which lays eggs in the nests of other bird species, including black-capped vireos (Kostecke et al. 2005). Although cowbird chicks don't usually oust vireo chicks from the nest, they outcompete them for food (Figure 6.1), and the vireo chicks thus fail to thrive. Although black-capped vireos used to coexist stably with brown-headed cowbirds, the ecological dynamic has shifted. When cowbirds aren't removed from vireo breeding grounds, vireo populations decline (Wilsey et al. 2014). And so, in an attempt to avoid this outcome, Texas Parks and Wildlife runs a cowbird trapping program, providing information to landowners about how to build effective traps and kill cowbirds via a method that is purported to be "humane, fast, and certain" (Texas Parks and Wildlife 2014).

Should cowbirds be killed to save vireos? In the eyes of many conservationists, there is no question here; it's obvious that this is the right course of action. However, some members of the general public have opposed the culling. One reason for opposition concerns disagreement about which values are most important; opponents to culling,

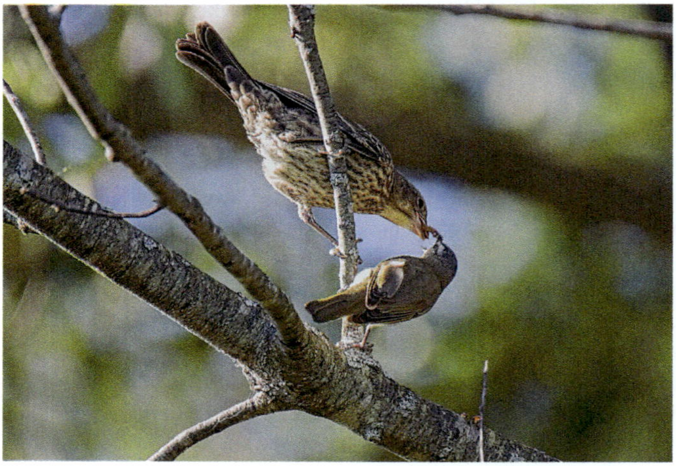

Figure 6.1 A brown-headed cowbird fledgling (the larger of the two birds) from Texas, USA, being fed by an adult black-capped vireo. An example of brood parasitism, a threat to the conservation of the vireo species. *Source:* Fiona M. Donnelly/Shutterstock.

for instance, may think that the lives of individual animals are more important than species persistence. In addition to conflicting answers to questions of "what matters," there may also be disagreement over *what one should do* about what matters. These disagreements take us into the domain of ethical theory.

To make this more concrete, let's consider some ethical questions raised by the cowbird culling proposals here, then explore how these questions would be addressed by different ethical theories.

- Clearly, the proposal involves *killing*. But here one could ask: is it permissible to kill some sentient animals to save others? Might killing individuals even be morally required if that would help to preserve an entire species?
- It's not only that the proposals involve killing; it's also likely that more adult cowbirds would be killed than vireo chicks would be saved. Could this too constitute grounds for opposition? That is, should the *quantity* of animal lives saved versus sacrificed be part of the equation?
- The killing of cowbirds could be done in a reasonably painless manner, whereas cowbird chicks likely cause vireo chicks a lot of suffering by depriving them of food. Should *aggregate suffering* be taken into account in our decision making?
- Is it fair to hold the cowbirds responsible for the decline in numbers of vireos? After all, humans destroyed vireo habitat and humans prevent the reestablishment of wildfire-dependent habitats in central Texas and beyond. Is the issue really a matter of failing to take full responsibility for human actions? Is the cowbird just a scapegoat?

Now, let's think about what major ethical theories would say about these questions.

6.2 Consequentialism

Consequentialism is best described as a family of ethical theories that's united by one key commitment: that actions should be evaluated solely on their consequences (as opposed to whether they were performed for the right reasons, whether it would be a problem if everyone acted that way, and so on). The most influential forms of consequentialism share a second commitment: that the goal is to bring about the *best* consequences (as opposed to consequences that are, say, better than some relevant alternative). Moreover, many of these theories understand the phrase "the best consequences" in terms of two related ideas: *aggregation* and *maximization*. Aggregation means that when considering an action or a policy, all its positive and negative consequences should be combined on a single scale, allowing them to be compared directly. Maximization means that the best action or policy – and so the one that ought to be selected – is the one that produces the greatest *net* good (positive features minus negative features, measured on a single scale).

Here, we'll look at two kinds of consequentialist theory that are particularly relevant to wildlife management and conservation: first, *utilitarianism,* understood as a view on which the welfare of human or all sentient beings is the primary concern; second, *ecocentric consequentialism*, where ecological collectives such as ecosystems and species have priority. So, in the vireo/cowbird case, utilitarians would ask "What would bring about the best outcomes in terms of welfare?" while ecocentric consequentialists would ask something like "What would bring about the best outcomes in terms of the biotic community, ecosystems, and species?."

6.2.1 Utilitarianism

Utilitarianism combines the view that what matters is the *welfare* of individuals (what is *good* for them, as discussed in Chapter 5) with *consequentialism*. A version of this idea has a long history in conservation. Gifford Pinchot, the founder of the US Forest Service, maintained that forests should be managed in the following way: "Where conflicting interests must be reconciled, the question shall always be answered from the standpoint of the greatest good of the greatest number in the long run" (Pinchot 1905, p. 1). This broadly captures a utilitarian approach, although Pinchot himself only counted the good for humans.

Indeed, as Pinchot (1905) illustrates, historically some utilitarian approaches to ethics have only taken into account the welfare of human individuals. This has usually been based on some form of what's called *human exceptionalism*: the view that humans are unique and more important than other living beings, sometimes to the point that humans are the only beings whose welfare has value (see the discussion of anthropocentrism in Chapter 2). However, welfare *isn't* confined to humans (as discussed in Chapter 5); there's little disagreement that sentient animals can have good or bad welfare, even if there's some disagreement about how welfare should be understood and about which animals are sentient. Moreover, it's difficult to explain why all humans' welfare matters but no animal's welfare does. So, extreme forms of exceptionalism appear arbitrary. Nevertheless, for the purpose of mapping the conceptual terrain, it's worth recognizing that people can endorse fully anthropocentric versions of utilitarianism, restricted to producing best outcomes in terms of human wellbeing. A weaker form of anthropocentric utilitarianism counts both human and animal interests but seriously discounts the latter (sometimes called "animal welfarism"; see Lund et al. 2021). This second position seems to be widespread. Even this weaker version, though, still needs to explain *why* human interests matter more than similar animal interests just because humans have them.

In any event, let's focus on a thoroughgoing welfare-centered utilitarianism that doesn't confine "the greatest good" to human beings but includes *sentient* animals as well. In this sense, it's egalitarian; it says that welfare *generally* should be maximized; that is, the interests of individuals are *considered equally*, regardless of species. As a result, this form of utilitarianism isn't vulnerable to the charge of inconsistency. The species of an individual is only relevant insofar as it makes a difference for that individual's welfare; according to utilitarianism, an individual doesn't count for less *simply* because the individual is a human or a cowbird.

Of course, many actions or policies will improve some beings' welfare while reducing the welfare of other beings. In this case, reducing the welfare of cowbirds through culling may benefit the survival and hence the welfare of vireos. So, utilitarians claim that the task is to identify what action (or policy) would produce more *net* welfare than any other option over time.

In one sense, this emphasis on net welfare is a strength of utilitarianism, because it allows (indeed, requires) a focus on just one value – namely, welfare. In principle, this should make working out policies and actions relatively straightforward. However, in practice, measuring net welfare (even in the human case) is hardly simple, since there are (as we saw in Chapter 5) different accounts of welfare, disagreement about how policies will affect welfare, and both practical and theoretical problems about how to aggregate welfare (see Sandøe et al. 2019). And when a policy involves aggregating welfare across members of wild species, about whose welfare we often know little, working out what actions would bring about best net welfare is even more difficult.

Basing wildlife policy on net welfare would likely look very different from most existing policies, as there's no guarantee human welfare will always outweigh aggregate animal welfare when measuring net welfare across human and wild animal species. For instance, the loss of welfare to many rodents from the use of anticoagulant poisons in human homes might well outweigh the welfare gains to the human communities administering it (see Fischer 2021).

What does this theory imply in the cowbird case? Here, the central question would be: what would bring about best welfare overall, taking into account vireo welfare, cowbird welfare, human welfare, and the welfare of any other sentient animals affected? Killing cowbirds would presumably improve vireo welfare: vireo hatchlings wouldn't starve to death because cowbird hatchlings outcompeted them for food. At the same time, killing cowbirds is arguably bad for cowbirds' welfare – although this would depend on whether killing in itself was seen, independently of the *process* of killing, as a welfare issue (as discussed in Chapter 5) and also on how the trapping was carried out. While the killing of trapped cowbirds can be very quick – cervical dislocation is recommended (Texas Parks and Wildlife 2014) – being caught in the trap itself (Figure 6.2) is likely to cause cowbirds distress. And given the scarcity of vireos and the high numbers of cowbirds, it's also likely that cowbird trapping will kill far more

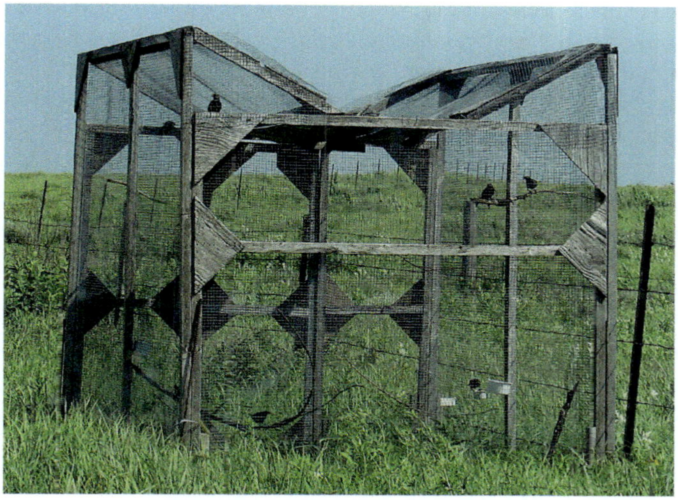

Figure 6.2 A brown-headed cowbird trap in Texas, USA. *Source:* Courtesy of Sarah Winnicki-Smith.

cowbirds than vireos saved. So, even if each trapped cowbird suffered less than each starved vireo chick, on balance, it at least seems plausible that killing cowbirds would cause more overall suffering than allowing cowbird chicks to cause the death of vireo chicks. It's likely, then, that utilitarianism would not support culling, though more details about the case would be needed to be sure.

Granted, the welfare of these two bird species is not all that's at stake; the welfare of members of other species is affected, most obviously humans. Some people really want the vireo species to survive and so those individuals' welfare is, in some small way, bound up with the vireos' success; others may be upset by the idea of killing cowbirds, or don't want the hassle of having to manage them, and so would have lower welfare if they had to participate in or hear about such conservation efforts. Moreover, there are various far-fetched risks. It's possible that if the vireo disappears, a previously innocuous insect population would explode, causing human health problems. There is concern that events like this may currently be occurring, linking human disease epidemics with declines in wildlife species (Springborn et al. 2022). Avian ecologists have given the ominous warning that "the societal importance of ecosystem services is often appreciated only during their loss" (Şekercioğlu et al. 2004).

However, utilitarians weigh such risks by multiplying their severity by their probability; as long as such disastrous outcomes are highly unlikely, they won't change the calculus when human welfare is incorporated. In any case, the important point is that all welfare impacts are being taken into account equally, regardless of who is being impacted and how impacts were caused; in particular, there's no distinction between welfare impacts on humans versus nonhumans or between anthropogenic and "natural" welfare impacts. So, if killing cowbirds causes more suffering than letting vireos die, cowbirds shouldn't be killed. Perhaps different land management patterns would be best, potentially including the use of fire; alternatively, it may be best to limit land development in vireo habitat.

It's important to note that utilitarianism doesn't factor in impacts on ecosystems, biodiversity, particular species, or the esthetics of a place – except insofar as any of those things can be linked to the welfare of individuals. If greater biodiversity makes no difference for welfare, then it doesn't matter. Obviously, this view is likely to be objectionable to many conservationists (after all, this doesn't really look like a conservation strategy at all). Some might even object on consequentialist grounds, pointing to other kinds of values that, in their view, ought to be maximized as well (we discuss this below).

Though applications of utilitarian thinking have been very important in policy making, including environmental policy (cost–benefit analysis, for instance, is widely used in economic assessments), utilitarianism has always been controversial. One key reason for this is that certain conceptions of *justice* have no obvious place. First, utilitarianism doesn't have a place for *inviolable rights*; there's nothing of value outside the welfare calculus. Killing cowbirds (or any other animal), for instance, is always, in principle, an option on the table. Second, what are sometimes called "backward-looking" concerns, ones that take into account past actions and the possibility of restitutive justice, also don't fit into a utilitarian approach. So, utilitarians won't find questions about *who's* responsible for the plight of vireos to be relevant to ethical decision making. What matters now is what should be done to bring about best welfare outcomes, not how the situation arose in the first place.

Another concern is that utilitarianism, as a wildlife management policy, seems very demanding, appearing to mandate high levels of intervention to reduce wild animal suffering. After all, it's likely that the welfare of wildlife could often be improved and that humans often have the means to help. From this perspective, the cowbird/vireo concern is just the tip of the iceberg; there may be many more severe cases of suffering in wild animals that also need attention if the goal is to maximize net welfare across all affected parties – including wild animals.

Utilitarianism, while the most popular form of consequentialism, is by no means the only one. Another kind of consequentialism that's particularly important in wildlife management and conservation – and that endorses very different values – is *ecocentric consequentialism*.

6.2.2 Ecocentric Consequentialism

In Chapters 3 and 4, we considered *ecocentric* positions, where value is located in states or properties of ecosystems, species, and/or biodiversity. When these values are embedded within a consequentialist ethical theory, the goal is to bring about the best outcomes with respect to those values – for instance, in terms of ecosystem preservation or species protection. On one interpretation of Aldo Leopold's statement of the Land Ethic (discussed in Chapter 4), it's broadly consequentialist, which is also the interpretation we'll explore here. (This is being used as a broad example; other readings of the Land Ethic are possible and Leopold's body of writing more generally is much more complex, if ethically unsystematic.) Leopold wrote "A thing is right when it tends to preserve the integrity, stability, and beauty of the biotic community. It is wrong when it tends otherwise" (Leopold 1949, p. 262). Understood as a form of ecocentric consequentialism, this view says what the key values are: the integrity, stability and beauty of the land community. And then it says what to do with them: do what "tends to preserve" the relevant features of the biotic community – that is, do what tends to bring about a certain good outcome. In that sense, the Land Ethic provides a test that allows determination of what should be done: does this action contribute to preserving the biotic community?

What would this Leopoldian form of ecocentric consequentialism have to say about the vireo/cowbird situation? What does it mean in practice to preserve the integrity, stability, and beauty of the biotic community? To work this out, more needs to be known about both the vireo's and the cowbird's importance to the biotic community. Since these are both native birds, the "integrity" of the biotic community might involve keeping these species in place. However, because the black-capped vireo is endangered (whereas the cowbird is plentiful), one could argue that there is more reason to protect vireos at the cowbirds' expense. Even though both have a place in the biotic community, the losses to the community from the extinction of the black-capped vireo would matter more than the loss of some cowbirds. All this indicates that a consequentialist Land Ethic would aim to protect the vireo against the cowbird. Like utilitarianism, though, the Land Ethic wouldn't narrow this choice to simply "killing the cowbirds, or no intervention." Other possible choices, such as managing land by fire (which also is an integral part of much conservation management in the US) to create better habitat, might be even better in terms of the integrity, stability, and beauty of the land community. After all, that might help many native species other than the black-capped vireo, thereby bringing about even better outcomes for the biotic community.

It's worth noting here that while the *values* of the Land Ethic are very different from utilitarianism (ecological values rather than welfare values), certain structural features of consequentialism remain the same. For instance, killing isn't ruled out in principle. Good and bad outcomes are still supposed to be aggregated to bring about the best net outcome overall. And the idea of "fairness" understood in terms of inviolable rights or restitutive justice has no obvious place. For this reason, consequentialism is viewed by some as unduly cynical (Nelson et al. 2016). However, the consequentialist interpretation of the Land Ethic raises complications that utilitarianism avoids, because it includes *multiple* values (Attfield 2013). How are we supposed to aggregate and maximize three entirely different values – integrity, stability, and beauty?

Protecting vireos may, in fact, protect all three values, but it's not hard to imagine cases where protecting integrity may not protect beauty or stability, making aggregation particularly difficult. This problem is acute where ecocentric consequentialists include multiple values such as ecosystems, species, and wildness. If those were at stake in the vireo case, it could be argued that an essentially permanent program to cull cowbirds reduces wildness value, even if it increases species protection. How should these values be aggregated?

Not all forms of ecocentric consequentialism, however, have multiple values; some just focus on one value, such as bringing about the best outcomes in terms of biodiversity (Attfield 2013). Again, in the vireo case, this is likely to require protecting the vireo, since loss of the vireo would mean a reduction in local and global species richness, one measure of biodiversity. Although, even here, since there are different measures of biodiversity (as discussed in Chapter 4), there could easily be policies that maximize biodiversity along one dimension while reducing it along another.

Consequentialist ethical theories – aiming to bring about the best outcomes in terms of one or more values – have long been a key part of policy and practice in wildlife management and conservation. Consequentialism may work better at the level of policy, though, than in terms of our everyday, individual decisions. One worry is that it's not possible to know many of the consequences of one-off, individual actions, which may be less predictable than policies, making it difficult to work out what to do. Worse, individual biases and cognitive shortcomings may mean that when trying to generate the best possible balance of good and bad consequences, serious mistakes and miscalculations are inevitably made (Nelson et al. 2016).

This criticism has led many adherents of consequentialism to adopt a more humble "two-level" approach. According to this view, at the level of everyday life, simple principles and straightforward virtues that are easy to understand should be adopted, on the assumption that this will normally bring about the best consequences (Hare 1982). The second level of explicitly consequentialist reasoning should only be undertaken in situations where everyday principles don't provide guidance, or when following this simpler approach will create severe negative consequences that could be avoided by a different decision. Explicit consequentialist reasoning is also well suited for the level of reflective policy making to govern complex situations, such as the case of vireos and cowbirds.

6.3 Rights Theory

Another leading ethical theory focuses on the idea of *rights*. Rights function as entitlements that confer a set of benefits to an individual: giving them certain freedoms to act, protecting their basic interests, and making claims on others to behave (or to refrain from behaving) in certain ways. Importantly, rights views generally reject the aggregation we saw in the two consequentialist views discussed above; according to rights views, the greater good can't justify sacrificing the basic interests of individuals. So, for instance, rights views deny that it's acceptable to kill a few individuals to produce small benefits for a great many others.

That human beings should be regarded as having certain fundamental rights is now widely (if not universally) accepted. It is, in fact, codified in the Universal Declaration of Human Rights, which has proven to be hugely influential in law and policy around the globe (UN General Assembly 1948). The most fundamental human rights are usually thought to be *negative* rights – that is, rights not to be interfered with in certain basic ways, for instance the right not to be killed, the right not to be unjustly imprisoned, the right not to be tortured. However, some argue that humans have *positive* rights too. A positive account of the right to life, for example, might entail the right to be provided with what's needed for life, such as food and water, rather than just the right not to be deprived of basic necessities.

From at least the late nineteenth century, when Henry Salt published *Animal Rights* (1892), there have been arguments that many animals also have basic rights. In brief, a leading version of the argument runs like this. The idea that humans are rights holders has traditionally rested on claims that humans are uniquely rational. However, many humans are not fully rational, including infants and people with severe cognitive disabilities. Surely, though, rights should be extended to these extremely vulnerable humans. After all, even if they aren't fully rational, many things matter to them, such as continuing to live, being free from serious suffering, and so on. Shouldn't the fact that they have fundamental interests be the basis for rights? But if the basis for rights isn't rationality but *interests*, then it isn't possible to consistently exclude animals that also have fundamental interests – in continuing to live and in being free from serious suffering – from being rights holders. Of course, this isn't to say that *all* their interests are the same as humans' interests. For instance, animals don't have a basic interest in education, and so don't have a right not to be deprived of it. But this wouldn't mean that they don't have *any* basic rights.

What does the rights view mean for wildlife conservation and management? Clearly, *human* rights play an important role. Most importantly, they serve as a constraint on the policies that ought to be adopted. For instance, creating wildlife reserves that exclude Indigenous peoples from their traditional lands would be unacceptable on a view that emphasizes human rights (see Chapter 8). Of course, there can be potential conflicts between particular ideas of wildlife management and conservation and the protection of human rights – for example, when it comes to the rights of Indigenous peoples to hunt animals of species that are endangered (see Chapter 13). However, in practice most of these conflicts seem, if not easily solvable, then at least manageable (as discussed in Chapter 9).

The situation is a lot more difficult in the case of animals' rights, however, because wildlife management practices commonly involve killing. And even when managers use nonlethal methods such as fertility control (Chapter 11) or translocation, that might involve violating different rights that animals have been argued to have: namely, either a right to reproduce or a right to their territory. So, if cowbirds have rights, then it's wrong both to kill individual cowbirds to pursue a conservation goal (saving the black-capped vireo species) and to manage them in at least some nonlethal ways.

This case also illustrates something particularly important about rights views. Most rights views only constrain the behavior of beings who can understand and recognize such moral claims – beings who have the capacities needed to function as *moral agents*. If cowbirds have rights, then they can make claims on humans that humans have duties to respect. But this is only possible because humans are, in the first place, moral agents who can *recognize* rights. This, however, cannot be said for vireos and cowbirds. Cowbirds and vireos aren't moral agents. So, when cowbirds starve vireo chicks, the cowbirds aren't violating rights and the vireos' rights aren't violated, any more than lightning would be violating rights if it were to strike a tree containing a vireo nest (see Hampton et al. 2019).

So, from a rights perspective, saving the black-capped vireo species by killing cowbirds wouldn't be acceptable because it would violate the cowbirds' rights. This doesn't mean that someone who accepted animal rights couldn't value whole species; the integrity, stability, and beauty of the biotic community; biodiversity; or wildness. Far from it. But they would not normally accept a wildlife management or conservation strategy that was pursued at the cost of rights violations.

There are, nevertheless, *some* circumstances in which some rights theorists will tolerate rights violations: namely, when confronted with a situation where there's no available alternative but to violate *some* rights. This is famously discussed by the animal rights philosopher Tom Regan (1983, p. 307). He proposed that such cases should be handled by following a principle he called "miniride": "When faced with overriding the rights of many innocent beings versus the rights of few innocent beings – when each individual involved would be equally harmed – we should override the rights of the few." This contrasts sharply with utilitarianism, according to which small harms to the many can outweigh significant harms to the few. On the rights view, by contrast, rights may only be violated where greater numbers of equally weighty rights would otherwise be violated.

But such circumstances are rare. Consider the kind of case to which it might seem to apply, such as hyperabundant deer that are facing starvation over winter (Chapter 11). A welfarist consequentialist might maintain that it's best to painlessly cull some small portion of the herd to ensure that there are more resources to go around; the aggregate welfare loss associated with many starving deer would be greater than the aggregate welfare loss of culling those few individuals. Someone might think that a rights theorist could agree by appealing to miniride, as all the individuals are facing equal harms – namely, death. But according to the rights view, the threat of starvation doesn't justify culling. Humans aren't entitled to take the lives of deer *even if* aggregate welfare would be higher as a result, since humans *would* be violating the rights of the deer they shoot whereas humans *wouldn't* be violating deer's rights by letting them starve. Humans are responsible for the harm they cause, not for all harm whatsoever.

There is one further point to make here. Even among those who accept that animals have rights, there's disagreement about *which* animals actually possess them. On some rights views, only members of species thought to be more cognitively and emotionally sophisticated have rights. The dominant view in recent discussions, though, is that merely being sentient is enough; rights holders are beings with subjective experiences of the world. This would include mammals and birds as rights holders (so cowbirds and vireos would both have rights) and probably reptiles, amphibians, and fish. If insects and plants aren't sentient, by contrast, then they don't have rights.

Clearly, adopting a rights view would impose significant constraints on wildlife management and conservation. While saving the vireo species would be a perfectly acceptable goal, it couldn't be pursued by means of killing cowbirds because cowbirds are rights holders. It also would preclude most wildlife research activities from occurring (see Chapter 15). In contrast, some relational views, to which we'll turn next, may accept cases where human historical responsibility for some past or ongoing harm permits actions that the rights view forbids.

6.4 Relational Theories

Utilitarianism, ecocentric consequentialism, and rights views share an important characteristic: namely, a focus on the intrinsic capacities or features of those entities concerned, such as sentience (in the case of animals) or integrity and stability (in the case of ecosystems). According to these theories, when deciding how to act, not much, if any, knowledge is needed about the histories of the entities that will be affected by an action, nor about their relationships with humans. All that needs to be known is what intrinsic capacities and features they have, how they ought to be treated in light of those features, and how the action might impact them. For some ethicists, however, this detached view of ethics, one that has no meaningful room for history or context, for special relationships and attachments, is worryingly incomplete. And it certainly doesn't map well onto the way people generally make their decisions.

For instance, most people feel that they have loyalties to family and community that override the reasons they have to help distant others, whether human or nonhuman. Suppose that a person's dog needs an expensive surgery and that the person has the means to pay for the surgery. If so, then they also have the means to euthanize the dog and donate the money they'd save to a highly effective nonprofit that restores injured wild animals to full health in their natural habitat. We can stipulate that the money would do more good if donated to the wildlife rescue charity. But many people are likely to judge that it's ethically permissible – and perhaps ethically required – for the person to take the dog to get surgery because he's *their* dog. On such a view, the person's special relationship with their dog means that they owe it to him to pay for the surgery.

Relational approaches to ethics can take many forms. One key distinction between them concerns the importance of moral emotions such as caring, compassion, and sympathy. Some relational approaches, most notably those associated with what's called an "ethics of care," emphasize the importance of attachment; they generally maintain that taking care of those to whom one is close should be the priority (Slote 2007). On this kind of view, the owner of a sick dog should take the dog to a veterinarian for surgery both because of her attachment to her dog and because caring for him is part of a trusting, interactive relationship between companion animals and their guardians.

On other relational approaches, emotions play a less central role, though such approaches don't necessarily reject the importance of attachment and sympathy. According to Clare Palmer (2010), for instance, the owner should take her dog to the veterinarian because she has taken on responsibility for the dog by adopting him, which gives her special obligations toward him that she doesn't have toward other dogs she hasn't adopted, or indeed toward wild animals. Sue Donaldson and Will Kymlicka (2011) take a different kind of relational approach, arguing that creating domesticated companion animals brings them into the human community, making them rather like animal citizens. Animal citizens, like human citizens, they argue, are owed access to health care. In another form of this view, Baird Callicott (2003) argues that humans generally have stronger duties to those in more intimate communities – including mixed communities of humans and companion animals such as dogs – than to those in more distant communities.

This dog case illustrates something else about relational obligations: they primarily concern what are thought of as *positive* obligations to assist rather than *negative* obligations not to harm. While a relationship may affect how far someone is obliged to *help* others, it's implausible that *all* obligations are based on relationships; relational views shouldn't be taken to imply that it's permissible for someone to seriously *harm* another individual with whom they don't have a relationship. The most important point here is that relational ethics tries, in various ways, to draw attention to the significance of context and relationships in the moral life. To see what this means in practice, let's just think about the kinds of questions that relational views raise with respect to vireos and cowbirds.

First, on an individual level, there's a question about what it means to *relate* to these animals in an appropriate way. The central idea here is that *any* relationship with another sentient being requires certain dispositions and skills, such as attentiveness, concern, and responsiveness. It's important to *notice* how individuals are doing, to be *concerned* about their wellbeing, and to be willing to *take action* for their sake. But here a problem may arise. In focusing on the vireo, these dispositions and skills seem to count in favor of culling cowbirds. But when thinking about how to respond to the cowbirds, what's required is less obvious. Will attentiveness to the cowbirds encourage acceptance of a policy that may lead to the vireo dying out?

Second, at a more collective level, a relational approach turns attention to *historical* relations between humans and relevant animals. There would still be wildfires in the vireo's range if there wasn't a human practice of preventing them; so, some humans, collectively, have a responsibility for vireos' precarious situation (both at the individual and species level). Since the lack of fire is a major, if unintended, contributing factor to the tension between the cowbirds and vireos that now exists, a case may be made that some humans bear special responsibility to the vireos. This is notably different from ecocentric consequentialism, utilitarianism, or rights theory; the idea of special responsibilities based on past relationships has no obvious place in any of these approaches.

Third, it can be asked what an appropriate human *role* with respect to these animals is. Someone might think, for instance, that humans ought to be in the position of *managing* nature, including wild animals. However, it isn't obvious what this unique role would involve. It wouldn't be like a traditional managerial relationship, where the aims of a for-profit business largely determine the responsibilities that a manager has with respect to the people she manages. Instead, the aims themselves are up for debate, as are the acceptable methods. And this isn't the only role humans might take to guide their interactions with these birds: another possible role might be as *caretakers* of both the cowbirds and the vireos, needing to promote their good.

However, another kind of relational view might take a very different approach here. While accepting that humans have special relations and therefore obligations toward domesticated animals, both cowbirds and vireo are *wild* animals, in the sense of being animals reasonably free from human constraints (see Chapter 2) to whom people have no special obligations. What happens between them is none of our business. On this view, killing cowbirds might not be permitted, either because it interferes with wild animals' autonomous lives or because it fails to respect the value of their wildness.

So, relational approaches to wildlife ethics may differ significantly from one another, but they all take the view that a being's intrinsic features are not all that needs to be known in order to make decisions about whether assistance or care is required.

6.5 Virtue Ethics

An alternative approach, one with a long history in ethics in general, and in environmental and conservation ethics in particular (Sandler and Cafaro 2005), is *virtue ethics*. As Ron Sandler (2013), a proponent of "environmental" virtue ethics, observes, leading environmental thinkers such as Henry David Thoreau (1854) and Rachel Carson (1962) espoused forms of virtue ethics, even if they didn't take themselves to be contributing to an ethical theory at the time. It might be argued that the virtue ethics approach could help in thinking more concretely about what it means to be a (morally) good person with respect to wildlife conservation and management or, perhaps more specifically, how to be a decent biologist, veterinarian, or wildlife manager.

Virtue ethics doesn't begin by asking how to act, nor what the best consequences are, nor what rules should be followed, nor whose rights are at stake. Instead, it's a theoretical approach that begins by asking "What sort of person should I be?" or, alternatively, asks what a virtuous person would look like – either as an individual or with respect to some professional role. While there are many different versions of virtue theory, most accounts take a virtue to be, as Sandler (2013, p. 3) puts it, a *well-justified character trait*, where a character trait is understood as "a disposition to take certain types of considerations as reasons (or as motivational) for action or emotion under certain types of circumstances." Virtues (and vices) are understood as having multiple aspects; they involve cultivating reasoning, desires, and emotions to respond in the right kinds of ways. Here there's a significant contrast with many other ethical theories: whereas emotions are an integral component of practical deliberation in virtue theory, in consequentialism and rights theory, for instance, emotions are often seen as troublingly likely to lead reason astray (Nelson et al. 2016). And virtues should be manifest in habitual actions; to be a kind person, for example, someone must both be kind in *practice* (not just in their imagination) and by *habit*, not just on one occasion.

Environmental virtue ethicists argue that key virtues, such as courage, have particular environmental applications; they also argue that there may be more specific environmental virtues and vices. Thoreau, for instance, advocated for simplicity in living, while Carson (1962) discussed the disposition to wonder at the natural world and to display humility in accepting humans' proper place in it. These sound like specifically environmental virtues. Tom Hill (1983) similarly argued that key human traits in the context of the environment recognize the need for "proper humility" and for appreciating one's (minor) place in the universe. More recently, Sandler (2013) discussed the role that cruelty, hubris, indifference, apathy, greed, wastefulness, and laziness play as environmental vices, and that care for living things, compassion, sensitivity, humility, courage, benevolence, temperance, perseverance, integrity, and wonder play as environmental virtues.

One attractive feature of virtue ethics is that it seems to reflect the way people often learn about living well. People can learn how to be good parents by watching good parents in action, thereby realizing that it's possible to handle difficult situations in surprisingly elegant ways. Likewise, by looking carefully at conservation professionals, it may be possible to identify exemplars who are doing a good job of navigating the moral complexities of dealing with wildlife. And by trying to be more like them – by cultivating admired character traits – perhaps individuals can do better when personally faced with similar challenges (Sandler and Cafaro 2005). So, for instance, in thinking about what it is to be a good wildlife manager, one starting place is to reflect on how those one already admires go about making decisions in practice.

However, this approach becomes more difficult when thinking about what should happen in particular cases. What would a virtuous person do in the case of the cowbirds and vireos? Because virtue ethics is somewhat contextual, there isn't a "one-size-fits-all" answer about how to manage interspecies conflicts that can be applied to this case. But it's possible to identify the kinds of questions that a virtue ethicist would recommend asking. Would a *compassionate* person kill cowbirds to save vireo chicks? Maybe, if the cowbirds can be killed painlessly and vireo chicks be saved from suffering. Otherwise, as in most real-world cases, probably not (see Wallach et al. 2018). Would a *benevolent* person kill cowbirds? Doing so certainly wouldn't be benevolent to cowbirds, even if it was to vireo chicks. What about displaying vices? Neither intervening nor standing back obviously seem to manifest cruelty, greed, or wastefulness. But a virtuous person might pause over hubris. Might it be hubristic to intervene to try to boost vireo populations at the expense of cowbirds? Possibly – but not necessarily. Again, it's going to depend on the details of the case and where serious reflection about it leads; decisions should be based on what's called, in the traditional language of virtue ethics, "practical wisdom" (*phronesis* in Greek), implying good judgment going beyond analytical knowledge and know-how, and excellence of character habitually manifested in practice, which, in combination, can lead to knowing what it's right to do in any specific situation.

The natural home of virtue ethics is at the level of developing *individual character* (either in general or in relation to some professional role). It's harder to see how it should be applied at the level of policy, and that's why we discuss virtue ethics less often in this book than consequentialism or rights theory, for instance. While it seems possible to assess a particular proposed conservation policy, strategy, or practice in terms of questions such as "Is this strategy fair?," "Is it cruel?," and "Is it humble?," this way of using virtue language seems less satisfactory when it's detached from the development of an individual character.

Having said this, one recent trend in conservation (which we'll discuss in more detail in Chapter 8) is a turn toward what is called "compassionate conservation" (see Wallach et al. 2018). Though compassionate conservation can take different forms, versions that are based on virtue ethics seem to suggest that a particular virtue – compassion – can be applied to the practice of conservation, and that this could go on to underpin a management policy. Compassionate conservationists would likely argue that cowbirds should not be culled to protect vireos, since this is hard to square with a compassionate practice (even though, it's worth noting, the vireo chicks themselves might also be appropriate subjects of compassion).

However, other conceptions of virtue in the context of wildlife could certainly allow for killing animals; the idea of a "responsible hunter" who, for instance, takes seriously the idea of a "fair chase," is widespread in hunting literature (Morris 2013). If hunting can be a virtuous pursuit, it seems likely that cowbird culling could also be virtuous, at least if carried out for the right reason and in the right way. This indicates, though, that even if virtue ethics is taken as the correct approach for our ethical engagement with wildlife, contrasting models of what virtue *is* in this domain are likely. Some people argue that this makes virtue ethics objectionably imprecise. It's true, of course, that it doesn't give the clear kind of guidance that utilitarianism and rights theories claim to offer. On the other hand, virtue ethicists argue that this approach interprets ethics plausibly and realistically as being more like learning and cultivating a skill, rather than like reading and applying an instruction manual. Clearly, as with all the other ethical theories we've considered here, virtue ethics has considerable appeal while also facing some significant challenges.

6.6 What to Do?

These ethical theories don't agree about what to do in many cases. Even when they do agree, they give very different accounts of what justifies particular actions. An ecocentric consequentialist approach would favor killing cowbirds; a rights theorist would oppose it. A virtue ethicist might oppose killing too, but for differing reasons – which means that they're likely to lead to diverging conclusions about other cases. What to do with all this disagreement?

Before we try to answer that question, however, we're going to make the problem harder – that is, we're going to expose even more disagreement. In the context of wildlife use, management, and conservation, people rarely apply moral theories directly. Instead, they tend to work with conservation "frameworks" or "paradigms" in which certain conservation values and ethical approaches are embedded (though not necessarily consciously or directly). Over the next two chapters, we will take a tour of these frameworks with an eye to their moral assumptions. As we'll suggest, they bear complex relationships to the values discussed in previous chapters, to the theories we explored in this chapter, and to one another.

Then, in Chapter 9, we'll come back to the question of what to do with moral disagreement. With a good sense of the breadth of values, moral theories, and management frameworks that people bring to the table, it's no wonder that such disagreements are difficult to resolve. Still, we'll suggest both some ways of understanding moral disagreement and strategies for navigating it transparently.

References

Attfield, R. (2013). Can biocentric consequentialism meet pluralist challenges? In: *Consequentialism and Environmental Ethics* (ed. A. Hiller, R. Ilea, and L. Kahn), 53–71. New York, USA: Routledge.

Callicott, J.B. (2003). The land ethic. In: *A Companion to Environmental Philosophy* (ed. D. Jamieson), 204–217. New York, USA: Routledge.

Carson, R. (1962). *Silent Spring*. Boston, USA: Houghton Mifflin.

Donaldson, S. and Kymlicka, W. (2011). *Zoopolis: A Political Theory of Animal Rights*. New York, USA: Oxford University Press.

Fischer, B. (2021). *Animal Ethics: A Contemporary Introduction*. New York, USA: Routledge.

Hampton, J.O., Warburton, B., and Sandøe, P. (2019). Compassionate versus consequentialist conservation. *Conservation Biology* 33 (4): 751–759.

Hare, R.M. (1982). Ethical theory and utilitarianism. In: *Utilitarianism and Beyond* (ed. A. Sen and B. Williams), 22–38. Cambridge, UK: Cambridge University Press.

Hill, T. (1983). Ideals of human excellence and preserving natural environments. *Environmental Ethics* 5: 211–224.

Kostecke, R., Summers, S., Eckrich, G., and Cimprich, D. (2005, 2005). Effects of brown-headed cowbird (*Molothrus ater*) removal on black-capped vireo (*Vireo atricapilla*) nest success and population growth at Fort Hood, Texas. *Ornithological Monographs* 57: 28–37.

Leopold, A. (1949). *A Sand County Almanac*. Oxford, UK: Oxford University Press.

Lund, T.B., Denver, S., Nordström, J. et al. (2021). Moral convictions and meat consumption – a comparative study of the animal ethics orientations of consumers of pork in Denmark, Germany, and Sweden. *Animals* 11 (2): 329.

Morris, S.P. (2013). Challenging the values of hunting: fair chase, game playing, and intrinsic value. *Environmental Ethics* 35 (3): 295–311.

Nelson, M.P., Bruskotter, J.T., Vucetich, J.A., and Chapron, G. (2016). Emotions and the ethics of consequence in conservation decisions: lessons from Cecil the lion. *Conservation Letters* 9: 302–306.

Palmer, C. (2010). *Animal Ethics in Context*. New York, USA: Columbia University Press.

Pinchot, G. (1905). *The Pinchot Letter*. Washington, D.C., USA: US Department of Agriculture, Forest Service.

Regan, T. (1983). *The Case for Animal Rights*. Berkeley, USA: University of California Press.

Salt, H. (1892). *Animals' Rights: Considered in Relation to Social Progress*. New York, USA: Macmillan.

Sandler, R. (2013). Environmental virtue ethics. In: *The International Encyclopedia of Ethics* (ed. H. Lafollette), 1665–1674. Hoboken, USA: Wiley.

Sandler, R. and Cafaro, P. (ed.) (2005). *Environmental Virtue Ethics*. Lanham, USA: Rowman and Littlefield.

Sandøe, P., Corr, S.A., Lund, T.B., and Forkman, B. (2019). Aggregating animal welfare indicators: can it be done in a transparent and ethically robust way? *Animal Welfare* 28 (1): 67–76.

Şekercioğlu, Ç.H., Daily, G.C., and Ehrlich, P.R. (2004). Ecosystem consequences of bird declines. *Proceedings of the National Academy of Sciences* 101 (52): 18042–18047.

Slote, M. (2007). *The Ethics of Care and Empathy*. New York, USA: Routledge.

Springborn, M.R., Weill, J.A., Lips, K.R. et al. (2022). Amphibian collapses increased malaria incidence in Central America. *Environmental Research Letters* 17 (10): 104012.

Texas Parks and Wildlife (2014). Cowbird trapping program. https://tpwd.texas.gov/huntwild/wild/nuisance/cowbirds/trappingProgram.phtml

Thoreau, H.D. (1854). *Walden*. Princeton, USA: Princeton University Press.

UN General Assembly (1948). *Universal Declaration of Human Rights*. New York, USA: United Nations www.ohchr.org/EN/UDHR/Documents/UDHR_Translations/eng.pdf.

Wallach, A.D., Bekoff, M., Batavia, C. et al. (2018). Summoning compassion to address the challenges of conservation. *Conservation Biology* 32 (6): 1255–1265.

Wilsey, C.B., Lawler, J.J., Cimprich, D., and Schumaker, N.H. (2014). Dependence of the endangered black-capped vireo on sustained cowbird management. *Conservation Biology* 28 (2): 561–571.

Wildlife Management and Conservation Models

7

7.1 Introduction

The American bison, colloquially but incorrectly known as the buffalo, is native to the Great Plains of North America. Males weigh close to a metric ton and stand two meters tall; nevertheless, they are agile and fast, capable of running at speeds of 60 km an hour, and so were once known as "the thunder of the plains." Prior to European settlement, bison inhabited much of North America, with estimates of bison numbers ranging from 25 to 60 million when Europeans first came to the continent. Bison were an important resource for many Native American tribes; their importance increased once tribes acquired horses in the early 1700s and could more easily participate in a market for cured bison hides (robes). Nonetheless, due to factors including a tribal common property regime, the lack of firearms, relatively low human population densities, and limited commercial use, estimates suggest that bison populations remained fairly stable when used primarily by Native American tribes (Lueck 2002).

As European settlers moved West, however, the expansion of railroads and the use of firearms made hunting much more efficient; in addition, bison occupied land wanted for grazing and crops. European settlers also perceived the bison as vital to the survival of the Plains Native American tribes; the extermination of bison, then, was also a strategy

Wildlife Ethics: The Ethics of Wildlife Management and Conservation, First Edition. Clare Palmer, Bob Fischer, Christian Gamborg, Jordan Hampton, and Peter Sandøe.

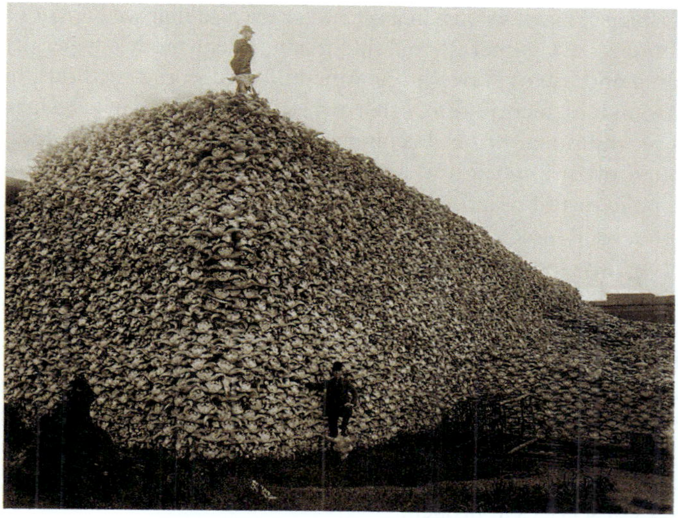

Figure 7.1 Photograph from 1892 of a pile of American bison skulls in Detroit (MI) waiting to be ground for fertilizer or charcoal. *Source:* Unknown author/Wikimedia Commons.

for defeating Native peoples. As harvesting costs fell and tanning techniques improved, bison were hunted at increasingly high rates for a fast-growing market in bison hides. Bison skulls were also utilized as a by-product to manufacture fertilizer (Figure 7.1). This decimated herds; fewer than 2000 bison were left by 1889 (Lueck 2002).

In the late 1700s, bison had seemed like an inexhaustible resource and there was general skepticism about humans' ability to cause extinctions. This idea was supported by European settlers who believed that species were immutable and permanent. In 1802, for instance, Thomas Jefferson, one of the founders of the US and its third president, wrote that "Such is the economy of nature, that no instance can be produced of her having permitted any one race of her animals to become extinct; of her having formed any link in her great work so weak as to be broken" (Jefferson 1955, p. 71).

But by the end of the 1800s, it became obvious that humans could, and very nearly did, eliminate bison entirely. Species no longer appeared to be stable features of the world. George Perkins Marsh, a US diplomat and author of the 1864 classic *Man and Nature*, wrote that "the myriad forms of animal and vegetable life, which covered the earth when man first entered [the theatre of nature], have been, through his action, greatly changed in numerical proportion, sometimes much modified in form and product, and sometimes entirely extirpated" (Marsh 1864, p. 140).

The well-known case of bison's near-extinction points toward one of the historically most important models of wildlife management, which is based on the idea of wildlife as a renewable but exhaustible resource. By "model," we mean a broad and multi-tiered approach to wildlife management that has several components, from the more conceptual to the more practical. At the heart of such models of wildlife management are commitments concerning (for instance) what values should be pursued or protected, what knowledge counts as relevant, and how it ought to be acquired. So, wildlife management models may reflect strong anthropocentrism or not be anthropocentric at all; they may endorse the high value of wildlife in itself and/or the idea that wildlife is of instrumental value as a resource (see Chapter 2). Wildlife management models generally depend on an understanding and use of Western scientific knowledge and methods, but they may also be built around, or incorporate, other ways of gaining knowledge about wildlife, such as forms of traditional or local ecological knowledge. Taken together, these commitments, though often implicit and assumed rather than explicitly affirmed, inform recommended policies and practices for wildlife management on the ground.

In this chapter, we'll look at three influential wildlife management and conservation models, exploring how they connect to the various values and ethical theories discussed in previous chapters. The first, as mentioned above, is a model based on seeing selected useful species – such as bison – as renewable but exhaustible resources; thus, it focuses on wildlife's instrumental value to humans. Here, management is necessary to restrain overexploitation, the aim being to ensure that these species can be used into the future. Although this broad model has various forms, we'll focus here on what's become known as the North American Model of wildlife conservation. We extend this discussion to take into account the idea of sustainable use of wildlife more broadly and to include the so-called ecosystem services approach.

The second model is the control of unwanted wildlife, where some wild animals are perceived to be of *disvalue* to humans, meaning that individuals, populations, or species are targeted for significant reduction or elimination (sometimes called "pest control"). This model has a long history, although it has been particularly prominent in the last few decades and has recently been extended to include "invasive" species.

The third model is conservation biology, a much more recent model founded in the 1980s, though one that draws on earlier ideas. Conservation biologists primarily see wildlife not as resources or pests, but as important contributors to biodiversity and as such *valuable in their own right.* (That said, if wildlife populations undermine biodiversity, as some nonnative species may, then conservation biology may borrow from the pest control model.)

What we present here is only a rough sketch. This is partly due to the limited space available, but also because wildlife management and conservation models shift in form and evolve over time (as argued, for instance, by Mace 2014). Moreover, there are complicated relationships between the models and the broader culture; conservation practices can shape cultural values and vice versa (Maller 2021). And, of course, these models can be rejected, in whole or in part. In the next chapter, Chapter 8, we'll look at some recent movements that, in various ways, push back against core theoretical tenets of these three models, or at least significantly adapt them. These movements focus on environmental justice, the long history of wildlife management by Indigenous peoples, and the value of individual animals' welfare and lives – all of which have been overlooked or even undermined by applications of the three models presented here.

7.2 The Overexploitation of Wildlife

We began this chapter with the rapid depletion of North American bison populations – a story that leads ultimately to what's probably the most well-known, and also widely adapted and applied, conservation model: the North American Model of wildlife conservation. According to the North American Model, "conservation" means preventing overexploitation of a resource (which might also be described as "sustainable use"). The North American Model is driven by the particular history of wildlife use in the US. For context, we'll look at a little more of that history.

Starting in the early seventeenth century, wild animals were trapped and hunted extensively by European settlers. Beavers, for instance, were trapped for their fur; birds – including swans, spoonbills, geese, and egrets – were killed for meat and plumage, for both North American and European markets. The consumption of wildlife largely continued without check among European settlers in North America well into the nineteenth century. However, as populations of many species began to decline, there was a realization that without legally enforced bag limits and other protections, these species would disappear. During the second half of the nineteenth century, some states began to create salaried game warden positions to control the numbers of game animals hunted and, in 1864, New York State introduced hunting licenses (Gray 1995). Movements to protect bird species became increasingly prominent and recreational hunters launched campaigns to protect game species from major losses due to commercial overexploitation. Restrictions on fishing were also put in place; Washington and Oregon states began regulating fishing equipment and having closed seasons in the 1870s (Merchant 2007).

These shifts in attitude were accompanied by a growing legal framework in the US for managing wildlife, in particular the development of what's now known as the Public Trust Doctrine. In 1896, the US Supreme Court judged that the states owned their fish and wildlife on behalf of their citizens. This developed into the broader idea that wildlife was publicly owned, should be preserved for public use, and should neither be destroyed nor passed into private ownership (Frank 2012). In an 1872 legislative development, Yellowstone was established as the world's first so-called National Park, designated to protect nature from development, to preserve natural beauty, and to serve as a refugia for harvested wildlife. At the same time, the Wildlife Refuge system was created, with the goal of preventing overexploitation of game. Around the world, wildlife protection societies were created, most prominently the Royal Society for the Protection of Birds (RSPB) in 1889 in Britain, and the National Audubon Society in the US (first founded in 1886 and reestablished in 1905) focusing on the protection of wild bird species.

By the early twentieth century, though, while wildlife conservation infrastructure was being built, it became clear that an emphasis on regulatory measures such as game laws was not enough to stop continuing wildlife decline. Aldo Leopold (see Chapter 3) began to develop a more comprehensive idea of game management, publishing his ground-breaking book of the same name in 1933. Here he famously maintained:

> The central thesis of game management is this: game can be restored by the creative use of the same tools which have heretofore destroyed it – ax, plow, cow, fire, and gun … Management is their purposeful and continuing alignment.
>
> (Leopold 1933, p. xxxi).

Leopold formulated the idea that an ecosystem has a carrying capacity for different species: that is, the maximum population size that the environment can sustain over time (see Chapter 11 for discussion of how this idea is currently applied). Once this carrying capacity was established, Leopold argued, a sustained yield harvest could be determined. However, determining such capacities took a long time. As Leopold put it:

> The early attempts to apply biology to the management of game as a wild crop disclosed the fact that science had accumulated more knowledge of how to distinguish one species from another than that of the habitats, requirements, and inter-relationships of living populations.
>
> (Leopold 1933, p. 22)

Tying all this back to work in preceding chapters, it's clear that the primary value of wildlife as understood in these growing ideas about game management is *instrumental*; wildlife is for human consumptive use. But there's a built-in recognition that while game is a renewable resource – animals, after all, can keep reproducing – it's a resource that can be destroyed, if populations become too small. So, if people wish to continue to use wildlife into the future, it must be used carefully; that is, use needs to be sensitive to the yield that can be maintained over time.

This brings us to the explicit formulation of the North American Model of wildlife conservation around 2001, which was intended to capture the basic principles of wildlife management in North America as they evolved over decades, if not centuries. As Peterson and Nelson (2017) point out, however, there's clearly some ambiguity about the function of the North American Model as currently articulated. It is not simply a descriptive account but a normative one: the principles concern not only how wildlife *has* been managed, but also how it *should* be managed. As such, the North American Model is a great example of the kind of value-laden model we are interested in here, and is particularly interesting because it's relatively formalized.

7.3 The North American Model

The fundamental goal of wildlife management in this model is to conserve and enhance nature's yield as a valuable resource for humans, present and future. The focus is on population "health," not individual welfare. The aim is to keep populations at levels suitable for harvesting by determining the right balance between reproduction and immigration rates in relation to death from diseases, starvation, predation, and, of course, human exploitation. Organ et al. (2012) pointed out that the model really has seven main components or principles.

1) *Wildlife is a public trust resource*: wildlife is not privately owned and landowners do not own the wildlife on their land. Wildlife is held in trust for the benefit of present and future generations by the state; population management should reflect this broad outlook.
2) *Elimination of markets for wildlife*: markets for game and nongame wildlife are normally unacceptable as they privatize a common resource (see #1); harvests should be regulated to avoid decline in wildlife populations.
3) *Allocation of wildlife by law*: wildlife should be accessible for all and regulated to that end; it should not just be allocated to those with special privileges (so, not based

on land ownership or the market). Allocation should take into account the scarcity (etc.) of particular species.

4) *Wildlife can only be killed for a legitimate purpose*: this principle seems primarily to concern good sportsmanship, in particular ensuring a "fair chase." Some interpretations take it as also expressing the concern that wildlife should not be wasted by killing without a serious intention for use.
5) *Wildlife is considered an international resource:* wildlife may migrate across borders and so the way one country manages its migrating wildlife has consequences for its neighbors, requiring international collaboration (this was reflected in the US in the 1918 Migratory Birds Act).
6) *Science is the proper tool for discharge of wildlife policy*: scientific research should be the basis for informed decision making in wildlife management, an idea to which Aldo Leopold significantly contributed (though this may not necessarily be rigorously applied in practice).
7) *Democracy of hunting*: there should be access for all to have the opportunity to hunt regardless of land ownership or wealth.

The North American Model has been lauded for giving wildlife high priority in a culture where private property rights and free enterprise otherwise ruled (Heffelfinger et al. 2013). Notably, hunting, rather than being seen as a threat to wildlife conservation, lies at its core. And in many ways, the North American Model has been successful, allowing for the recovery of many once diminishing species, such as white-tailed deer (Chapter 11), wild turkeys, and black bears. However, the model and its principles, as described above, also raise ethical questions.

Before exploring these questions further, we should note that although the broad idea of "sustainable use" at work here can be found internationally, in many other respects the North American Model is geographically bound and unique to European settler North America, depending on an interplay between natural conditions, social and cultural contexts, and the evolution of highly specific regulatory frameworks, established over decades. In many European countries, for instance, landowners *do* own the wildlife on their land and hunting is not "democratic" in the sense outlined here. And in most locations, including countries across Asia, Africa, Australasia, and Europe, markets for hunted wild animals are permitted. Indeed, it's sometimes argued that markets actually help to ensure rather than undermine sustainable use (see Chapter 10). However, this geographic specificity should not stop us from looking more closely at the values embedded in the North American Model.

These values relate both to human access to wildlife and to the wild animals themselves. Perhaps the most important human value concerns distributive justice, understood in terms of equal opportunity to access wildlife both within and across generations. In principle, at least, this model contends that everyone, not just the wealthy or privileged, should have access to wildlife as a resource (though we'll raise questions about this shortly). In the case of the animals themselves, wildlife is valued as a resource, and interpreted solely at the level of populations, species, and ecosystems.

As such, the North American Model raises ethical questions about historical justice, instrumentalization of wildlife, inclusivity, and selectivity of species conservation (Mahoney and Geist 2019). Let's begin with an issue relating to its origins.

The North American Model emerged from a European settler culture that had tried to eliminate Native Americans, people who previously occupied territory now annexed for the "public trust." Critics such as Eichler and Baumeister (2018) argue that the North American Model legitimized settler colonialism, including the expropriation of Native American lands and the setting aside of Indigenous worldviews and values, thus perpetuating the "logic of elimination." So, the "equal access" of the North American Model actually renders invisible the prior claims of Indigenous people to lands they occupied for hunting and fishing – claims that predate the "democratization" of hunting established by European settlers.

The orientation of wildlife management around hunting and fishing has, more recently, also been subject to critical scrutiny. One objection is that where wildlife management focuses almost entirely on hunting (largely practiced in this context by white men), it ignores the (much more diverse) environmental movement and the importance of legislation such as the Endangered Species Act (Nelson et al. 2011).

Another closely related set of concerns is that the focus on game species has not prevented *other* species declining towards extinction, nor does the North American Model necessarily protect biodiversity more generally (nor other values, such as wildness). Examples include long-term declines in taxa lacking in obvious instrumental usefulness, such as amphibians. In some cases, the focus on heathy populations of game species has *hastened* the decline of nongame species. An especially well-studied example is that of introduced trout (a recreational angling species) and the decline of mountain yellow-legged frogs in California (Knapp and Matthews 2000). Another worry is that the emphasis on hunting and fishing does not appropriately represent the interests of those who value wildlife nonconsumptively (birdwatchers, for instance). This seems particularly troublesome as the number of hunters and anglers declines (see Chapter 8). Having said this, it should be noted that funding derived from hunting – for instance, from hunters purchasing "duck stamps" and taxes on the sale of firearms – has played an important role in protecting and expanding wetlands in the US National Wildlife Refuge system. Those wetlands have broader benefits not just for conservation, but also for nonconsumptive users such as birdwatchers (Vrtiska et al. 2013).

Another set of concerns about the North American Model focuses on the assumption that wildlife is a *resource*, which is plainly anthropocentric. As we saw in earlier chapters (and as is defended by the conservation biology model below), on some non-anthropocentric ethical views, ecosystems and species are morally important in their own right, not just as human resources. And those concerned about *individual* sentient animals are critical of the model too. On their view, wild animals are neither mere resources nor species representatives. Instead, individual sentient animals have moral significance in themselves.

Finally, some object to the North American Model's commitment to science as the proper basis of wildlife decision making. First, it does not take into account the rather different kinds of knowledge that Indigenous Americans may have in terms of the land and management of wildlife (see Chapter 8) And second, as Peterson and Nelson (2017) point out, while science may *inform* certain kinds of decision making, ultimately decisions about wildlife management depend on values and ethical choices, rather than being exclusively the domain of science.

We'll revisit several of these objections to the North American Model in the next chapter. For now, though, we'll look at how the basic idea of conservation as "sustainable use," which underpins the North American Model, has become more broadly important in wildlife management internationally.

7.4 Sustainable Use of Wildlife and the Idea of Ecosystem Services

The idea of "sustainable use" depends on how "sustainability" is defined – a term that's widely used but also hotly contested. The basic idea has a long history in a European context, apparently originating in a Saxon forest regulation in 1560, gaining traction as "sustained yield" at least since in the beginning of the eighteenth century, and later adopted by some fisheries in the middle of the nineteenth century.

But more recently and most famously, the notion figures in the 1987 World Commission on Environment and Development report *Our Common Future* – chaired by Norway's former prime minister Gro Harlem Brundtland, and now generally known as the Brundtland Commission. In that report, sustainable development was described as: "development that meets the needs of the present without compromising the ability of future generations to meet their own needs" (Brundtland 1987, p. 16). Strictly speaking, the Commission gave a sufficient condition for development being sustainable, not a definition of sustainability in general, but the line now has a life of its own; it is now widely (though certainly not universally) seen as a good way of capturing sustainability's central meaning. In theory, it connects environmental, economic, and social concerns, suggesting that it's possible to use resources wisely in the present while conserving nature for the future.

Like the North American Model (which is a manifestation of a similar idea), the Brundtland definition of sustainable development is anthropocentric. The "needs of the present" are *people's* needs, not the needs of nonhuman nature; likewise, the "future generations" in question are future *human* generations. The definition is certainly concerned about poverty and poor welfare among current human generations; the needs of the poor should be met. But this should be done in ways that are also fair to future people, so that they are able to meet their needs too. The rest of the world, including its wildlife, is a resource that should make this possible, and should be managed sustainably in order to achieve this goal.

The model of managing wildlife for fair and sustainable use within and across generations has been important across the globe. Consider, for instance, the definition of sustainable ("wise") use in the book *Wildlife Conservation by Sustainable Use*, which focuses on the possibilities of sustainable wildlife use in African rangelands (Prins et al. 2012). There, the authors define sustainable use in a way that echoes the Brundtland definition:

> Wise use of an animal assemblage means to utilise an animal population, that is neither endangered or vulnerable, in an optimum and wholly sustainable fashion for the benefit of the stakeholder; and in such a manner as to maintain ecological processes, to preserve genetic diversity and to accommodate the optimum sustainable utilisation of all other non-vulnerable renewable natural resources in that area.
>
> (Prins et al. 2012, p. 5)

Key characteristics are shared here with the North American Model, in particular the idea that wildlife is a resource for "the benefit of the stakeholder." But there are also two key differences. First, sustainable use is placed in the broader context of biodiversity and species protection, unlike the North American Model; second, though this is not explicit in the quotation above, the monetization of wildlife and wildlife markets are key to this form of sustainable use.

Indeed, in the African rangelands, an important argument for sustainable use is that wildlife will be squeezed out if it is *not* monetized, thanks to competition for land between humans and wildlife. The editors of *Wildlife Conservation for Sustainable Use* put the idea bluntly: "We are not interested in measuring quite arcane concepts such as existence value or replacement value, but we are interested in the financial value of this wildlife" (Prins et al. 2012, p. 46). If wildlife can be sustainably used for economic benefit by stakeholders such as landowners, then the landowners do not need to make income in some *other* way that threatens the land tenure of wildlife. So, it may be claimed that in at least some situations, sustainable use may be the best or even the only way of protecting wildlife, especially where there is land use competition. As such, assigning economic value could be a way of protecting the other kinds of values we have discussed (see Chapter 2), including esthetic value, the intrinsic value of species, and so on (see Chapter 10).

Other populations of wild animals, though, aren't competing for land. But these populations may still be targets of human consumption, especially for food. "Sustainable yield" models of wild populations have been developed to make this possible, trying to find harvesting rates that do not result in declines in the resource over time (like living off the interest of a savings account, not the principal). In fisheries, the goal of maximum sustainable yield is to sustain the highest possible catch consistent with the population persisting in perpetuity (Barber 1988). This idea has been extended to populations of marine mammals, game, and subsistence wildlife hunting (see, for instance, Wilkie et al. 2019).

Models based around maximum sustainable yield raise in-practice questions about their sustainability and, therefore, their ability to meet the needs of future generations. However, the idea of maximum sustainable yield – along with other sustainable use models – also raises a significant in-principle concern, just as the North American Model did but on a much broader scale. Sustainable use – especially where that use is consumptive – treats many sentient beings as interchangeable, replaceable units. For those concerned about individual wild animals, this population-level focus misses the moral importance of suffering and killing.

However, we should also note that wildlife management for sustainability does not need to take the strongly anthropocentric form we have considered so far (which has been the dominant version to date). Basically, what counts as sustainable wildlife management is going to depend on what's to be sustained; in principle, the goal could be to sustain nonanthropocentric values, such as ecosystem "health." And sustainability may be only one among several values. As Vucetich and Nelson (2010) point out, there's no reason why concern for sustainability *must* be paired with concern for social justice, but nonetheless, most modern accounts maintain that a sustainable society should *also* care about social welfare. Likewise, sustainability could be paired with concern for *animal* welfare. In practice, though, the most common reasons for protecting wildlife are linked to long-term human interests and the welfare of future human generations. Insofar as wildlife is a resource that contributes to these goals, it's positively – and instrumentally – valued.

A related idea or perhaps an expansion of the sustainable use approach has been developed in the *ecosystem services* model. The term was coined in the early 1980s in a seminal book by Ehrlich and Ehrlich (1981) on the causes and consequences of the disappearance of species. However, related ideas have been around for decades. Indeed, some point to George Perkins Marsh's 1864 book, *Man and Nature* (mentioned above), as the starting point of the history of modern concern for ecosystem services, since he maintains that America's resources are not infinite (Gómez-Baggethun et al. 2010). In any case, although several definitions exist, ecosystem services can be described as the "… processes and functions that benefit people, consciously or un-consciously, directly or indirectly" (Costanza et al. 2017, p. 3). This approach has a disciplinary background in both economics and ecology (which is why some also link the notion to conservation biology) and was synthesized in an integrating discipline "ecological economics" in the 1990s (Braat and de Groot 2012). In keeping with sustainable use, the idea is that species and biodiversity make essential contributions to human wellbeing; hence, they should be conserved (see Chapter 2). Some of the key proponents of the approach have tried to resist labeling it as an anthropocentric view of nature, instead arguing that the concept is a "whole system aware view of humans embedded in society and embedded in the rest of nature" (Costanza et al. 2017, p. 3).

Unlike the North American Model or a commitment to sustainable use, an ecosystem services approach does not say anything in particular about how to conserve and manage wildlife. Instead, it's a way of recognizing the value of ecosystems, species, and populations. Essentially, it's important to limit consumption of and damage to these entities in order to gain certain benefits, such as water filtration and carbon cycling (Lele et al. 2013). Moreover, the "services" here may be very wide-ranging, including, for instance, cultural and spiritual values. Ecosystem services approaches see wild animals as members of valuable species and as contributors to the "functioning" of the ecosystem, thus providing "services"; but like the idea of sustainable use, such approaches have little room for valuing wild animals as individual beings.

All these approaches – the North American Model, sustainable use, and ecosystem services – positively value at least some wildlife for the important benefits wildlife brings people. Now, however, we'll briefly move to a rather different model of wildlife management: where wildlife is *negatively* valued, and rather than being a resource, is seen as in some way a threat. Here, the goal is to control wild animals by repelling, deterring, reducing, or eradicating their populations.

7.5 Controlling Unwanted Wildlife Populations

Let's briefly return to the American bison. Perhaps surprisingly, there was active resistance to protecting bison in the nineteenth century, even among those who had no objection to bison being used as resources. Here's an argument that US Representative Omar Conger made in 1874 concerning a bill that would have banned bison hunting by white settlers:

> There is no law that Congress can pass that will prevent the buffalo from disappearing before the march of civilization. There is no law which human hands can write, there is no law which a Congress of men can enact, that will stay the disappearance of these

> wild animals before civilization. They eat the grass. They trample upon the plains upon which our settlers desire to herd their cattle and their sheep. They range over the very pastures where the settlers keep their herds of cattle. They destroy the pasture. They are as uncivilized as the Indian.
>
> (United States Congress 1874, p. 2107)

We will return to the history of ethnocentrism and colonialism in the next chapter. The important point here, however, is that animals do not fall neatly into one human category or another; they can be both resources *and* pests, as they were for nineteenth-century settlers.

With that in mind, we can observe that wildlife control goes far back into human history; humans have been trying to eradicate wild animals regarded as "pests" in and around their settlements since human settlements existed. Animals might be competing for, or damaging, resources such as crops (Chapter 11); threatening humans indirectly, for instance by being reservoirs for infectious diseases (Chapter 16); or threatening them directly by attacking them (Chapter 19). Alternatively, they may just be regarded as a nuisance. In this sense, wildlife control is something with which most people are familiar, even if it's just at the level of setting mousetraps or poison bait in or around their homes. Some groups of animals have been targeted for population control either because they are hyperabundant (see Chapter 11 on hyperabundant native animals) or nonnative (see Chapter 12 on Predator Free New Zealand) and are believed to be threatening native species, ecosystems or populations.

In many cases, wildlife control is driven by straightforwardly human-centered reasons either about eliminating direct threats to human lives or resources or more indirect threats to ecosystem services. But wildlife control can also be squarely ecological, for instance if an introduced species is threatening a species or ecosystem thought to be morally considerable. It's even possible that population control could be carried out to improve animal welfare. Take, for instance, the case of introduced mice on Gough Island in the South Atlantic. These mice have been eating the chicks of Tristan albatrosses alive (Wanless et al. 2009). One argument for eliminating these island mouse populations is the amount of suffering caused to the albatross chicks, not only the threat to the whole Tristan albatross species.

Unlike the North American Model, there's no widely formalized model of wildlife control. The nearest to such a model is integrated pest management, which was developed during the 1970s in response to public concerns about the use of pesticides and their broader impacts on populations of birds and nontarget wild animals, as well as on human health. One of the goals of integrated pest management was to develop a more holistic approach to managing insect pests, one that was integrative (using different methods harmoniously), had a set of decision rules, and a level of "economic injury" at which pest management activities were triggered. Specifically, in the case of insect pests, integrated pest management tried to move away from the use of pesticides as the first step in pest control, allowing that while pesticides could be part of the picture, they should be used more sparingly and in a more targeted way (Elliott et al. 1995).

Integrated pest management wasn't designed with vertebrate animals in mind as target species, but a variety of versions of vertebrate pest control have since been developed, sometimes drawing on integrated pest management (DuBois et al. 2017). When applied to native species, these vertebrate pest management approaches generally ratchet up from deterrence (such as scaring devices) through trapping and relocating, to lethal management, which in the case of mammals often entails the use of poisons such as anticoagulants with significant animal welfare implications (Russell et al. 2016). When applied to introduced species, lethal control methods generally take priority, as options such as relocation are not normally desirable (Chapter 12).

These versions of vertebrate pest control suggest that trapping and relocation is to be preferred to lethal control, presumably for welfare reasons (though in welfare terms this may be misguided, given potentially severe welfare impacts of relocation, especially if animals are relocated to unfamiliar areas lacking in unoccupied territory and with predator activity). And more generally, issues about animal welfare are becoming increasingly prominent in vertebrate pest control, though often this discussion is couched in terms of "social acceptability" (e.g., Koichi et al. 2013). Some public surveys also show more support for nonlethal control methods (such as deterrents and repellants) than for lethal methods, especially when applied to native species (e.g., in Greece; Liordos et al. 2017).

Such worries about methods of vertebrate pest control do seem to take animal lives and suffering to count for something, at least in theory. However, in most forms of vertebrate pest control, animals' lives and welfare are still of much less importance than humans' interests. Perhaps this could be thought of as a weakly anthropocentric framework, something like "animal welfarism" (see Chapter 6). Recent concerns about the impact of poisons on nontarget organisms also reflect concern for various *ecological* values, such as the protection of particular states of ecosystems, species and populations; this could reflect an ecocentric, not just an anthropocentric orientation.

Growing controversies about the necessity for, and the methods of, wildlife control, and how far humans and wild animals should coexist in particular areas, are likely to lead to the development of new models of wildlife control (Linnell et al. 2020). We'll say more about this in Chapters 8, 11, 12, 19, and elsewhere. In the present context, such controversies also remind us about tensions between viewing animals as resources and/or problems, on the one hand, and as valuable dimensions of biodiversity on the other.

Accordingly, we'll now consider a final and highly influential model of wildlife management in this chapter: conservation biology. This model, at least to some degree, takes a less anthropocentric approach than sustainable wildlife use and wildlife control. This is not to say that conservation biology has no place for either use or control. But the primary values at stake are not human interests, but rather values such as species, biodiversity, ecosystem flourishing, and wildness.

7.6 Conservation Biology

Formally founded by Michael Soulé and colleagues in the 1980s, although drawing on ideas from the 1960s and earlier, conservation biology is what Soulé called a "mission-oriented crisis discipline" (Soulé 1985). It is multidisciplinary, drawing on research from a range of scientific, social scientific, and, in Soulé's original model, humanities fields (he includes "ecophilosophy" as a component) and attempts to integrate these multiple disciplinary approaches into conservation policy (Gerber 2010).

The primary goal of conservation biology is to develop management methods to try to protect species and biodiversity, and where possible to restore some of what has already been lost. In practice, pursuing these goals may involve both hands-off or "passive" activities, such as setting aside protected areas to safeguard biodiversity, and more hands-on activities, such as ecological restoration and *ex situ* captive breeding of endangered species (see Chapter 14).

These goals are, in turn, underpinned by values. For Soulé, the values here (as we noted in Chapter 2) are intrinsic. Soulé maintains that "diversity is good" and has "intrinsic value" (Soulé 1985,p. 731). Evolution is also good. Species "have value in themselves, a value neither conferred nor revocable, but springing from a species' long evolutionary heritage and potential or even from the mere fact of its existence" (Soulé 1985, p. 731). These values mean that "the untimely [anthropogenic] extinction of populations and species is bad" (Soulé 1985, p. 730) and that "there's an ethical imperative to conserve species diversity" (Soulé 1985, p. 731).

Conservation biology, then, at least in Soulé's original model, expands upon, or perhaps reframes, two key ideas found in the North American Model. The North American Model focuses on the value of *game* species, while passing over all the other species without comment; conservation biology, in contrast, expands its concerns beyond game species to include, in principle, *all* wild species. Second, conservation biology does not see wildlife protection as being mostly about *use,* as does the North American Model; it's also about conserving species that are *not* useful to humans; species and biodiversity are taken to be independently valuable in themselves.

In theory, conservation biology could defend the valuation of wildlife, ecosystems, species, and biodiversity both intrinsically (in themselves) and instrumentally (for other services they bring humans). In practice, though, these two value approaches have been the cause of tension in conservation biology, especially in the early twenty-first century. Those primarily defending an intrinsic value basis for conservation biology were concerned that a shift in focus to instrumental values would undermine the ethical reasons for protecting biodiversity and, what's more, they worried that it opened the gates to destroying what wasn't obviously useful (Tallis and Lubchenco 2014). On the other hand, those defending the importance of including or focusing on use values of wildlife and ecosystems argued that "intrinsic value" positions had not to date actually been effective in protecting biodiversity, and that collaborating with key stakeholders, including businesses, could effectively develop support for conservation, as could emphasizing human ecosystem services such as clean water or tourism (Figure 7.2). Abstract ideas about "intrinsic value" were, on this argument, less practically effective (Tallis and Lubchenco 2014).

Growing tensions between these two perspectives led to a petition published in *Nature*, led by Tallis and Lubchenco (2014). The petition argued that conservation biology needed to listen to more diverse voices and to accept broader philosophical positions. The goal, the petitioners argued, was "a unified and diverse conservation ethic; one that recognizes and accepts all values of nature, from intrinsic to instrumental, and welcomes all philosophies justifying nature protection and restoration, from ethical to economic, and from aesthetic to utilitarian" (Tallis and Lubchenco 2014, p. 27). The thought here seems to be that conservation biology can be supported by many different underlying values, provided they all converge on conservation.

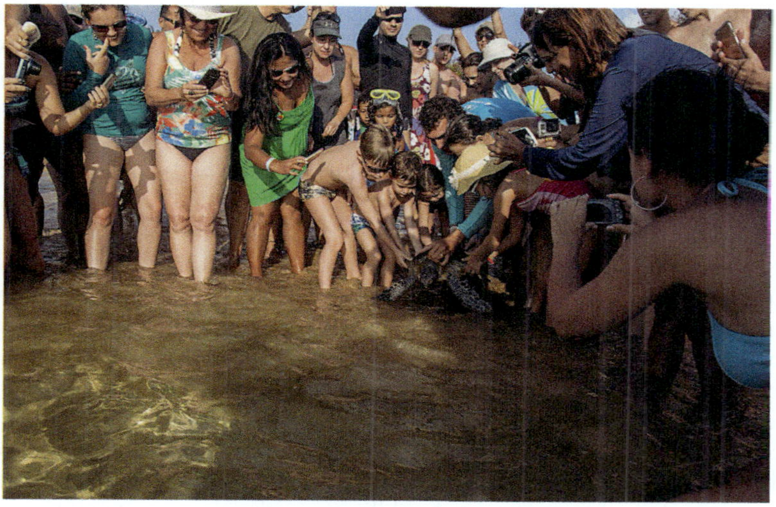

Figure 7.2 Releasing a tagged sea turtle in front of a crowd of "eco-tourists" in Pernambuco, Brazil. *Source:* Fernando de Noronha/Dreamstime LLC.

This might be seen as an appealing vision, but there's still likely to be significant divergence in practice over what to conserve and how to conserve it. The petitioners in *Nature* present the difficulties here as though there is not disagreement about what to *do*; decisions merely concern what arguments to use with which audience to get broad support for any particular conservation decision. However, there are surely cases where intrinsic value arguments will diverge from instrumental value arguments about actually what to do; if that's right, the way forward is much less obvious – an issue we considered in Chapter 2 in the context of Bryan Norton's convergence hypothesis (Norton 1986).

Despite the differences between an intrinsic or instrumental value-focused approach to conservation biology, there are some values that all "traditional" conservation biologists share – and indeed, also share with the North American Model. One value is the fundamental importance of scientific research in understanding and shaping conservation policy. Another is that wildlife should be theoretically and ethically approached in the evolutionary context of species and populations, not as individuals. This means that conservation biologists generally also accept wildlife control in certain contexts, including lethal control of wildlife that's perceived to threaten native populations, species or systems that are the target of conservation.

We can see how these values play out in the kinds of projects supported by conservation biologists. The "Half Earth" project, for instance, was proposed by prominent conservation biologists, most notably E.O. Wilson (2016), and has been supported by many conservation organizations. The project describes itself as having science at its core and our "transcendent moral obligation to the rest of life at its heart" – locating itself within the intrinsic value tradition of conservation biology and also emphasizing the importance of science. Its goal is to designate half the Earth's surface, including the oceans, as interconnected protected areas. Currently, approximately 16% of terrestrial areas and little more than 8% of the oceans are protected areas (UNEP-WCMC & IUCN 2022), so this is a sizeable expansion. While there's no suggestion that these protected areas should be uninhabited, clearly such a designation would have a significant impact on very many people who live in or use these areas – Schleicher et al. (2019) estimate as many as a billion. This has the potential to raise wide-ranging environmental justice issues, of the kind we'll return to in Chapter 8.

Many conservation biologists have also supported ecological restoration and rewilding projects, alongside more hands-off, preservationist ones. Indeed, Soulé (with Reed Noss) published one of the founding papers in the field, "Rewilding and biodiversity: complementary goals for continental conservation" (Soulé and Noss 1998). Restoration – currently defined by the Society for Ecological Restoration (2021) as "the process of assisting the recovery of an ecosystem that has been degraded, damaged, or destroyed" – could be based on intrinsic or instrumental values, or both, but it clearly has a focus on the application of scientific knowledge and works at the level of ecosystems and populations rather than individuals. Restoration projects may also involve the removal, perhaps lethally, of unwanted wildlife (see Chapter 12). *Rewilding* (an idea that has many interpretations) in this context can be understood as a form of restoration that focuses on introducing wildlife to perform particular functions as part of creating or recreating ongoing and independent ecosystems. This may mean reintroducing top predators (such as wolves) and ecosystem "engineers" (such as beavers) to areas from which they have declined or disappeared, or introducing functional grazers or browsers to prevent afforestation. Again, the focus is at system and species level – and as we saw in the case of Oostvaardersplassen in Chapter 4, such system restorations may cause welfare issues for the individual animals involved.

Popular though it is, the conservation biology model has also run into objections. Movements that push back against some of its core value commitments have recently emerged, in particular those arguing that conservation biology in practice has led to environmental injustices, that the dependence on "western" scientific knowledge ignores the traditional knowledge of Indigenous peoples, and that the focus at the level of ecosystems and species leaves out the welfare of individual animals. We'll turn to these concerns in Chapter 8.

7.7 Conclusion

In this chapter, we have looked at three models of wildlife management and conservation: the North American Model (including the broader idea of sustainable use into which the North American Model fits, and the ecosystem services approach); wildlife control; and conservation biology. These models are all value laden and, as we have seen, vary considerably in their approaches. The North American Model, for instance, was wholly anthropocentric and focused primarily on selected valued game species. Wildlife control was also primarily anthropocentric – focused on eliminating or reducing populations of disvalued animals – but at least in some recent forms, may have basic consideration for animal welfare, and in some cases also undertakes wildlife control for ecocentric reasons. Conservation biology, on the other hand, at least in its earlier forms, was ecocentric (see Chapter 4) rather than anthropocentric, maintaining that biodiversity and wild ecosystems have intrinsic value, independently of any usefulness to human beings. All three models share one value in common: the value of grounding their activities in scientific research.

The next chapter explores several more recent prominent movements that, in various ways, reject either the values or practices endorsed by the models we have discussed here.

References

Barber, W.E. (1988). Maximum sustainable yield lives on. *North American Journal of Fisheries Management* 8 (2): 153–157.

Braat, L.C. and De Groot, R. (2012). The ecosystem services agenda: bridging the worlds of natural science and economics, conservation and development, and public and private policy. *Ecosystem Services* 1 (1): 4–15.

Brundtland, G.H. (1987). *Report of the World Commission on Environment and Development: Our Common Future*. New York, USA: United Nations.

Costanza, R., de Groot, R., Braat, L. et al. (2017). Twenty years of ecosystem services: how far have we come and how far do we still need to go? *Ecosystem Services* 28 (A): 1–16.

Dubois, S., Fenwick, N., Ryan, E.A. et al. (2017). International consensus principles for ethical wildlife control. *Conservation Biology* 31: 753–760.

Ehrlich, P. and Ehrlich, A. (1981). *Extinction: The Causes and Consequences of the Disappearance of Species*. New York, USA: Random House.

Eichler, L. and Baumeister, D. (2018). Hunting for justice: an Indigenous critique of the North American model of wildlife conservation. *Environment and Society* 9 (1): 75–90.

Elliott, N.C., Farrell, J.A., Gutierrez, A.P. et al. (1995). *Integrated Pest Management*. New York, USA: Springer Science & Business Media.

Frank, R. (2012). The public trust doctrine: assessing its recent past & charting its future. *UC Davis Law Review* 45: 665–692.

Gerber, L. (2010). Conservation biology. *Nature Education Knowledge* 3 (10): 14.

Gómez-Baggethun, E., De Groot, R., Lomas, P.L., and Montes, C. (2010). The history of ecosystem services in economic theory and practice: from early notions to markets and payment schemes. *Ecological Economics* 69 (6): 1209–1218.

Gray, G. (1995). *Wildlife and People: The Human Dimensions of Wildlife Ecology*. Champaign, USA: University of Illinois Press.

Heffelfinger, J.R., Geist, V., and Wishart, W. (2013). The role of hunting in North American wildlife conservation. *International Journal of Environmental Studies* 70 (3): 399–413.

Jefferson, T. (1955). *Notes on the State of Virginia*. Chapel Hill, USA: University of North Carolina Press (original work published 1785).

Knapp, R.A. and Matthews, K.R. (2000). Non-native fish introductions and the decline of the mountain yellow-legged frog from within protected areas. *Conservation Biology* 14 (2): 428–438.

Koichi, K., Cottrell, A., Sangha, K.K., and Gordon, I.J. (2013). What determines the acceptability of wildlife control methods? A case of feral pig management in the Wet Tropics World Heritage Area, Australia. *Human Dimensions of Wildlife* 18 (2): 97–108.

Lele, S., Springate-Baginski, O., Lakerveld, R. et al. (2013). Ecosystem services: origins, contributions, pitfalls, and alternatives. *Conservation and Society* 11 (4): 343–358.

Leopold, A. (1933). *Game Management*. New York, USA: Scribner, Armstrong & Company.

Linnell, J.D., Cretois, B., Nilsen, E.B. et al. (2020). The challenges and opportunities of coexisting with wild ungulates in the human-dominated landscapes of Europe's Anthropocene. *Biological Conservation* 244: 108500.

Liordos, V., Kontsiotis, V.J., Georgari, M. et al. (2017). Public acceptance of management methods under different human–wildlife conflict scenarios. *Science of the Total Environment* 579: 685–693.

Lueck, D. (2002). The extermination and conservation of the American bison. *Journal of Legal Studies* 31 (S2): S609–S652.

Mace, G.M. (2014). Whose conservation? *Science* 345 (6204): 1558–1560.

Mahoney, S.P. and Geist, V. (ed.) (2019). *The North American Model of Wildlife Conservation*. Baltimore, USA: Johns Hopkins University Press.

Maller, C. (2021). Turning things around: a discussion of values, practices and action in the context of social-ecological change. *People and Nature* https://besjournals.onlinelibrary.wiley.com/doi/10.1002/pan3.10272.

Marsh, G.P. (1864). *Man and Nature, or Physical Geography as Modified by Human Action*. London, UK: Sampson Low, Son and Marston.

Merchant, C. (2007). *American Environmental History*. New York, USA: Columbia University Press.

Nelson, M.P., Vucetich, J.A., Paquet, P.C., and Bump, J.K. (2011). An inadequate construct? North American model: what's flawed, what's missing, what's needed. *Wildlife Professional* 5: 58–60.

Norton, B. (1986). Conservation and preservation: a conceptual rehabilitation. *Environmental Ethics* 8: 195–222.

Organ, J.F., Geist, V., Mahoney, S.P. et al. (2012). *The North American Model of Wildlife Conservation*. Bethesda, USA: Wildlife Society.

Peterson, M.N. and Nelson, M.P. (2017). Why the North American Model of Wildlife Conservation is problematic for modern wildlife management. *Human Dimensions of Wildlife* 22: 43–54.

Prins, H.H., Grootenhuis, J.G., and Dolan, T.T. (ed.) (2012). *Wildlife Conservation by Sustainable Use*. New York, USA: Springer Science & Business Media.

Russell, J.C., Jones, H.P., Armstrong, D.P. et al. (2016). Importance of lethal control of invasive predators for island conservation. *Conservation Biology* 30 (3): 670–672.

Schleicher, J., Zaehringer, J.G., Fastré, C. et al. (2019). Protecting half of the planet could directly affect over one billion people. *Nature Sustainability* 2 (12): 1094–1096.

Society for Ecological Restoration (2021). Mission and Vision. www.ser.org

Soulé, M.E. (1985). What is conservation biology? *BioScience* 35 (11): 727–734.

Soulé, M. and Noss, R. (1998). Rewilding and biodiversity: complementary goals for continental conservation. *Wild Earth* 8: 18–28.

Tallis, H. and Lubchenco, J. (2014). Working together: a call for inclusive conservation. *Nature News* 515: 27–28.

UNEP-WCMC & IUCN (2022). Protected Planet: The World Database on Protected Areas. www.protectedplanet.net

United States Congress (1874). Congressional Record. www.google.com/books/edition/Congressional_Record/ltQjYA0IcQoC?hl=en&gbpv=0

Vrtiska, M.P., Gammonley, J.H., Naylor, L.W., and Raedeke, A.H. (2013). Economic and conservation ramifications from the decline of waterfowl hunters. *Wildlife Society Bulletin* 37 (2): 380–388.

Vucetich, J.A. and Nelson, M.P. (2010). Sustainability: virtuous or vulgar? *BioScience* 60 (7): 539–544.

Wanless, R.M., Ryan, P.G., Altwegg, R. et al. (2009). From both sides: dire demographic consequences of carnivorous mice and longlining for the critically endangered Tristan albatrosses on Gough Island. *Biological Conservation* 142 (8): 1710–1718.

Wilkie, D.S., Wieland, M., and Poulsen, J.R. (2019). Unsustainable vs. sustainable hunting for food in Gabon: modeling short- and long-term gains and losses. *Frontiers in Ecology and Evolution* 7: 357.

Wilson, E.O. (2016). *Half-Earth: Our Planet's Fight for Life*. New York, USA: W.W. Norton.

Recent Movements in Wildlife Management

8

8.1 Introduction

In Chapter 7, we outlined three broad, influential, value-laden models of wildlife management and conservation: the North American Model together with sustainable use and ecosystem services; wildlife control; and conservation biology. These approaches differed in some significant ways. Most obviously, traditional wildlife control and sustainable use are broadly anthropocentric; conservation biology, at least in many forms, accepts nonanthropocentric ecological values such as species value. But as we noted at the end of the chapter, all share an explicit grounding in western science, and all work at the level of populations, species, and systems, rather than focusing on individual wild animals. In addition, as we'll shortly discuss, all (perhaps with the exception of wildlife control) have been argued to have emerged from a largely white, wealthy, postindustrial understanding of wildlife management.

In this chapter, we'll consider some significant current movements in, or impacting on, wildlife management and conservation, that to a greater or lesser extent push back against the approaches we considered in Chapter 7. We'll look at important questions raised by *environmental justice* as it relates to the more traditional approaches to

Wildlife Ethics: The Ethics of Wildlife Management and Conservation, First Edition. Clare Palmer, Bob Fischer, Christian Gamborg, Jordan Hampton, and Peter Sandøe.

wildlife conservation and management in Chapter 7. Then we'll discuss the movement to foreground *Indigenous peoples'* land and wildlife management, emphasizing the importance of traditional and Indigenous knowledge as well as western science. Lastly, we'll look at *wildlife mutualism* and *compassionate conservation*, which we've already mentioned several times and which, it might be argued, shift the conversation about justice to a different location: the place of *individual* wild animals. First, however, we'll introduce a case that helps to illustrate important issues for the movements we'll discuss in this chapter: the management of Addo Elephant Park in South Africa.

8.2 Addo Elephant National Park

Addo Elephant National Park is the third largest national park in South Africa. It was originally established in 1931 to protect African elephants, whose populations had been decimated by hunting; only 11 elephants remained in the area at the time the park was established. Once the park was established, the elephant population significantly expanded (Figure 8.1). Until part of the park was fenced in 1954, this increase in elephant abundance led to friction with local farmers, owing to the elephants' capacity to disrupt agriculture and threaten humans (for further discussion of cases like this, see Chapter 11).

Addo has, more recently, shifted from being managed just for the protection of elephants to (according to South Africa National Parks) conserving the "rich biodiversity of the area" (South Africa National Parks n.d.). Lions and spotted hyenas, which had become locally extinct, were reintroduced in 2003–4. The presence of the Big Five (originally a term used by big game hunters, but now used by tour operators and national

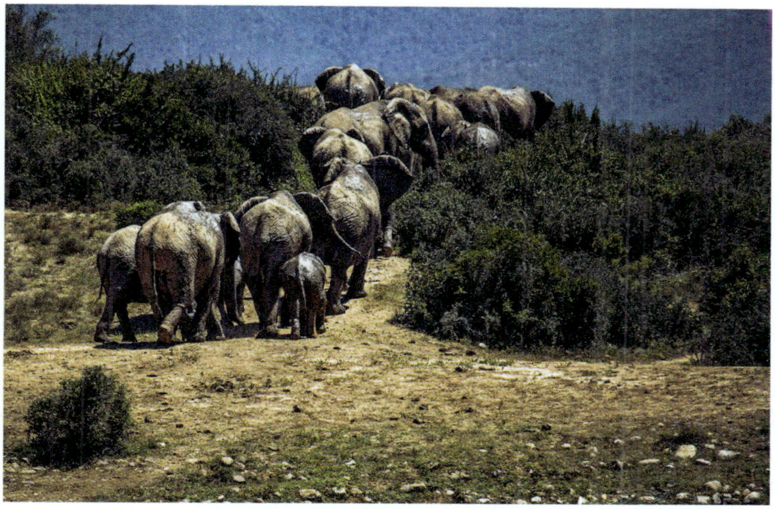

Figure 8.1 A herd of African elephants in Addo National Park, South Africa. *Source:* Francesco Valenti/Dreamstime LLC.

parks in relation to observing these animals in their natural habitat) – elephants, lions, black rhinoceroses, Cape buffalo and African leopards – make this park particularly attractive to tourists. Indeed, Addo has recently expanded to the Eastern Cape coast of South Africa, and now advertises the Big Seven – the Big Five, plus the southern right whale and the great white shark. Features such as an artificially lit drinking hole near the main tourist area make it easy for tourists to see the land-based wild animals.

Despite recent expansions, however, Addo is a relatively small (178 918 ha or 1789 km^2) fenced reserve. Protecting species diversity through wildlife management in such reserves is far from straightforward (Tambling et al. 2013). The expanded elephant population, while fundamentally important both for the conservation of the species and for tourism, poses significant problems for other species in the park. In particular, the park is the location of the endangered Sundays Spekboom Thicket vegetation type, to which the elephants have been causing significant damage (Lombard et al. 2001). This in turn affects the habitat of other animals, such as the Cape grysbok and the bushpig. Some areas of the park have now been fenced off from elephants.

But the impacts of large numbers of elephants on park ecosystems have led to debates about culling, immunocontraception (which is practiced, at the time of writing, with some populations in the park), relocation, and removing park boundary fences to create more space for elephants to roam (Marris 2008). Removing park fences, however, would be likely to bring back conflicts between humans, especially farmers, and the elephants. And further park expansions, though they are planned, are also likely to be contested, since they occur in a place where human populations are growing and land shortage and poverty are significant concerns.

Addo thus raises wide-ranging issues for wildlife management and conservation, in particular about conflicts between wildlife and local human populations around the park; the treatment of the animals themselves, including highly sensitive, intelligent, and social animals like elephants in the context of threatened ecosystems; and the predominance of wealthy, majority-white visitors to the park. The management of Addo, and many other national parks and/or nature and wildlife reserves, also has a role in ongoing debates about fairness and justice in the context of conservation values and community livelihoods. This discussion is part of a much bigger, global movement – the environmental justice movement.

8.3 Environmental Justice

The environmental justice movement emerged in the US during the 1980s, originally as a protest against the disproportionate burden of environmental risk carried by minority and low-income groups with respect to toxic waste and pollution (Bullard 2019). Since then, environmental justice has become a global movement, rooted in several importantly different senses of justice. First, environmental justice concerns *distributive* justice, here understood in terms of fair access to goods and benefits related to the environment (including land) and/or the bearing of proportionate environmental burdens or risks. Second, environmental justice concerns *participative* justice – the meaningful involvement by all groups in the political and social processes that determine and impact on their environments (Shlosberg 2004). And third, environmental justice includes *recognition* justice, where "policies and programs must meet the standard of fairly considering and representing the cultures, values, and situations of all affected parties" (Whyte 2011, p. 200). Taken together, these justice commitments constitute a significant challenge to aspects of the wildlife management and conservation paradigms we considered in Chapter 7; we'll outline just some of these concerns here.

The most significant justice issue relates to Indigenous peoples (and other tribal and traditional peoples in countries that were not formerly colonized). As we noted in Chapter 7, the North American Model of wildlife use failed to acknowledge the prior claims of Native American tribes in the United States. In addition, the development of national parks and wilderness areas in the US, seen as critically important for the development of conservation, involved actively expelling native peoples from the land. The most famous example was the expulsion of the Miwok people from Yosemite Valley in the late nineteenth century in order to create Yosemite National Park; indeed, this episode led to the coining of the term "Yosemite model" for the creation of conservation areas from which human residents had been excluded (Dowie 2011).

The practice of separating local tribal and Indigenous people from their traditional lands to create land dedicated to conservation (and more recently, biodiversity more specifically) was exported from North America to Asia, Africa, and South America. Given the goal of keeping local people out, and frequently using park rangers to patrol the borders, the practice has been dubbed "fortress conservation" (Brockington 2002). The only acceptable uses of such conservation "fortresses" were taken to be tourism, safari hunting, and scientific research. So, it's not difficult to see how such practices could manifest all three forms of environmental injustice mentioned above. Local Indigenous and traditional peoples have been unfairly deprived of access to traditional lands while others (tourists, scientists, and nonlocal hunters) can benefit from the land: that seems to be distributive injustice. Historically, there has rarely been meaningful consultation with the local communities affected, leading to participatory injustice, and the cultures, values, and relationships of local communities with the land were rarely recognized so there's also recognition injustice. And although estimates vary, it's likely that, globally, many millions of people have been displaced from their homes and the land that previously sustained them in the name of conservation alone.

Indigenous and traditional people's territories may also be in demand by outsiders for other purposes, for instance logging, mining, and cattle farming. In attempting to defend their lands from illegal land grabs, land activists and environmental defenders have suffered physical attack and been killed; between 2002 and 2018, at least 1734 were killed, one-third of whom were Indigenous people, principally in Brazil, the Philippines, Colombia, Honduras, Mexico, and Peru (Le Billon and Lujala 2020). Evictions and physical attacks are two of many current concerns in the long story of attempts to part Indigenous people from their lands, whether for the purpose of protecting and conserving the land or for exploiting the land or the wildlife the lands contain.

Addo is an interesting example to consider in this context. The land from which the park was originally created had been occupied by the amaXhosa, amaFengu, and Khoekhoe peoples, but by the 1910s, they were largely dispossessed of land in the area (Skotnes-Brown 2021). Initially, the creation of national parks in South Africa did not wholly exclude local African communities. However, over the course of the twentieth century this changed: "Through removals, fences, game guards and laws against poaching and trespassing, reserves and parks became highly secured areas to be kept safe from threatening outsiders, i.e. the local black people" (Dahlberg et al. 2010, p. 212). Local people were denied access to Addo, despite the important role it played for them in terms of cultural as well as physical resources, and the park was widely regarded as "primeval bush," becoming a popular tourist location for white South Africans seeking "wilderness experience" (Brooks 2005). It seems likely, then, that this situation manifested multiple forms of injustice, as discussed above: distributive, participative, and in terms of recognition.

Since democratic elections in 1994, achieving environmental justice has been part of the agenda of South Africa National Parks. This has involved, depending on the case, co-management with communities, financial compensation, the allocation of land near parks to local communities, and giving local communities access to parks for a number of purposes (though not normally including hunting terrestrial wildlife). So, the current management plan for Addo allows community access to parts of the park for subsistence fishing, for carrying out rituals, and for visiting established graveyards (South Africa National Parks n.d.). Local school groups are brought to the park, and there's community outreach; one of the goals is to "provide socio-economic empowerment opportunities associated with the Addo brand" (South Africa National Parks n.d.). This includes the creation of local jobs, internships, skills development opportunities, and supporting bee-keeping and the processing of nonnative fish. Where the park has expanded into land that was previously used for farming, there's a commitment by South Africa National Parks that "all these workers have the same or better housing, salary and benefits (e.g. rations, right to keep livestock on land, etc.). Either the worker moves to a new farm with the original landowner or SANParks must give the worker employment – permanent or, if this is not available, contractual" (South Africa National Parks n.d.).

How far these commitments really work out on the ground, and whether these kinds of commitments constitute an adequate response to past injustice in the name of conservation, are, of course, contested. But more generally, concern about situations where generally poorer, rural populations are negatively affected by conservation initiatives without being offered appropriate alternatives or adequate compensation has become increasingly important in wildlife management and conservation. One well-known expression of this worry has emerged within what's become known as the "new conservation" movement (Minteer and Miller 2011).

The new conservation movement is highly contested, starting with its name. On the one hand, it might be argued that what's said, in the context of environmental justice at least, is not all that "new." Since the late 1980s, Indigenous scholars, anthropologists, geographers, and other social scientists have voiced their concern about the ways in which western ideas of wilderness – in particular, the idea of nature as separate from human culture – have led Indigenous and traditional peoples to be dispossessed of their land (Colchester 1994), and have defended more community-based conservation (e.g., Brockington 2002). And on the other hand, it's been argued that this movement is not really "conservation" either. Michael Soulé – whose work we discussed in the context of conservation biology in Chapter 7 – maintained in a strongly worded editorial in the journal *Conservation Biology* that owing to its prioritization of human interests, new conservation "does not deserve to be labelled conservation" (Soulé 2013, p. 893).

The new conservation movement is also rather diverse, and different figures associated with it champion a variety of distinct ideas (for instance, concerning the meaning and value of wildness). However, one key set of ideas is that traditional conservation, structured around parks and preserves, is failing, even on its own measure of biodiversity protection (Kareiva et al. 2012). Rather than centering conservation around setting land aside, the authors argue, conservation needs to be more "people friendly" and to focus on working landscapes, and local and Indigenous people need "to be trusted to care for their land" (Kareiva et al. 2012). The authors argue that the creation of parks and protected areas is anyway counterproductive, since if local people lack the resources to survive, especially if they have been excluded from the land, they will see nature as "the enemy" and, understandably, poach wildlife and use protected areas in other potentially damaging ways (Kareiva et al. 2012). Conversely, if local communities have opportunities for income growth and a higher standard of living, so that they are freed from such pressing economic worries, they will be able to develop an attachment to nature and ultimately welcome attempts to protect it. The authors conclude their argument in this way:

> Protecting biodiversity for its own sake has not worked. Protecting nature that is dynamic and resilient, that is in our midst rather than far away, and that sustains human communities – these are the ways forward now. Otherwise, conservation will fail, clinging to its old myths.
>
> (Kareiva et al. 2012)

Not surprisingly, this approach has not been welcomed by some members of the conservation biology community, who contend that the emphasis on human development over biodiversity protection "would hasten ecological collapse globally, eradicating thousands of kinds of plants and animals and causing inestimable harm to humankind in the long run" (Soulé 2013, p. 896).

In the next section we'll look further at arguments that Indigenous and other traditional and tribal communities should have much more significant involvement in land and wildlife management. Before moving to that, though, we'll briefly consider some rather different ways in which concerns about environmental justice can impact on wildlife management and conservation. These focus on participative justice, specifically in terms of the lack of diversity in conservation organizations, and in decision making about wildlife conservation and management policy.

In 2014, Dorceta Taylor published a US-based report called *The State of Diversity in Environmental Organizations* (Taylor 2014). This report looked at employee diversity in 191 conservation and preservation organizations, 74 governmental environmental agencies, and 28 environmental grant-making foundations. It found that while there had been progress on *gender* diversity, most positions had gone to white women, and white men were still more likely to occupy the most powerful positions. Although the employment of individuals from ethnic minority groups had increased over time, ethnic minority employees were "severely underrepresented" in the environmental workforce, and concentrated in the lower ranks in all kinds of environmental organizations.

The lack of diversity in conservation organizations isn't just a problem confined to North America. A 2020 report on the conservation site Mongabay, for instance, investigating inclusiveness and diversity in conservation work across the African continent, highlighted numerous instances of white employees being brought in from outside to run conservation projects, research teams from overseas replacing local researchers, and local workers being sidelined or ignored, in episodes of what Resson Kantai Duff, the author, calls "subtle racism" (Duff 2020). In general, Duff points out, there's a lack of African leadership in African conservation. Illustrating this pattern, recent research at Addo found that "local people were only employed as administration clerks, drivers, gate guards, receptionists, room attendants, trade workers, general workers, horse guides, handy men, people and conservation officers, fuel pump attendants and switchboard attendants. None of them had a managerial position" (Fezeka and Kwizera 2020, p. 8).

This discussion, both of injustice in land distribution and the involvement (or otherwise) of diverse ethnic groups, Indigenous and local peoples in wildlife management, leads directly to the next concern we'll discuss in this chapter: Indigenous and traditional wildlife management and conservation.

8.4 Indigenous Wildlife Management and Conservation

Over the past two decades, a growing movement has advocated for the extension of Indigenous people's wildlife management, including returning land to the stewardship of Indigenous peoples and other local and traditional land-owners, and the adoption of co-management strategies with Indigenous peoples (Butler 2021).

These proposals appear to target all three kinds of environmental injustice we've just discussed. First, in terms of distributive justice, they assert that Indigenous peoples have a right to their traditional lands, and that these rights should have legal protection (now enshrined in the UN Declaration on the Rights of Indigenous Peoples). In terms of participative justice, Indigenous peoples should be free to be decision makers with respect to the management of their lands and wildlife, and in terms of recognition justice, the cultures, values, and special relations of Indigenous and other local peoples to their traditional lands should be recognized as central.

Let's look a bit more closely at what's being proposed here. First, Indigenous peoples already have rights to, or actually manage, a good deal of land and wildlife globally that's critical for conservation. Although mapping and identifying this land are difficult, the UN Environment Programme (UNEP) has estimated that "at least a quarter of the world's land area is owned, managed, used or occupied by Indigenous peoples and local communities" (UNEP 2020). Second, much of this land is in areas of high biodiversity; a 2019 study found that vertebrate biodiversity on Indigenous-managed lands (without other forms of protection) in Australia, Canada, and Brazil was as high as vertebrate biodiversity in formally protected lands (Schuster et al. 2019). And this high biodiversity, other research suggests, hasn't come about by chance; the ways in which Indigenous peoples have managed the land over generations have helped to maintain or bring this about (e.g., Ellis et al. 2021). Given this apparent success in terms of high biodiversity and wildlife flourishing, proposals for Indigenous land management argue that the land tenure of Indigenous peoples should not only be protected because it's *just* to do so, but also for conservation reasons, because Indigenous peoples are largely successful at caring for the land and for wildlife.

This success in managing traditional lands shouldn't be taken to mean that Indigenous and traditional peoples do, or should, reject the use of modern technologies for land management; the organization Conservation International in partnership with NASA, for instance, is currently teaching Indigenous groups to use geospatial technology to help protect their land (Conservation International n.d.). Nor does it mean that Indigenous and traditional peoples don't or shouldn't join partnerships with scientists from outside their communities to develop strategies of coexistence with, or comanagement of, wildlife. Many examples of cooperation and partnership exist. For instance, in the Kimberley region of Australia, a group of Indigenous leaders brought together an Indigenous-led working group to manage what was called the Kimberley Indigenous Saltwater Science Project, working with selected researchers from western science-based institutions (Austin et al. 2019).

However, such partnerships do face what Austin et al. (2019, p. 582) call "the challenge of working with radical difference." This difference is particularly striking in terms of what counts as "knowledge." Local ecological knowledge, traditional ecological knowledge, and Indigenous knowledge are crucial to these groups' understandings of their environments, but differ significantly from scientific knowledge in the western tradition, pushing back against assumptions of the wildlife management paradigms we looked at in Chapter 7 and the methods widely adopted by western scientists (Berkes 1999). As noted by Agrawal (1995) and other scholars, this doesn't mean that there are two very rigid categories of "knowledge" here; there's variety among Indigenous, traditional, and local groups and, as philosophers and sociologists of science have long argued, there's no monolithic "scientific method" for producing knowledge either. Unsurprisingly, then, arguments for pluralism – using both scientific and traditional knowledge – are increasing within conservation science (Pascual et al. 2021).

Definitions of "local ecological knowledge," "Indigenous knowledge" or "traditional ecological knowledge" vary; for simplicity, we'll focus on traditional ecological knowledge here. Kyle Powys Whyte (2013, p. 2) suggests that no definition of traditional ecological knowledge can "satisfy every stakeholder in every context." Some definitions treat traditional ecological knowledge as a body of knowledge that, while embedded within communities and their relationships, could, albeit with difficulty, be catalogued and used in management practices, including by scientists and external agencies. According to that conceptualization, traditional ecological knowledge is understood as information that Indigenous peoples possess about the local ecosystems in which they live – that is, information about the properties, behaviors, and locations of particular plants and animals, the signs of healthy and unhealthy plant life, how the local environment has changed and is changing, and much more. Indigenous knowledge understood in this sense, Whyte (2018) argues, is seen as having "supplemental value" – it's used to *enrich* scientific research by providing information to which scientists wouldn't otherwise have access (see also Tomaselli et al. 2018).

Other definitions, however, often proposed by Indigenous scholars but increasingly accepted more widely, take traditional ecological knowledge to be about *active engagement*: "to speak of a society's Traditional Ecological Knowledge is to speak of ongoing activities expressive of responsibilities" (Whyte 2013, p. 4). In this sense, traditional ecological knowledge is *normative*, relating to systems of responsibilities and the development of character. Seen in this way, traditional ecological knowledge looks much less easily accessible to those who are not members of the relevant traditional communities. For instance, Pierotti and Wildcat (2000, p. 1336) focus on participation in and respect for the nonhuman world as key to understanding traditional ecological knowledge, arguing that connections "based on a mixture of extraction, e.g. animals are taken as prey, combined with recognition of the inherent value and good of non-human lives" are crucial.

In terms of managing wildlife, recognition that Indigenous knowledge is not just a body of information but a *lifeway* has become increasingly important, and has a number of ethical implications. One is that sharing knowledge can impose risks on Indigenous peoples, and for this reason, they should be able to withhold knowledge in some circumstances. So, for instance, the Climate and Traditional Knowledges Workgroup (CTKW) formed under the auspices of the US National Oceans and Atmosphere Administration notes that:

> Sharing traditional knowledges may also disclose the fact that Indigenous peoples have plants, animals and sacred places in locations that are part of their ancestral territory. Sharing traditional knowledges could disclose the location and importance of these areas, which can encourage other people to ignore the priority of Indigenous practices and to infringe on Indigenous use by over-consuming or misusing plants and animals in these areas.
>
> (CTKW 2015)

Another ethical implication, as Whyte (2018) makes clear, is that traditional knowledges have "governance value" for Indigenous peoples; this knowledge forms part of the way in which Indigenous communities organize and imagine themselves, and what they are trying to achieve in their own right, and these community goals may diverge from those being pursued by scientists trying to use Indigenous knowledge. So, the interface between Indigenous groups and scientific researchers can be a difficult one.

Western researchers and Indigenous and traditional groups may also understand human relationships with animals and other living things very differently. Few Indigenous groups take a wholly anthropocentric perspective (for instance, of the kind that underpins the idea of sustainable use or much wildlife control discussed in Chapter 7) but neither are their views very close to those of conservation biologists. Many Indigenous perspectives are much more relational and reciprocal, seeing living things as fellow beings, with whom they have ongoing and significant relationships. However, this doesn't mean that hunting is unacceptable (see Chapter 13). As Pierotti and Wildcat (2000) note above, many Indigenous groups see animals as offering themselves to hunters as a gift. Here's an example, from the report of an anthropologist (Nadasdy 2007) who was working with the members of the Kluane First Nation peoples in Alaska. He was learning how to trap rabbits, and came upon one still alive in his snare. He had never killed an animal with his bare hands before, but now needed to do exactly that. Unsurprisingly, the rabbit suffered in the process, and the anthropologist felt guilty about the pain he'd caused. When he told the chief of the tribe, he was told that he was making a mistake:

> The proper reaction, [the chief] said, is simply to say a prayer of thanks to the animal; it is disrespectful to think about an animal's suffering when you kill it. [... Another person explained] that .... If they give themselves to you, you say a prayer of thanks

and accept the gift of meat you have been given. To think about the animals' suffering, she said, is to find fault with the gift, to cast doubt on whether the animal should have given itself to you in the first place …

(Nadasdy 2007, p. 27)

This understanding differs significantly from three other ideas that have a role in this book: the anthropocentric idea that humans are entitled to use animals as human resources; the idea that, as animals are sentient beings with their own inner lives, we shouldn't normally harm them (as is defended by compassionate conservationists, below); and the idea that wild animals are primarily important as members of valuable species and ecosystems. Here, the animal is understood as having a mind, as being some kind of self (since the animal has the conception of offering itself as a *gift* – though not clear from whom or what) but this isn't seen as reason to refrain from hunting.

This means, therefore, that there may be a value conflict between Indigenous and traditional perspectives on and methods of hunting, and the perspectives of people for whom animal welfare (understood in terms of subjective experience) and animal lives are of high moral significance. There may also be conflicts with conservationists, if the animals hunted are members of protected species (such as whales or dugongs; we'll explore this conflict further in Chapter 13). This potential disagreement leads us to consider approaches to wildlife conservation in which *individual* wild animals are of high significance.

8.5 The Growth of Mutualism and Compassionate Conservation

So far, we haven't considered any frameworks in which the value of *individual* wild animals has particular significance. None of the approaches we considered in Chapter 7 emphasized the value of individual animals; many forms of environmental justice don't explicitly do so either. However, research from the first two decades of the twenty-first century in postindustrialized countries suggests that there are now broader shifts in public views about wildlife in which individual animals *do* matter. Research into wildlife value orientations – that is, the fundamental values and beliefs people hold about wildlife, which to some degree ground attitudes and behaviors – shows that, at least in some countries and regions of the world, individual wild animals are, or are becoming, more socially significant and increasingly valued.

After the Second World War, many (although by no means all) nations underwent social modernization, a process characterized by increased affluence, better educational systems, more urbanization, and shifting social values (Inglehart 1997). Among these value shifts seems to have been a movement toward "wildlife mutualism." To see what this means in context, it's helpful to get a sense of the four types of wildlife orientations researchers have identified. These are *utilitarian* (high utilitarian, low mutualism), *mutualist* (high mutualism, low utilitarian), *distanced* (low mutualism, low utilitarian), and *pluralist* (high mutualism, high utilitarian). For our purposes here, utilitarian and mutualist are the two most important orientations. However, it's worth recognizing that in several (mainly European) countries, there are also many individuals who display a *distanced* orientation – not particularly interested in wildlife at all.

Utilitarian (or *domination*) orientations understand wildlife as to be used and managed primarily for the benefit of humans ("utilitarian" here shouldn't be confused with the ethical theory of the same name, discussed in Chapter 6, most forms of which take the interests of sentient animals and humans to be of equal ethical importance). Humans are taken to be highly distinct from, and superior to, nonhuman animals. Thus, this is a broadly anthropocentric orientation. A person with a strong utilitarian orientation is likely to find sport hunting and culling acceptable, and (more specifically) to be on board with something like the North American Model of wildlife management discussed in Chapter 7.

Mutualists, on the other hand, "adopt a view that wildlife are part of one's social network and worthy of care and compassion" (Manfredo et al. 2020, p. 1549). This orientation is obviously in tension with the idea of "sustainable use" and with many forms of wildlife control. It may even be in conflict with conservation biology, inasmuch as conservation biology prioritizes ecological values over caring for individual wild animals, and emphasizes the reduction or eradication of undesired introduced species. Michael Manfredo et al. (2020), however, found that wildlife mutualism is also positively associated with concern for endangered species, habitat protection, and maintaining natural conditions (Figure 8.2). Given that these values could conflict with care for individuals, there's likely to be a need for wildlife mutualists to deal with inner conflicts over prioritizing values.

The research carried out by Manfredo et al. (2020) found a significant increase in mutualist orientations and a reduction in utilitarian orientations over time in the US (2021) and other postindustrialized countries (2020), especially in more urban populations. Among more prominent reasons proposed to explain this shift are a lack of actual

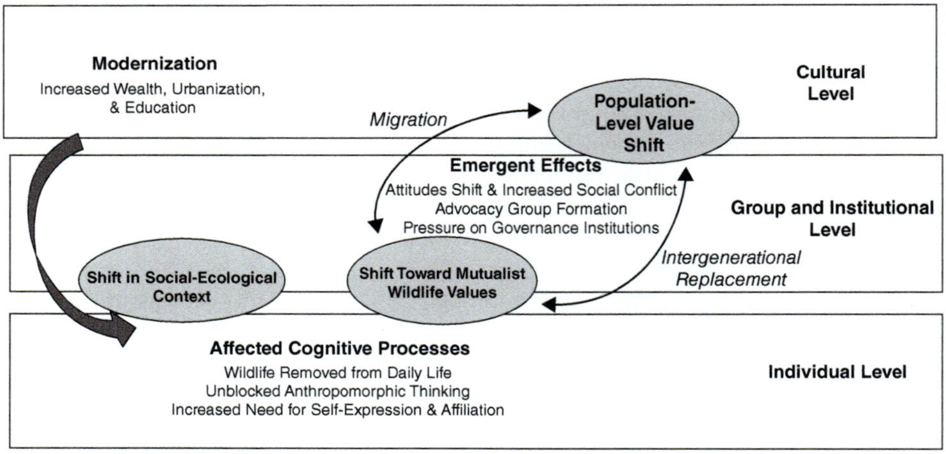

Figure 8.2 Multilevel model of the changing sociocultural context of wildlife conservation in the USA. It illustrates how cultural-level processes, driven by increased wealth, urbanization, and education, affect changes in cognition at the individual level, leading to a shift from domination to mutualist wildlife values – a shift which is likely to be applicable to many modernized countries. *Source:* Manfredo et al. (2020)/with permission of John Wiley & Sons.

engagement with wildlife and so a lower risk of having negative wildlife encounters; an increased desire for social affiliation and companionship that's extended to include wildlife; and learning about wildlife through media sources rather than through direct encounters, where the images of the wild animals portrayed are positive and humanized (Manfredo et al. 2020).

This shift toward wildlife mutualism has been identified in countries from several continents. However, Manfredo et al. (2020) do sound a note of warning about too much generalization. For instance, while their US survey found that states with higher income and higher education levels had higher levels of wildlife mutualism (fitting the postindustrial shifting values hypothesis), another survey in China found that while wildlife consumption had dropped slightly between 2004 and 2012 (and more significantly in Beijing), overall, higher education levels and higher income were actually associated with *higher* wildlife consumption (Zhang and Yin 2014). Moreover, this bimodal representation and explanation of people's views toward wildlife is inevitably somewhat oversimple; the divide between mutualism and utilitarianism may not be so clear. For instance, this divide doesn't map at all well onto the ways in which, as we've seen, some Indigenous peoples view wildlife; at the same time, in the same person, in the same community, wildlife can be seen both as valuable and worthy of care, and as available for hunting and use. So obviously, caution is needed when trying to apply frameworks like these, as they only capture part of the complexity found in different cultures and traditions toward wildlife.

In general, though, shifts toward mutualism and away from utilitarian and dominance orientations to wildlife seem to be widespread. And this has led to significant pushback against some of the management practices embedded in the frameworks discussed in Chapter 7. After all, the North American Model was designed to manage wildlife for sustainable hunting and fishing. But mutualists are much less interested in hunting and fishing – a change that, along with increasing urbanization, may underpin the decline of those practices in the US. And mutualists are also generally opposed to predator control – for instance, wolf culling – not just because of worries about the persistence of a wolf species, or because wolves are crucial to maintaining ecological communities, but because of concern about individual wolves in the context of a sense of social affiliation with wild animals. As such, they perceive wildlife as part of an "extended family" where animals are ascribed something like rights (e.g., the right not to be killed by humans; Dayer et al. 2007).

The growth in wildlife mutualism is a social shift that has important ramifications in terms of support (or otherwise) for the adoption of particular wildlife management policies. However, the *compassionate conservation* movement is attempting to make a more systematic intervention into wildlife management, by deliberately bringing attention to harms to individual animals caused by conservation practices. The title "compassionate conservation" was first used at a symposium organized by the Born Free Foundation in 2010, and was subsequently adopted as the name of the Centre for Compassionate Conservation at the University of Technology, in Sydney, Australia. The movement endorses four principles: first, do no harm; individuals matter; inclusivity; and peaceful coexistence (Wallach et al. 2018). In endorsing these principles, compassionate conservation is pushing back not only against models of human–wildlife relations centered primarily around use, but also against conservation biology, inasmuch as compassionate conservation objects to policies that focus on saving valued species and populations at the expense of the lives and welfare of individual animals, for instance from more abundant or nonnative species. The approach "aims to safeguard Earth's biological diversity while retaining a commitment to treating individuals with respect and concern for their wellbeing" (Wallach et al. 2018, p. 1260).

A key strand of compassionate conservation is the use of a science base that hasn't featured strongly to date in the science of conservation: that of *animal minds*, *emotions*, and *cognition*. Compassionate conservationists argue that this scientific base needs to be considered alongside the sciences of biology and ecology, given that some wild animals are sentient (see Chapter 5), can think and feel, and have their own inner lives. Accordingly, compassionate conservationists argue that the impact of wildlife management on the individual animals being managed needs to be taken much more seriously than has historically been the case.

However, it's not yet completely clear what this means in practice; compassionate conservation is a relatively young movement with more and less radical forms and different theoretical grounds. In relation to the ethical theories discussed in Chapter 6, for instance, some forms of compassionate conservation emphasize "compassion" and other *virtues* in terms of engaging with wild animals. Other forms seem much closer to an animal *rights* view. But in all forms of compassionate conservation, there's either a rejection of, or a very high threshold for adoption of, policies that require killing sentient animals. It's unlikely that any form of compassionate conservation, for instance, would accept painful, drawn-out killing, such as from the use of anticoagulant poisons typically used as rodenticides (see Chapter 12). But some forms of compassionate conservation – though not normally those that endorse animal rights theories – may accept quick and painless killing as a last resort. Concern is also expressed about conservation practices such as captive breeding and translocation that may cause suffering to individual animals in the process of trying to protect species.

Returning to Addo Elephant Park, it's interesting to consider what compassionate conservation might look like in such a management context. Some aspects of current population management of the elephants, involving fertility control rather than culling, fit fairly well with the goals of compassionate conservation. However, the lethal management of introduced mammals, which is currently practiced, seems ethically problematic from this perspective. One relevant point here is that compassionate conservation doesn't generally consider the welfare of animals indirectly or unintentionally affected either by particular management practices or by not managing in particular ways (Johnson et al. 2019). So, in the case of Addo, intentional killing of elephants would be highly ethically problematic for compassionate conservationists but the welfare of *other* wild animals in the ecosystem that may suffer from declining or degraded habitat due to overbrowsing by elephants – such as the Cape grysbok and the bushpig – wouldn't normally attract ethical concern (Hampton et al. 2019). Addo also has a program to reintroduce predators. It's not at all clear what compassionate conservationists would have to say about this, given that such reintroductions are likely to cause suffering to the prey (as well as to the predators during transport) but the human involvement in causing the suffering to prey is somewhat indirect. Compassionate conservation, then, certainly seems to open up some of the questions raised by wild animal suffering more generally (as discussed in Chapters 5 and 6).

Unsurprisingly, compassionate conservation has provoked concern (and in some cases, alarm) among the broader conservation community. One point of contention is the role that animal welfare already has in conservation practice. Some have argued against the claim that the welfare of individual animals has been neglected by traditional wildlife management and conservation, pointing to several decades of integration of animal welfare science into conservation practices (Hampton et al. 2020). This is reflected in statements such as: "Compassion (or, less specifically, concern for individual animal welfare) has already become an important aspect of best practices in conservation" (Hayward et al. 2019, p. 762). Certainly, if one took the view that killing itself is not a welfare issue (discussed in Chapter 5) and accepted a more consequentialist approach to suffering reduction, including suffering that occurs if humans *don't* act (rather than doing *no* harm), animal welfare *does* already play a role in current mainstream conservation practices in countries such as Canada, Australia, and New Zealand (Stephen et al. 2018).

Some criticism of compassionate conservation has gone further and questioned whether this approach would actually create benefits for the welfare of animals or people. These criticisms were prominent in debates during 2019 in the journal *Conservation Biology* (Oommen et al. 2019). A second, more acute concern for conservation biologists is that, given the rise in wildlife mutualism, compassionate conservation is likely to attract popular support. As such, conservation biologists worry, it might prevent the enacting of projects designed to protect endangered *species* and *ecosystems*, especially from undesired introduced species – such as the Predator Free New Zealand plan discussed in Chapter 12:

> Ultimately we fear that a world of "Compassionate Conservation" could stymie the global conservation efforts required to meet international biodiversity targets derived from evidenced based practice, such as the Aichi targets developed by the Convention on Biological Diversity and adopted by the International Union for the Conservation of Nature and the United Nations
>
> (Callen et al. 2020, p. 2)

Probably the views here fall along a spectrum; virtually no one in this debate thinks that animal suffering and animal lives don't matter at all, and virtually no one thinks that conserving biodiversity, species, and ecosystems doesn't matter at all. However, compassionate conservationists (and many wildlife mutualists) prioritize avoiding causing intentional suffering and killing, while more traditional conservationists instead emphasize the ecological values we discussed in Chapters 3 and 4. This can lead to value conflicts that are difficult to resolve.

8.6 Conclusion

Chapters 7 and 8 have walked through a variety of value-laden different paradigms, models, and movements that have shaped wildlife management and conservation. In Chapter 7, we outlined traditional management models dominated by wild animals as game, as pests, and as members of valuable species and ecosystems. In this chapter, we explored movements that in various ways critique, reject or expand on these traditional models, by emphasizing environmental justice, the importance of the land management of Indigenous and traditional peoples, and the welfare and lives of individual animals. To a large extent, these models draw on and reflect the different values and ethical theories presented in Chapters 2–6, but also, notably, when it comes to issues of justice, supplement these. The presented competing values and ethical views mean that ethical decision making can be difficult to achieve and lead to conflicts. We'll look in more detail at the management of ethical conflicts over wildlife in Chapter 9.

References

Agrawal, A. (1995). Indigenous and scientific knowledge: some critical comments. *Antropologi Indonesia* 3 (3): 3–6.

Austin, B.J., Robinson, C.J., Mathews, D. et al. (2019). An indigenous-led approach for regional knowledge partnerships in the Kimberley region of Australia. *Human Ecology* 47: 577–588.

Berkes, F. (1999). *Sacred Ecology. Traditional Ecological Knowledge and Resource Management*. Philadelphia, USA: Taylor and Francis.

Brockington, D. (2002). *Fortress Conservation: The Preservation of the Mkomazi Game Reserve, Tanzania*. Bloomington, USA: Indiana University Press.

Brooks, S. (2005). Images of 'Wild Africa': nature tourism and the (re) creation of Hluhluwe game reserve, 1930–1945. *Journal of Historical Geography* 31 (2): 220–240.

Bullard, R.D. (2019). *Dumping in Dixie: Race, Class, and Environmental Quality*, 3e. New York, USA: Routledge.

Butler, R. (2021). *Securing Indigenous Guardianship of Vital Ecosystems*. https://news.mongabay.com/2021/02/securing-Indigenous-guardianship-of-vital-ecosystems-qa-with-nia-tero-ceo-peter-seligmann

Callen, A., Hayward, M.W., Klop-Toker, K. et al. (2020). Envisioning the future with 'compassionate conservation': an ominous projection for native wildlife and biodiversity. *Biological Conservation* 241: 108365.

Climate and Traditional Knowledges Workgroup (CTKW) (2015). The Ethics of Traditional Knowledge Exchange in Climate Change Initiatives. https://earthzine.org/the-ethics-of-traditional-knowledge-exchange-in-climate-change-initiatives

Colchester, M. (1994). *Salvaging Nature: Indigenous Peoples, Protected Areas and Biodiversity Conservation*. Geneva, Switzerland: United Nations Research Institute for Social Development.

Conservation International (n.d.). Earth Observations for Indigenous-Led Land Management. www.conservation.org/projects/earth-observations-for-Indigenous-led-land-management

Dahlberg, A., Rohde, R., and Sandell, K. (2010). National parks and environmental justice: comparing access rights and ideological legacies in three countries. *Conservation and Society* 8 (3): 209–224.

Dayer, A.A., Stinchfield, H.M., and Manfredo, M.J. (2007). Stories about wildlife: developing an instrument for identifying wildlife value orientations cross-culturally. *Human Dimensions of Wildlife* 12 (5): 307–315.

Dowie, M. (2011). *Conservation Refugees: The Hundred-Year Conflict between Global Conservation and Native Peoples*. Cambridge, USA: MIT Press.

Duff, R.K. (2020). Building a Road to Recovery for Subtle Racism in Conservation (Commentary). https://news.mongabay.com/2020/11/building-a-road-to-recovery-for-subtle-racism-in-conservation-commentary

Ellis, E.C., Gauthier, N., Goldewijk, K.K. et al. (2021). People have shaped most of terrestrial nature for at least 12,000 years. *Proceedings of the National Academy of Sciences* 118 (17): e2023483118.

Fezeka, M. and Kwizera, A.S. (2020). Assessment of the socio-economic impacts of tourism on three rural communities neighbouring Addo Elephant National Park, Eastern Cape, South Africa. *African Journal of Hospitality, Tourism and Leisure* 9: 1.

Hampton, J.O., Warburton, B., and Sandøe, P. (2019). Compassionate versus consequentialist conservation. *Conservation Biology* 33 (4): 751–759.

Hampton, J.O., Baker, S.E., Beausoleil, N.J. et al. (2020). Animal welfare science aids conservation. *Science* 370 (6513): 180–181.

Hayward, M.W., Callen, A., Allen, B.L. et al. (2019). Deconstructing compassionate conservation. *Conservation Biology* 33 (4): 760–768.

Inglehart, R.F. (1997). *Modernization and Postmodernization*. Princeton, USA: Princeton University Press.

Johnson, P.J., Adams, V.M., Armstrong, D.P. et al. (2019). Consequences matter: compassion in conservation means caring for individuals, populations and species. *Animals* 9 (12): 1115.

Kareiva, P., Lalasz, R. and Marvier, M. (2012). *A New Conservation Ethics for the 21st Century*. www.triplepundit.com/story/2012/new-conservation-ethic-21st-century/67946

Le Billon, P. and Lujala, P. (2020). Environmental and land defenders: global patterns and determinants of repression. *Global Environmental Change* 65: 102163.

Lombard, A.T., Johnson, C.F., Cowling, R.M., and Pressey, R.L. (2001). Protecting plants from elephants: botanical reserve scenarios within the Addo Elephant National Park, South Africa. *Biological Conservation* 102 (2): 191–203.

Manfredo, M.J., Teel, T.L., Don Carlos, A.W. et al. (2020). The changing sociocultural context of wildlife conservation. *Conservation Biology* 34 (6): 1549–1559.

Marris, E. (2008). Africa conservation: making room. *Nature* 448 (7156): 860–863.

Minteer, B.A. and Miller, T.R. (2011). The new conservation debate: ethical foundations, strategic trade-offs, and policy opportunities. *Biological Conservation* 144 (3): 945–947.

Nadasdy, P. (2007). The gift in the animal: the ontology of hunting and human-animal sociality. *American Ethnologist* 34 (1): 25–43.

Oommen, M.A., Cooney, R., Ramesh, M. et al. (2019). The fatal flaws of compassionate conservation. *Conservation Biology* 33 (4): 784–787.

Pascual, U., Adams, W.M., Díaz, S. et al. (2021). Biodiversity and the challenge of pluralism. *Nature Sustainability* 4 (7): 567–572.

Pierotti, R. and Wildcat, D. (2000). Traditional ecological knowledge: the third alternative (commentary). *Ecological Applications* 10 (5): 1333–1340.

Schlosberg, D. (2004). Reconceiving environmental justice: global movements and political theories. *Environmental Politics* 13 (3): 517–540.

Schuster, R., Germain, R.R., Bennett, J.R. et al. (2019). Vertebrate biodiversity on indigenous-managed lands in Australia, Brazil, and Canada equals that in protected areas. *Environmental Science & Policy* 101: 1–6.

Skotnes-Brown, J. (2021). Domestication, degeneration, and the establishment of the Addo Elephant National Park in South Africa, 1910s–1930s. *Historical Journal* 64 (2): 357–383.

Soulé, M. (2013). The "new conservation". *Conservation Biology* 27 (5): 895–897.

South Africa National Parks (n.d.). Addo Elephant National Park. www.sanparks.org/parks/addo

Stephen, C., Wittrock, J., and Wade, J. (2018). Using a harm reduction approach in an environmental case study of fish and wildlife health. *EcoHealth* 15 (1): 4–7.

Tambling, C.J., Minnie, L., Adendorff, J., and Kerley, G.I.H. (2013). Elephants facilitate impact of large predators on small ungulate prey species. *Basic Applied Ecology* 14: 694–701.

Taylor, D. (2014). The State of Diversity in Environmental Organizations. http://orgs.law.harvard.edu/els/files/2014/02/FullReport_Green2.0_FINALReducedSize.pdf

Tomaselli, M., Kutz, S., Gerlach, C., and Checkley, S. (2018). Local knowledge to enhance wildlife population health surveillance: conserving muskoxen and caribou in the Canadian Arctic. *Biological Conservation* 217: 337–348.

UN Environment Programme (UNEP) (2020). Indigenous Peoples and the Nature they Protect. www.unep.org/news-and-stories/story/Indigenous-peoples-and-nature-they-protect

Wallach, A.D., Bekoff, M., Batavia, C. et al. (2018). Summoning compassion to address the challenges of conservation. *Conservation Biology* 32 (6): 1255–1265.

Whyte, K.P. (2011). The recognition dimensions of environmental justice in Indian country. *Environmental Justice* 4 (4): 199–205.

Whyte, K.P. (2013). On the role of traditional ecological knowledge as a collaborative concept: a philosophical study. *Ecological Processes* 2 (1): 1–12.

Whyte, K.P. (2018). What do indigenous knowledges do for indigenous people? In: *Traditional Ecological Knowledge: Learning from Indigenous Practices of Environmental Sustainability* (ed. M. Nelson and D. Shilling), 57–84. Cambridge, UK: Cambridge University Press.

Zhang, L. and Yin, F. (2014). Wildlife consumption and conservation awareness in China: a long way to go. *Biodiversity and Conservation* 23: 2371–2381.

Moral Disagreement about Wildlife

9

9.1 Introduction

In the first half of this book, we've identified several ways of valuing and disvaluing wildlife. Wild animals can be appreciated as constituents of an important ecosystem, as dimensions of biodiversity, and as subjects of welfare; they can be disvalued as pests, as physical threats, and as disease vectors. We've also mapped out moral theories and conservation models that offer different rankings of these values. With all this complexity on the table, two challenges emerge. First, individuals need to make up their own minds about some of these issues. Second, diverse groups need tools to navigate disagreements about values, theories, and frameworks that inform wildlife management and conservation decisions.

Moral disagreement can be about moral judgments in *specific* cases, such as whether it's acceptable to kill seals in a particular place if they're perceived to have a negative impact on salmon stocks; alternatively, it can be about general moral issues such as whether lethal wildlife control is permissible as such. Making progress on such disagreements is an important step toward resolving conflicts, or at least lessening their severity. This chapter introduces some ways of approaching ethical decision making

Wildlife Ethics: The Ethics of Wildlife Management and Conservation, First Edition. Clare Palmer, Bob Fischer, Christian Gamborg, Jordan Hampton, and Peter Sandøe.

and dealing with moral disagreement. We consider how individuals might think through specific issues to make up their own minds. We then turn to the even more complex task of justifying decisions to others and making collective decisions sensitive to diverse ethical views. We'll begin with the contentious case of recreational hunting.

9.2 Moral Disagreement: Recreational Hunting

People hunt for many reasons, including subsistence, to manage animals regarded as "pests" (as discussed in Chapter 7), and for recreation. Recreational, or sport, hunting may provide game that's eaten or sold by the hunters; it may have the effect of reducing numbers of animals regarded as pests (such as red foxes in Australia) or hyperabundant native animals (such as white-tailed deer in the US) (Chapter 11). However, recreational hunters don't *depend* on hunting for subsistence, nor are they primarily concerned to manage wildlife. Instead, recreational hunters enjoy hunting in itself. They value the skills and challenges involved, they enjoy the time outdoors, and they often view hunting as part of their own, their families', or their culture's identity, especially in more rural areas. In some cases, they also seek a trophy – for example, a set of antlers or a picture of themselves with the animal they've killed.

However, recreational hunting also generates ongoing controversies; consider, for instance, trophy hunting in southern Africa (Figure 9.1), bear hunts in the US state of Colorado, gamebirds released for hunting in Europe, and the use of dogs to hunt wild

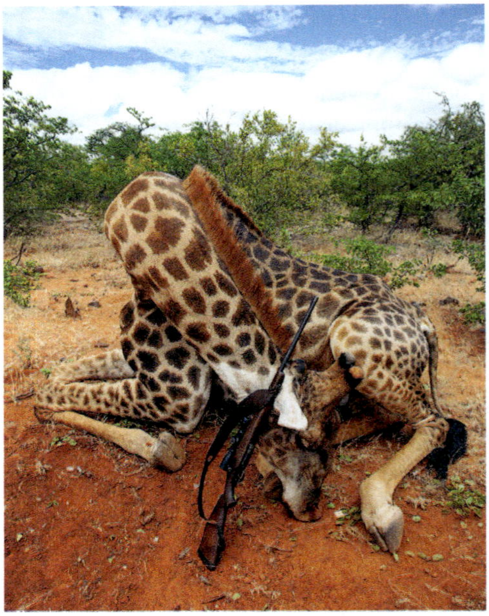

Figure 9.1 An African giraffe killed by a hunter during a licensed trophy hunt in South Africa. *Source:* Okyela/Shutterstock.com.

pigs in Australia. Critics raise concerns about the welfare of the hunted animals, the nontarget wildlife species that may be affected, the animals used in hunting, such as dogs, and they challenge the idea that recreation is an adequate justification for taking animals' lives. Moreover, critics who aren't generally opposed to recreational hunting may still object to some forms of it.

The use of nonnative and farm-reared gamebirds, for instance, can raise serious *conservation* issues. In the UK, significant tracts of land are controversially managed by fire for gamebirds, mainly red grouse habitat, which can have impacts on nonavian wildlife species. There have also been instances where protected predators, especially birds of prey, have been illegally killed to reduce predation on gamebirds. There are also persistent controversies about whether trophy hunting contributes to, or detracts from, the abundance of the species being hunted, especially in southern Africa.

Some people also object to particular *ways* of hunting, such as gamebirds being made easily available for shooting or "canned" hunts where exotic animals are contained in high-fenced areas (Feber et al. 2020). Here, the concern is that such hunts violate the ethic of fair chase, according to which animals should be given a reasonable chance of escaping hunters, discussed in a well-known paper by Posewitz (1994). Indeed, some extend this objection even further. A keen hunter himself (Figure 3.2), Leopold (1949, p. 285) noted that "very intensive management of game or fish lowers the unit value of the trophy by artificializing it."

Hunters, of course, often reply by emphasizing the social and cultural reasons already given for hunting, as well as its ostensible instrumental benefits: food, pest control, significant economic benefits, and, in some locales, substantial funds for conservation, whether through the purchase of hunting licenses and taxes on hunting equipment or (more controversially) through hunting safaris and other kinds of hunting tourism (Feber et al. 2020). In any event, our aim here is not to settle the disputes between recreational hunters and their critics. Rather, it's to consider how these disputes can be approached thoughtfully.

In part, how to tackle such conflicts depends on whether the focus is on *individual* moral decision making (for instance, where individuals are torn between different values) or *collective* decision making. And, of course, there are various collective levels. There are community councils and municipalities that have to decide how to deal with animals that are seen as nuisances by some community members. There are federal or state agencies that must decide whether – and if so, how – to control undesired introduced species or hyperabundant native species, and how far to protect traditional hunting freedoms. There are politicians drafting national legislation to compensate farmers for livestock losses due to wildlife attacks. Additionally, collective decisions are made at the international level, including treaties, such as the Bern Convention on the Conservation of European Wildlife and Natural Habitats, managed by the Council of Europe, and the Habitats Directive, which is the EU's legal instrument for wildlife conservation.

At every collective level, the issue of navigating moral disagreement is made more complex by differences in the *relationships* between decision makers and stakeholders. It's one thing, for instance, to address moral disagreements between members of a decision-making body and a nongovernmental organization (NGO) that has been hired as a consultant; it's quite another to address moral disagreements between members of a decision-making body and the participants in a grassroots social media campaign. So, we can only sketch some general considerations here in the hope that they can be adapted to the specific needs of particular contexts. We also refer the reader to the massive literature in the field of addressing wildlife-related conflicts (e.g., Redpath et al. 2015), much of which is based on the assumption that while such conflicts will never cease to exist, they can be productively managed (Clarke and Peterson 2015).

Before considering these *collective* challenges, though, let's think through *individual* decision making.

9.3 The Individual's Perspective: Making Up One's Mind

As individuals, we may feel the pull of different values, different conservation and management paradigms, and different ethical theories. Suppose, for instance, that we value animal welfare intrinsically. However, we may also think that hunting traditions are important; that firearms cause less pain than predation and parasitism; and that while being hunted is stressful for animals, it's stress that they'd experience regardless (i.e., if not due to human predators, then due to nonhuman ones). If we're drawn to utilitarianism, then we may conclude that there's nothing wrong with recreational hunting per se. But suppose we're also drawn to the principle that we shouldn't cause pain unnecessarily. Since killing is almost never completely painless and since recreational hunting involves causing pain unnecessarily (by definition, no one *needs* to do it to survive), this principle indicates that recreational hunting is indeed objectionable. What to do?

A traditional and widely accepted answer is that individuals should begin working toward *reflective equilibrium*, a goal made famous by John Rawls. See Daniels (2016) for an accessible presentation of the theory; see Haslett (1987) for criticisms. We offer a simple model of reflective equilibrium in Figure 9.2.

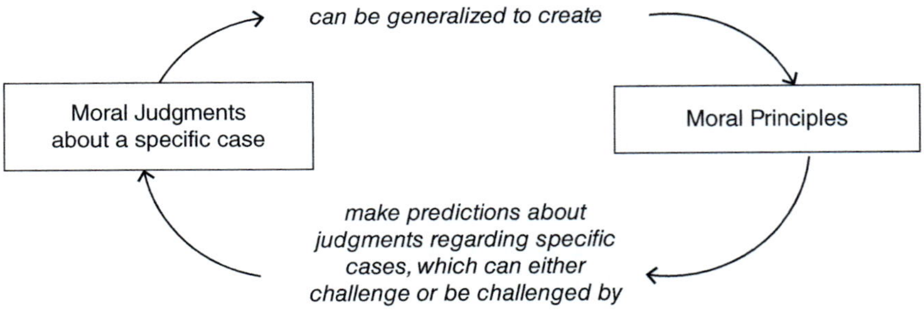

Figure 9.2 A simple version of the model for moral thinking called reflective equilibrium. According to the model, we should go back and forth between particular judgments and principles, trying to improve the overall coherence of our moral outlook. Figuratively, this could be seen as reducing the "distance" between the boxes representing judgments and principles. Though they may never completely overlap – which would represent perfect consistency – the number and severity of the tensions can probably be reduced.

The basic idea here is that we should try to make our moral views more consistent. The method for doing this involves starting with either our moral judgments about particular cases (e.g., "it's wrong to confine lions in a small space for canned hunting") or moral principles that apply generally (e.g., "it's morally good to alleviate suffering"). If, for instance, we start with moral judgments, then it might be possible to generalize to get moral principles. (If it's wrong to confine lions in a small space for canned hunting, it's probably wrong to confine *any* animal in a small space for canned hunting. Or to generalize further, perhaps canned hunting is *always* wrong, even if the fenced area is large.) Then, those moral principles can be applied to new cases to assess their implications. If a principle's implications fit with our intuitive moral judgments, that provides some reason to hang on to the principle; if it doesn't, then we need to decide whether the intuitive moral judgment or the principle is more plausible. If the intuitive moral judgment is more plausible, then the principle should be revised or rejected; if the principle is more plausible, then the moral judgment should be revised or rejected.

The process is roughly the same if we begin with moral principles, though without the step of generalizing from particular moral judgments. Either way, we go back and forth between particular judgments and principles, trying to improve the overall coherence of our moral outlook. Figuratively, this could be seen as reducing the "distance" between the boxes representing judgments and principles in Figure 9.2. Though they may never completely overlap – representing perfect consistency – the number and severity of the tensions can probably be reduced.

This process involves scrutinizing all our values carefully. We might conclude that while we thought we valued getting a trophy over the ideal of so-called fair chase, we don't in fact. Likewise, we might have thought that we were opposed to causing unnecessary harm, but given our attachment to recreational hunting, we realize that we don't accept that principle in its fully general form. Instead, we find that we're willing to cause unnecessary harms to animals under certain conditions, such as giving an animal a decent chance of eluding us.

Alternatively, we might conclude that we were wrong about *how* we value something. For example, we may discover that while we thought we cared about biodiversity intrinsically, we only value it instrumentally – say, insofar as it promotes wildness. When biodiversity conflicts with wildness – as it does in cases where it's possible to save species by breeding animals for canned hunts – we don't think that biodiversity deserves much consideration at all.

Achieving reflective equilibrium also involves coming to terms with the implications of various moral theories. Utilitarianism, for instance, allows the sacrifice of some individuals' rights to pursue the common good. This might lead us to abandon the theory in favor of an alternative. Or it might lead us to refine the theory, moving toward the "two-level" utilitarianism mentioned in Chapter 6. In any case, the hope is that as individuals refine their values and their judgments about cases, they also come to better understand what their moral theory needs to explain. Likewise, as people consider and refine their respective moral theories, they move toward more consistent and systematic understandings of their moral responsibilities.

Unsurprisingly, this is a lengthy process. It takes time to consider all the arguments for and against particular moral theories, not to mention all the ways in which these theories might be modified in response to criticisms or improved in light of relevant knowledge from biology, psychology, sociology, economics, and so forth. So, we may never reach a perfectly consistent moral outlook; we may never find decision procedures to guide every action. Still, we can reduce the arbitrariness in our moral outlook, we can make it more consistent, and we can increase both its explanatory power and usefulness. This may also help when it comes to understanding and appreciating the moral views of others. When we realize how hard it is to make up our own minds, we may better understand why others reach different conclusions.

The upshot is that we can move closer to the ideal of being able to give clear and consistent rationales for our views about particular practices and policies. As the remainder of this chapter explains, though, reflective equilibrium may be less useful when whole communities and societies need to deliberate. Let's now turn to the challenges of collective decision making.

9.4 Collective Decision Making

In collective decision making, stakeholders make decisions in a participatory or nonparticipatory way. *Stakeholders* are persons or organizations with an interest in or concern about the issue being decided. There are narrower and broader groups of stakeholders, ranging from those with a material interest in the outcome of a decision (in the case of recreational hunting, that might mean hunters and landowners) to those with nonmaterial interests (such as animal welfare or rights organizations and members of the broader public, all of whom may be concerned about hunting for one reason or another). Decisions are *participatory* where stakeholders are consulted or involved in decision making; they're *nonparticipatory* when a government or an agency makes a decision alone. We're particularly interested here in *participatory* approaches, given that they often create contexts where disagreements about wildlife are most visible.

Regardless of how decisions are made, there are almost always disparities in power: governments and agencies often have a disproportionate influence on outcomes (Redpath et al. 2013). In addition, members of certain groups – such as scientists, landowners, nature protection NGOs, and corporations – can also be particularly influential. These power differentials can raise the concern that those with less power are being marginalized, that their inclusion in decision making is just to placate them or to legitimize the outcome to the general public. If more powerful parties don't take steps to address these concerns, deliberative processes are unlikely to alleviate conflict or reach politically stable decisions.

As we noted at the beginning of the chapter, decision-making collectives operate at different levels and within different legal frameworks. In some countries, formal stakeholder consultation processes are required to pass laws and other types of wildlife-related regulation (to ensure a just and fair decision-making process). In others, deliberations are far less participatory or not participatory at all – at least officially. After all, in many countries and at many decision-making levels, lobbying and advocacy (and in some cases, bribery) play huge roles in policy processes.

Nevertheless, larger (and diverse) groups of stakeholders and the public are often brought together to work out disagreements. This isn't an easy task. First, stakeholder meetings don't just happen; someone has to bring the interested parties and stakeholders together. This is often the mandate of local, regional, or national governments or organizations commissioned by those governments. Second, in terms of achieving inclusiveness and procedural justice (see Chapter 8), a wide variety of stakeholders must be brought into the conversation. A thorough process would also locate "hidden stakeholders" – groups that may be dependent on wildlife but who wouldn't normally be consulted (perhaps because they are on the fringes of or even outside the law, such as local poachers and squatters) (Vogler et al. 2017).

Once these groups have been gathered, participants face the complex task of trying to *understand* their disagreements – a prerequisite for actually resolving them. Unfortunately, disagreements concerning wildlife management and conservation can be difficult to disentangle. Are they "really" differences regarding *values* and how to prioritize them? Or are they competing *interests*, not so much driven by moral concerns as by aversion to personal losses or desire for personal gain? From a tactical point of view, it can be a good rhetorical trick to "upgrade" an interest to a value. That is, one way to "hide" a personal interest is to frame it as a value, signaling that others ought to care about the issue too.

Differences may also be about *empirical* questions rather than about values, regarding, say, the most likely implications of two different policy options. For example, based on one ecological study, members of a group might think that a population of wolves is likely to grow if a particular hunting or conservation policy is implemented; others might think, based on a different study, that the population is likely to decline. In principle, empirical disagreements could be resolved by sorting through the relevant evidence. But reaching agreement even about empirical matters can be extremely difficult, often reaching an impasse mired in further disagreements about whom to trust. Traditional ecological knowledge or local landowner perceptions of a situation, such as the relative abundance or scarcity of a species in a particular area, may be at odds with the data produced by scientists, for example in the harvest of dugongs in the Torres Strait between northern Australia and New Guinea (Butler et al. 2012). In addition, people's views about how things *ought* to be can affect their judgments about how things *are* or *will be*. This bias can affect what people take to be relevant facts or appropriate evidence. So, even where disagreements are empirical, values are often lurking in the background.

Having said all this, a great deal of collective decision making is based on the assumption that there is *reasonable* disagreement among many parties to the conversation. That is, while some views may simply be dismissed out of hand, the assumption is that the main stakeholders have views that can't simply be set aside as "crazy" or otherwise irrelevant to decision making; the premise of the discussion is that those taking part have the kinds of views that deserve some consideration.

Finally, there is the question of what, exactly, decision making aims to achieve. Typically, collective decision making strives for some degree of consensus. However, there's not always agreement about the amount or kind of consensus that's desirable and/or feasible (Sidaway 2005). Below, we'll consider different approaches to try to deal with moral disagreements. First, we consider attempts either to reach full agreement or to agree to accept a compromise about a particular wildlife management question. Second, we look at pure procedural approaches, where the agreement concerns only fair ways to reach decisions and the fair treatment of special interest groups.

9.4.1 Full Agreement and *Modus Vivendi*

Ideally, people would work toward full and genuine agreement about the values, ethical convictions, and empirical facts that are relevant to a given decision. This might occur via a collective version of the reflective equilibrium process that we described earlier. Groups of individuals would get together and deliberate about a wildlife management or conservation issue, eventually agreeing on the best set of moral commitments to have – whether that happens to be one already represented in the group or a novel alternative. In some cases, it could turn out that people share the same values but prioritize them differently, perhaps due to being differently located with respect to the issue at hand. For instance, a farmer in Brazil losing livestock to jaguar predation might have different priorities compared to a foreign conservationist interested in protecting jaguars (Marchini and Macdonald 2018). If that's right, then they could work out a fair policy that's sensitive to their identities and histories. As we describe this ideal, however, striving for a full agreement process is invariably very time-consuming. In any case, it's unlikely to produce the desired consensus when people are entrenched in their views. Some question the wisdom of even trying, as the failure might legitimize current power relationships (Peterson et al. 2005).

Let's assume, then, that in a diverse society, there won't be full agreement at the level of values and ethical theories. Still, agreement might be achieved about *some* values, practical questions, and policies. The aspiration here is for a *modus vivendi*, or an arrangement where all parties agree that they ought to get along by acting in a particular way or adopting a particular policy. Ideally, a *modus vivendi* involves a kind of minimal consensus: people agree about what to do or what policy to set, though they may disagree about why that action or policy is the right one. For instance, there may be cases where animal welfare organizations and ecocentric-inclined conservationists can agree that white-tailed deer should be culled during a hard winter (see Chapter 11), though they justify the decision in very different ways. For animal welfare organizations, it may be understood as a case of mercy killing, akin to euthanasia, to prevent suffering due to starvation. For conservationists, by contrast, it may be about protecting native flora from rapidly growing deer populations.

Unfortunately, however, even a minimal consensus can't always be achieved. The details of the situation need to be just right, and the values of the various stakeholders just right, to produce practical agreement despite disagreement about underlying reasons. However, there are other forms that a *modus vivendi* can take, such as brokering a *compromise*. Compromise is about finding some sort of middle ground between competing viewpoints, which typically involves the various parties making concessions, giving up part of what they want. The various stakeholders may not believe that the agreed-upon solution is the best one, but the hope is that they will think that this solution is the best available at the time, given competing values and interests.

Let's return to recreational hunting. At least three groups – hunters, conservationists, and those concerned about the animals as individuals – have deeply held values about wildlife and hunting (there may be some overlap between the groups; hunters might also be conservationists, of course). It's difficult to get these groups in the same room for a discussion. However, some countries have set up fora where representatives can have a structured dialogue. There are different models but Denmark offers a well-functioning example (Jensen et al. 2011). There, a governmental advisory council includes nine of the major hunting and wildlife management-related stakeholder groups, including a hunters' association, farmers' and forestry organizations, animal protection groups, and environmental NGOs. This council is key to brokering compromises on wildlife-related issues. However, a politically defined premise for the discussion is that some forms of hunting are acceptable. Such a premise obviously makes compromises easier to reach. Nevertheless, the council is open to critical input on hunting practices and regulations, albeit in terms that are, in principle, compatible with hunting. So, while some stakeholders are effectively excluded from making the arguments they would prefer to make, they are not excluded from the conversation entirely. If they can find other ways to argue for more restrictive hunting regulations – say, on the basis of animal welfare, public safety, or environmental considerations – hunters would have no right to ignore them and would instead have to address their concerns.

Another strategy for achieving a *modus vivendi* is *deliberative democracy*, the proponents of which claim that sincere, reasonable dialogue is necessary for legitimate decision making. Many advocates for this view see it as being especially important that such dialogue occurs among ordinary citizens in groups sometimes called "deliberative mini-publics." The aim is to encourage public-spirited perspectives on relevant issues, promote mutually respectful decision making, and help correct previous decision mistakes (Gutmann and Thompson 2009).

Methods of deliberative democracy are plentiful. They include *citizen juries*, which gather representative groups of citizens to consider expert testimony, deliberate about its implications together, and ultimately make a joint recommendation; *twenty-first century town meetings*, which can include thousands of people (albeit broken into groups of 10–12) engaging in structured online conversations; *citizens' councils*, designed to operate alongside elected chambers (a model recently adopted in Belgium); and *deliberative community forums*, where participants have an opportunity to develop more reflective opinions about issues after learning the relevant facts, hearing a range of perspectives from experts and peers, and having opportunities to discuss all this information in small groups (Gastil and Levine 2005). For example, citizen juries were used to achieve wide agreement on how to protect the Cienega Corridor lands in Arizona in the US. These lands are important movement corridors for "Sky Island" mountain mammals, especially black bears, mountain lions, coatis, and mule deer (Hanson and Brott 2005).

Many of these methods of deliberative democracy have mainly been applied in western countries or countries with similar political systems and political cultures. In many other countries, different educational or cultural foundations and mixed literacy rates may make the methods just mentioned more challenging (Maynard and Jacobson 2017). Here, other approaches such as the nominal group technique – using ranking cards with different colors, sizes, and symbols, as used in five conservancies in Maasai group ranches in the Rift Valley of Kenya – may be a better option (Maynard and Jacobson 2017).

9.5 Procedural Approaches

None of the methods, however, is guaranteed to produce consensus, as deliberation cannot make incompatible views compatible. In many circumstances, it's effectively impossible to achieve even a minimal consensus or a compromise between stakeholders.

In democratic societies, however, there's a standard method for dealing with such cases: namely, to shift the goal. Instead of trying to achieve consensus about the merits of the decision, people can try to achieve consensus about the legitimacy of the decision-making *process*.

The proceduralist tradition claims that democracy is a *decision procedure* whose goal is to ensure a fair distribution of political power. In principle, there are few limits regarding what a majority can legitimately decide by using the agreed-upon procedures. In cases of moral disagreement, a majority can legitimately dominate a minority. Procedural approaches only require agreement about a fair way of adjudicating disputes; they don't require agreement that the result of the process is the correct one, except in the sense that the parties should agree it was produced via a fair process. The insistence that this process should be fair reveals that even procedural approaches involve certain value commitments; they just happen to be minimal relative to the alternatives considered. It's expected that at the end of the process, at least some of the parties to the dispute will be left with substantive objections to the course of action that's chosen.

9.5.1 Majority Rule

The simplest kind of procedural approach is a familiar one: voting. Modern western-style democracies mainly function as some type of representative democracy; citizens vote for representatives who then make decisions on their behalf. There are also examples of more "direct" democracy where citizens vote directly for certain decisions (e.g., whether to leave an economic and political union). The number of referenda may vary and so may the types of issue put up for direct vote. In some places, such as Switzerland, ordinary citizens vote directly about the kinds of issues addressed here. Voting is not trying to reach consensus about which policy is best, nor is it trying to achieve consensus about values and moral principles. Rather, it requires agreement about one relatively modest point: namely, that in this context, it's fair to settle the question by casting ballots.

Voting is normally premised on the idea that everyone's vote counts equally and that (by whatever electoral system is selected) the majority rules. A distinction is often made, however, between the responses of the less affected "general public" and "relevant communities" who will actually feel the effects of a decision. This leads to the ethical question whether it's fair for the members of these groups to have votes that count the same as anyone else's. Should they get more say?

9.5.2 Fair Treatment of Special Interest Groups

People aren't affected equally by conservation and wildlife management policies. Some people are benefitted, while others stand to be made significantly worse off, including people in communities that are already poor and marginalized. This can happen when, for conservation purposes, some people are excluded from lands they have traditionally used for hunting and gathering (as discussed in Chapters 8 and 13). Such concerns are especially salient in the context of Indigenous or traditional communities that have had communal ownership of land for generations; these concerns are amplified further by past injustices.

To navigate these disproportional impacts, there's increasing interest in a procedural approach called FPIC: free, prior, and informed consent. (This is also used as a principle

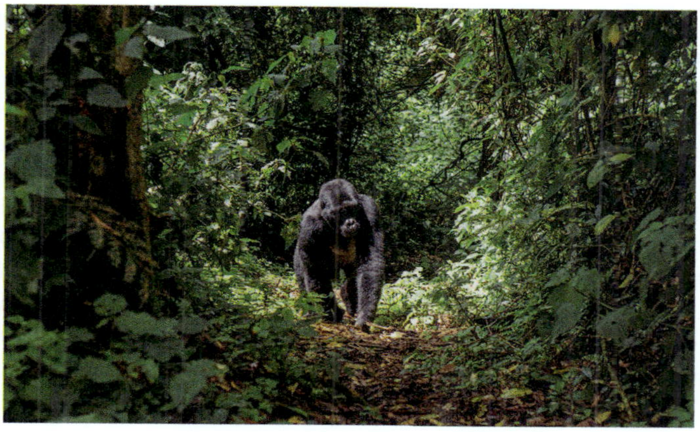

Figure 9.3 A mountain gorilla in Bwindi National Park, Uganda. The Batwa People were evicted from the area in 1994 to prioritize the flourishing of the gorillas. *Source:* Andrey Gudkov/ Dreamstime LLC.

guiding the involvement of individual participants in scientific research.) Historically, Indigenous peoples have been excluded from decision-making processes affecting them, such as the 1994 Ugandan eviction of the Batwa People from an area that was turned into Bwindi National Park. This decision gave priority to protecting half of the world's population of mountain gorillas (Figure 9.3) over the land use traditions of local Indigenous peoples (Ampumuza et al. 2020).

According to the United Nations Permanent Forum on Indigenous Issues, when development proposals are made for Indigenous lands, Indigenous communities must be consulted in good faith and not coerced or manipulated. They must be given time to find out what's being proposed and to review all relevant factors, they must be provided with all the necessary information to understand all the impacts of the proposal, and consent must be given by legitimate representatives (Macdonald and Zezulka 2015). Thus, FPIC is a process that implies an ongoing set of discussions, consultations, meetings, and agreements in which relevant issues may be revisited. Essentially, this may give Indigenous peoples a veto over proposals (such as development proposals) that relate specifically to land to which they have title. This right to veto is built on the UN Declaration of the Rights of Indigenous People, which emphasizes both the historical injustices suffered by Indigenous peoples and the need to protect their rights – especially their land rights.

From some ethical perspectives, concerns about procedural justice stretch to include certain *nonhumans*, especially sentient animals. Standard decision-making procedures identify only *humans* as the relevant community or group of stakeholders, no matter how much is at stake for wild animals. Wild animals have no representation at all in decisions about their own environments. This concern has led to arguments that particular nonhuman beings or things – including wild animals, rivers, and mountains – should be permitted to bring legal actions to enforce their own protection; that is, to have standing in the courts, an argument made famously in the book *Should Trees Have Standing?* (Stone 1972). Recent legal cases in the US and India have argued that individual wild animals, including captive chimpanzees and elephants, should be seen as legal persons or entities with rights (although only a few of these cases have been successful; Staker 2017). More generally, there's debate about the idea that nature *as such* has legal personhood and rights. This sometimes takes the form of a critique of the anthropocentrism of current legal systems or, more pragmatically, some argue that nature has rights because human wellbeing depends on "healthy" ecosystems. Ecuador first included the rights of nature in its 2008 constitution (Republic of Ecuador 2008). At the time of writing, rights of nature laws exist in 17 countries (many in South America), while a number of municipalities and states – in the US, New Zealand, and elsewhere – have attributed legal rights to particular natural features (Staker 2017).

9.6 Achieving Justice

These considerations about fairness in terms of procedure highlight a need to distinguish between *procedural* justice and *substantive* justice. Procedural justice is achieved when decisions are made using fair procedures that were agreed on by relevant stakeholders in an appropriate way. Substantive justice, however, is achieved when the outcome reflects whatever justice – as interpreted by different theories – actually demands. There's no guarantee that fair procedures will deliver substantive justice, as legal examples make plain. Consider a case where a trial goes just as it should, but due to some technicality, a guilty person isn't convicted. Procedural justice was achieved; substantive justice wasn't. Equally, stakeholders could agree using perfectly fair procedures to pursue some policy that's seriously unjust in terms of its outcomes. While including multiple stakeholders with diverse values may make such outcomes less likely, it doesn't rule them out.

Ideally, resolving conflicts would involve procedural justice delivering substantive justice. In some cases, as we've noted, concerns about substantive justice may form the basis for giving some groups, such as Indigenous communities, special status in making particular kinds of decisions. In other cases, views about substantive justice or other conservation values can be built into the decision-making procedure, thereby blocking certain outcomes in advance. For example, in a case discussed by Vucetich et al. (2018), the US Fish and Wildlife Service developed a mediated process including many stakeholders to create a recovery plan for Mexican wolves. To join this process, stakeholders had to accept that recovery would happen; what was up for debate was how it should be done.

Obviously, it's difficult to decide when substantive justice concerns should restrict what options or outcomes are on the table or when some groups should have special status or be represented in decision-making procedures. And further complications may be raised where significant conservation, nonhuman, and human justice issues are in conflict, forcing decision-making constraints and/or considerations about special status in opposite directions. While these issues can't be resolved here, ethical decision making ought to take these concerns into account (see Chapter 13).

9.7 Conclusion

While procedural approaches are available as fallbacks for handling moral disagreement, it's usually best to employ deliberative methods. Deliberative methods help people to understand views with which they agree, to recognize the merits of those views, and to better understand (and perhaps refine or change) their own moral commitments. Accordingly, these methods can, when employed well, move people toward otherwise unlikely compromises and partnerships. Practically speaking, results from public participation in wildlife management in the US suggest that quality stakeholder involvement processes are those that use scientific information, have genuine influence on decisions, treat citizens fairly, and promote informative communication and learning (Chase et al. 2004).

As we noted in the beginning of the chapter, many disagreements about wildlife are proxies for deeper social conflicts. Accordingly, there's a growing discipline that studies how to deal with such conflicts (Maser and de Silva 2019). For instance, conflicts between ranchers and environmentalists over predators concern deep issues of identity, not covered just by measuring the economic losses of livestock predation from wolves. Moreover, there might be skewed or directly undemocratic political systems that give rise to conflicts (some of which are violent), activism, protest, and civil disobedience (again, see Chapter 13). This is a major barrier to stable, long-term solutions, causing people to see one another as adversaries and making conflicts appear intractable (Lewicki et al. 2003). In situations like these, better understanding and compromise, rather than reconciliation, may be the best one can hope to achieve. Mediation can encourage mutual understanding, relationship building and collaboration, trying to transform the disagreement into a shared – and addressable – problem (Madden and McQuinn 2014). In this way, community building can, in time, help to navigate moral disagreements.

In public debate, it's often most important to be transparent, clearly providing the evidence for a conclusion and the justifications for holding particular positions. Transparency is itself a method of inclusivity: it ensures that anyone can engage in the deliberative process, as there's no question about why an individual or organization takes a particular view and what it would take to get them to change their position. Transparency is also crucial in terms of public accountability, providing a common ground of claims and evidence that people can draw on, test, and challenge. In Part 2 of this book, we'll try to model that transparency, making it as clear as possible how people might think through the ethical issues in particular cases.

References

Ampumuza, C., Duineveld, M., and van der Duim, R. (2020). The most marginalized people in Uganda? Alternative realities of Batwa at Bwindi impenetrable National Park. *World Development Perspectives* 20: 100267.

Butler, J.R., Tawake, A., Skewes, T. et al. (2012). Integrating traditional ecological knowledge and fisheries management in the Torres Strait, Australia: the catalytic role of turtles and dugong as cultural keystone species. *Ecology and Society* 17 (4): 34.

Chase, L.C., Decker, D.J., and Lauber, T.B. (2004). Public participation in wildlife management: what do stakeholders want? *Society and Natural Resources* 17 (7): 629–639.

Clarke, T. and Peterson, T.R. (2015). *Environmental Conflict Management*. Thousand Oaks, USA: Sage Publications.

Daniels, N. (2016). *Reflective Equilibrium. The Stanford Encyclopedia of Philosophy*. Stanford, USA: Stanford University.

Feber, R.E., Johnson, P.J., and Macdonald, D.W. (2020). Shooting pheasants for sport: what does the death of Cecil tell us? *People and Nature* 2 (1): 82–95.

Gastil, J. and Levine, P. (2005). *The Deliberative Democracy Handbook: Strategies for Effective Civic Engagement in the Twenty-First Century*. San Francisco, USA: Jossey-Bass.

Gutmann, A. and Thompson, D.F. (2009). *Why Deliberative Democracy?* Princeton, USA: Princeton University Press.

Hanson, R. and Brott, E. (2005). Citizens' council protecting Sky Island wildlife corridor. In: *Connecting Mountain Islands and Desert Seas: Biodiversity and Management of the Madrean Archipelago* (ed. G.J. Gottfried, B.S. Gebow, L.G. Eskew, and C.B. Edminster), 327–329. Fort Collins, USA: US Department of Agriculture.

Haslett, D.W. (1987). What is wrong with reflective equilibria? *Philosophical Quarterly* 37 (148): 305–311.

Jensen, K.K., Gamborg, C., and Sandøe, P. (2011). The social dimension of pluralism: democratic procedures and substantial constraints. *Ethics, Policy and Environment* 14 (3): 313–327.

Leopold, A. (1949). *A Sand County Almanac*. Oxford, UK: Oxford University Press.

Lewicki, R., Gray, B., and Elliott, M. (ed.) (2003). *Making Sense of Intractable Environmental Conflicts: Concepts and Cases*. Washington, D.C., USA: Island Press.

MacDonald, G. and Zezulka, G. (2015). *Understanding Successful Approaches to Free, Prior and Informed Consent in Canada. Part I*. http://borealcouncil.ca/wp-content/uploads/2015/09/BLC_FPIC_Successes_Report_Sept_2015_E.pdf

Madden, F. and McQuinn, B. (2014). Conservation's blind spot: the case for conflict transformation in wildlife conservation. *Biological Conservation* 178: 97–106.

Marchini, S. and Macdonald, D.W. (2018). Mind over matter: perceptions behind the impact of jaguars on human livelihoods. *Biological Conservation* 224: 230–237.

Maser, C. and de Silva, L. (2019). *Resolving Environmental Conflicts: Principles and Concepts*. Boca Raton, USA: CRC Press.

Maynard, L. and Jacobson, S.K. (2017). Stakeholder participation in wildlife management: adapting the nominal group technique in developing countries for participants with low literacy. *Human Dimensions of Wildlife* 22 (1): 71–82.

Peterson, M.N., Peterson, M.J., and Peterson, T.R. (2005). Conservation and the myth of consensus. *Conservation Biology* 19 (3): 762–767.

Posewitz, J. (1994). *Beyond Fair Chase: The Ethic and Tradition of Hunting*. Helena, USA: Falcon Press.

Redpath, S.M., Young, J., Evely, A. et al. (2013). Understanding and managing conservation conflicts. *Trends in Ecology and Evolution* 28 (2): 100–109.

Redpath, S.M., Gutiérrez, R.J., Wood, K.A. et al. (2015). An introduction to conservation conflicts. In: *Conflicts in Conservation: Navigation towards Solutions* (ed. S.M. Redpath, R.J. Gutiérrez, K.A. Wood, and J.C. Young), 3–18. Cambridge, UK: Cambridge University Press.

Republic of Ecuador (2008). Constitution of the Republic of Ecuador. https://pdba.georgetown.edu/Constitutions/Ecuador/english08.html.
Sidaway, R. (2005). *Resolving Environmental Disputes: From Conflict to Consensus*. New York, USA: Routledge.
Staker, A. (2017). Should chimpanzees have standing? The case for pursuing legal personhood for non-human animals. *Transnational Environmental Law* 6 (3): 485–507.
Stone, C. (1972). *Should Trees Have Standing? Toward Legal Rights for Natural Objects*. Oxford, UK: Oxford University Press.
Vogler, D., Macey, S., and Sigouin, A. (2017). Stakeholder analysis in environmental and conservation planning. *Lessons in Conservation* 7: 5–16.
Vucetich, J., Burnham, D., Macdonald, E.A. et al. (2018). Just conservation: what is it and should we pursue it? *Biological Conservation* 221: 23–33.

PART

2

THE PRACTICE OF WILDLIFE ETHICS – CASE STUDIES

10 Conservation via Commodification: A Legal Trade in Rhino Horn?

10.1 Introduction

Despite the efforts of conservationists over several decades, Africa's rhinoceros species ("rhinos") may be headed for extinction. About 25 000 rhinos remain in Africa, including about 19 000 white rhinos in South Africa and about 5630 black rhinos across the southeastern portion of the continent. The western black rhino was declared extinct in 2011 and the world's last remaining male northern white rhino died in 2018. With the exception of products from a few trophy hunts, international trade in rhino parts became illegal in 1977 under the Convention on International Trade in Endangered Species (CITES). Nevertheless, the main driver of rhino population decline has been illegal killing (poaching) to harvest rhino horn, a valued black market product.

Many policies have been tried to prevent poaching of rhinos for their prized horns, including better fencing, drone surveillance, education campaigns, and dyeing horns (Eikelboom et al. 2020). But even policies enacted by wildlife managers that allow rangers to shoot to kill poachers have failed to stop all illegal rhino killing. The intractable combination of economic need in sub-Saharan Africa and lucrative international

Wildlife Ethics: The Ethics of Wildlife Management and Conservation, First Edition. Clare Palmer, Bob Fischer, Christian Gamborg, Jordan Hampton, and Peter Sandøe.

markets for rhino horn seems to be conspiring to mean that Africa will lose these species. What can be done? One bold, and much contested, proposal to save Africa's rhinos is to allow *legal* international trade in their horn.

Skepticism is understandable. After all, isn't the desire to purchase rhino horn what threatened the rhinos in the first place? However, the logic is that a trade ban limits supply, which raises prices and drives black market poaching. A regulated legal trade would in theory do the opposite, rapidly increasing supply, reducing prices, and reducing incentives for poaching (Biggs et al. 2013). This is a *market-based* conservation strategy.

Many critics of this approach recognize the importance of innovative methods to address the biodiversity crisis; they just question whether "the market" is the answer (Büscher et al. 2014). More specifically, in this case, there are considerable uncertainties about the level of demand for rhino horn in a legal market and whether supply would, or even could, sustainably increase to meet demand (and thereby effectively reduce poaching). There are also ethical concerns. Even if commercializing rhino horn might make economic sense, is it the right thing to be doing? What would this mean for the welfare and lives of individual rhinos? Does it raise concerns about a potential loss of the wildness of rhinos? Would a legal market create or exacerbate justice concerns between humans? And is the "commodification" of nature or individual animals itself ethically troubling?

In this chapter, we will explore these issues by taking a closer look at the proposal to use a rhino horn market to protect the rhino species.

10.2 Rhinos in Sub-Saharan Africa

Rhinos can be valued in multiple ways, both as individuals and as a species. They are often considered to be a keystone species, making important contributions to the maintenance of savanna grasslands. They are valued for their contribution to biodiversity, as the last remaining members of a clade, representing unique genetic information and manifesting unique morphological features. They are valued intrinsically, as sentient individuals. And, as we noted in Chapter 8, they are one of the Big Five species, at the heart of the southern African safari industry. However, despite their importance, it has been difficult for conservationists to stop poachers. During the nine-year period between 2008 and 2016, an estimated 7124 rhinos were poached for their horns in Africa, with most of that killing occurring in South Africa. An estimated 1054 rhinos were poached there during 2016 alone (Taylor et al. 2017).

Poaching is driven by demand for rhino horns, used in traditional medicine in China and Vietnam, for dagger handles in Yemen (Hanley et al. 2018), as well as for investment and for money laundering. It's a lucrative business. In some markets, rhino horn is worth more by weight than diamonds or cocaine. If poaching continues at a high level, or even accelerates, Africa's remaining rhino populations may become extinct in the wild around 2030 (Biggs et al. 2013).

An obvious thought is that more draconian anti-poaching measures and better judicial prosecution are needed. In countries such as Botswana, shoot-to-kill policies have been enacted against poachers, effectively rendering this form of wildlife use punishable by the death penalty – a form of "green militarization" (Lunstrum 2014). Aside from ethical worries about the extreme nature of such policies, maintaining them on the ground is very expensive. Since many of South African's rhinos (>42%) are privately owned (Chapman and White 2020), this creates immense financial burdens for private conservation projects. And even the threat of death hasn't deterred all poachers, a fact that has encouraged conservationists to question the effectiveness of CITES's ban on international rhino horn trade. (The *international* qualifier matters here, as there is already a legal domestic market in South Africa.) Given the location of the vast majority of the demand – mostly in Southeast Asia and Yemen – the international market is what matters.

10.3 Legal Trade in Wildlife

We opened this book with the impact of the pet trade on parrots in Peru (Chapter 1). It's an example of one of the most challenging ethical dilemmas in conservation – where and when should the sale of wildlife as commodities be permitted? South American parrots and African rhinos are by no means alone in this regard. Efforts to establish legal trade in wildlife have a rich history. Australia's kangaroos (Chapter 5), one of the nation's faunal emblems, for example, are shot and killed for their meat every year by the millions. To explain why some people are optimistic about the prospect of a legal rhino horn market, let's take a brief detour to consider what's often proclaimed as a conservation success story: the American alligator.

American alligators are native to the southeastern states of the mainland US. Indigenous Americans hunted these alligators as a food source for thousands of years. Colonial Americans started harvesting alligators commercially in the early 1800s – mostly for their skin (leather), but also for oil made from their fat, which was used as a lubricant in steam engines. The US Civil War drove up demand, as US Southerners wanted alligator skins to make saddles and shoes for Confederate soldiers. By the late 1800s, Americans were killing tens of thousands of alligators per year, causing the population to decline precipitously. In the mid-1900s, US states recognized this fact and, in keeping with the North American Model of wildlife management (see Chapter 7), tried to manage alligator harvests more actively. Still, illegal harvesting (poaching) continued, forcing the State of Louisiana to ban alligator hunting entirely in 1962 (Barrow 2009). Unfortunately, there is nothing unique about the story of the American alligator; when the IUCN eventually formed the Crocodile Specialist Group in 1971, all 23 crocodilian species were either endangered or threatened.

By the 1980s, however, many crocodilian species were faring much better. The change? Researchers at Louisiana's Rockefeller Refuge started collecting alligator eggs, raising the young alligators for two years in captivity (Figure 10.1), and then returning a small percentage to the wild. This radically increased alligator survival rates, as the animals were protected from predators during the most vulnerable period of life. But if only a small percentage of alligators were being returned to the wild, what was happening to the rest of them? In short, they were farmed for their skins – wild animals were being raised in captivity in order to produce a valuable commercial commodity. The strategy of the Rockefeller Refuge was to align market interests with conservation goals.

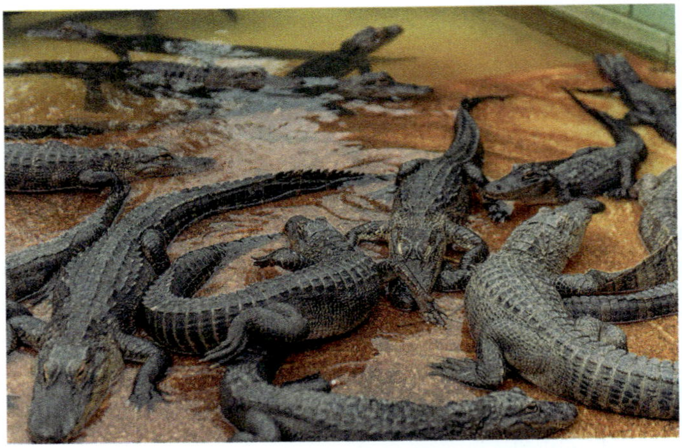

Figure 10.1 Juvenile American alligators farmed in Florida, USA. *Source:* Mindaugas Dulinskas/ Dreamstime LLC.

There are now "sustainable harvest" strategies for alligators in Texas, Florida (Figure 10.1), and Louisiana, with farming and ranching at a large scale. In 2016, there were over 932 000 alligators on ranches in Louisiana alone (Woodward and Elsey 2019) and a statewide hunting season was reintroduced in Louisiana in 1981. This approach caught on elsewhere (Rice et al. 1999) and today the IUCN considers nearly half of crocodilian species to be in its "least concern" conservation category.

From some perspectives, this is one of the great success stories in the history of conservation (Thorbjarnarson 1999). Of course, the moral premise of such a strategy is that it's acceptable to bring wild animals into captivity and kill them for human use. Humans can have their alligators and wear (and eat) them too. The American alligator species once more flourishes in the wild and performs an important ecosystem role as a top predator.

The story for *individual* alligators is a bit more complicated. Those who were released into the wild seem to do well, since they were protected on the farm during the most vulnerable period of their lives. Assuming that the captive alligators are kept in reasonable conditions and are killed quickly, their lives could be perceived to be worth living, and at least would be likely to be longer and less stressful than if their eggs hatched in the wild, given the mortality rate of baby alligators. Therefore, the only obvious ethical grounds for objecting to this market seem to be based on rights arguments, where purposely killing the alligators and treating them as market commodities is morally unacceptable even if they would otherwise have had worse lives in the wild.

10.4 A Legal Trade in Rhino Horn

There have, then, been at least some past cases where market-based approaches have been successful from a conservation perspective (that is, in preventing extinction). Is this idea equally plausible for rhinos? Here's the basic argument for a legal market.

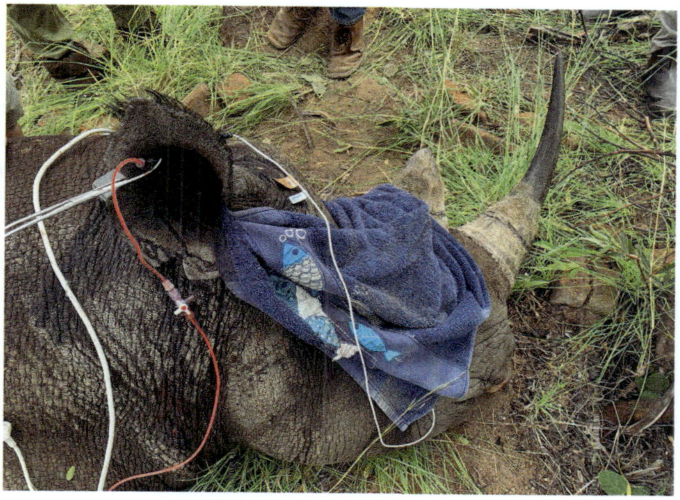

Figure 10.2 A black rhinoceros anesthetized for horn removal to discourage poaching in South Africa. *Source:* Courtesy of Leith Meyer.

Rhinos don't need to be killed for their horns: the animals can be anesthetized and their horns removed with a saw (Figure 10.2). This is known as "de-horning" (Brown et al. 2019) and shouldn't cause long-term harm to rhinos. Moreover, their horns are almost entirely composed of keratin, the same material that makes up human fingernails and hair, which grows back over time. It's possible therefore to obtain rhino horn sustainably. If those who own rhinos privately could sell that product, they would be in a better financial position to breed more rhinos and protect them from various threats (Biggs et al. 2013). There are also significant stockpiles of rhino horn that could be released for sale (or into the market). And if legal producers could generate enough rhino horn to reduce the price of the product – supplemented, perhaps, with synthetic rhino horn, which is chemically identical and can made to look exactly like the original, then that should reduce the incentive to poach.

Many economic commentators claim that a legal trade in rhino horn is feasible. Following the logic mentioned earlier, a legal trade would increase supply, reduce prices, and reduce incentives for poaching. This theory holds that the ban is failing because it artificially restricts supply in the face of persistent and growing demand. The alternative option is a carefully regulated legal trade based on the renewable harvesting of horn from live rhinos (Biggs et al. 2013). Horns typically grow back in 18–36 months (though there are cases of it taking as much as eight years). However, this idea has yet to be tested in an international marketplace, so there have been no opportunities thus far to check these assumptions by monitoring conservation outcomes (rhino abundance) as a product of legal trade. Given the longevity and low fecundity of rhinos, any such monitoring would likely require decades after the beginning of a legal trade to yield answers.

There are some reasons to doubt that a legal market will achieve its goal, largely related to the significant uncertainty about what a legal market would do for demand. First, while it's clear that a legal market in rhino horn would increase the incentive for producers to breed and protect rhinos, surveys in China and Vietnam suggest that the demand for rhino horn is much larger than predicted, based on the current demand for *illegal* rhino horn (USAID Wildlife Asia 2018). Moreover, while some of these consumers would probably be satisfied by synthetic horn, it would be surprising if others weren't. Indeed, this raises a separate problem, which is that the availability of synthetic horn may actually increase the demand for the wild product, with the latter fetching a premium as the "highest quality" version – only exacerbating the problem that synthetic horns are designed to solve (Chen 2017).

Second, while it's true that those who own rhinos would have an incentive – and more resources with which – to breed and protect rhinos, producers can't scale up their production faster than horns regrow and new rhinos are born. Again, synthetic horn can help with this problem, but only insofar as consumers accept it as a substitute.

Third, given the extraordinary prices that rhino horn fetches, poaching operations would still be profitable even if the product were only worth a fraction of its current price. As it is, poachers will even kill rhinos for the horn stub that's left *after* harvesting – which is no more than 7–10% of the total horn mass (Biggs et al. 2013). Jointly, these considerations indicate that those who own rhinos probably may not be able to produce enough rhino horn to discourage poaching. And given how few rhinos there are, even low rates of poaching are unsustainable.

If a legal market in rhino horn wouldn't save rhinos, then there is no *conservation*-based argument for it – even if there are other economic or political considerations in its favor. But let's just suppose, for the sake of argument, that there *is* a good case to be made that a legal market in rhino horn would indeed save certain rhino species. Are there any remaining ethical concerns? In what follows, we will consider several possible ethical worries.

10.5 What about Rhino Welfare?

Three welfare-related concerns might be raised about a legal market in rhino horn.

The first is that horns have a useful function for rhinos, and that removing the horn is therefore detrimental to rhino welfare:

> The rhino uses its horn for protection and defense, mark territory, display, digging, pushing, lifting and carrying, breaking branches, rolling etc. The rhino mother uses her horn to protect, defend, guide, lift and break branches for the calf.
>
> (Trendler 2014, p. 60)

However, as Trendler (2014) also notes, there's little research into negative welfare effects of de-horning in the wild, and these effects don't seem especially significant in captivity; so, there's not much to go on here.

Second, rhinos have to be anesthetized to have their horns removed, and as well as risks from the anesthetic, the surgery itself carries postoperative risks, such as infection. In most cases, rhinos recover quickly, but medical complications are possible and some mortalities inevitably occur (Derkley et al. 2019). However, it's worth noting that this concern isn't generated by the legal market specifically. Even if there were no legal market, conservationists may, at least in some cases, remove the horns of rhinos to discourage poaching. Equally, the rhinos may be anesthetized in the same manner for research projects or translocation efforts (Penny et al. 2020). Nonetheless, though, since in a commercial setting we'd expect rhino populations to increase, the number of potentially risky surgeries would also increase.

A third welfare-related issue concerns the constraints on the lives of rhinos if there's a commercial market in rhino horn (Brown et al. 2019). Rhinos are likely to be kept in highly controlled environments where they can easily be monitored and managed. They are unlikely to be free to roam where they choose – a worry that seems especially significant on conceptions of welfare that emphasize natural behavior (Chapter 5). And also there's a risk, as with any farmed animals, that those managing them might mistreat them. But as with the previous worry, without a commercial market, remaining rhinos are also likely to be kept under tight security anyway to protect them from poachers.

These worries about welfare may be grounds to hesitate about accepting a legal market in rhino horn. But the worries could also be seen as reasons to promote high welfare standards as industry norms, backed up by enforced regulations where possible. If, overall, rhino welfare is better with a commercial horn industry than in the current poaching situation, and there's no alternative way of improving rhino welfare within practical reach, then rhino welfare doesn't look like a decisive objection to a legal market in rhino horn (Derkley et al. 2019) – at least from consequentialist perspectives on which the main concern is optimizing rhino welfare.

10.6 Is Commodification an Ethical Problem?

Proponents of animal rights, however, might raise a concern about a market in rhino horn that's independent of concerns about animal welfare. If sentient animals have rights, perhaps it is wrong to commodify them – to treat them merely as means rather than as ends in themselves. This might be taken to suggest that it's wrong to have a legal market in rhino horn.

However, this is not a market in rhinos themselves. Nor is it a market in the meat or skins of rhinos, or any commodity requiring them to be killed. It is a market in rhino *horns*. And it is not clear that conservationists are failing to treat rhinos as ends in themselves by cutting off their horns, since conservationists are doing it to save their lives.

Proponents of animal rights might make two possible replies. First, they could say that while it isn't *necessary* that people treat rhinos as mere means in a market for rhino horns, *in practice* they are likely to do exactly that. Once there is enough money at stake, people's priorities will shift. This, however, is an empirical prediction, and while it might be plausible, it simply isn't possible to say whether it would happen. Given the stakes, morever, it seems reasonable to give conservationists the benefit of the doubt.

Second, though, proponents of animal rights might argue that there is a sense in which individual rhinos *are* being commodified even though, strictly speaking, rhinos aren't for sale. The thought might be that, in establishing such a market, conservationists are treating individual rhinos as mere means because they are saving individuals not for their own sake but to save the *species*. As evidence for this, proponents of animal rights might say that if there were millions of rhinos, conservationists wouldn't worry about people killing a few thousand rhinos here or there for their horns. So, in essence conservationists are commodifying individual rhinos to save the rhino species.

One possible reply is that de-horning individual rhinos also protects the *individual* de-horned rhinos from poaching, as well as helping to protect the species, so concerns about individuals and the species coincide here. Second, if the *only* way to save individual rhinos is for people to commodify them, then while commodification may be morally objectionable, it can't be a decisive objection. Presumably, animals' lives shouldn't be sacrificed for their rights not to be commodified. While it might be far from ideal to have a market in rhino horn, that may be the best rights-respecting option.

Whether that's so depends on whether there are any available alternatives. For instance, some have defended herding rhinos like cattle to protect them from poachers, though others worry that this would habituate them to humans, which may increase their risk of being poached at a later time (Fàbregas et al. 2021). This may also compromise their wildness, about which we'll have more to say below. As mentioned earlier, another possibility is to flood the market with a cheaper, synthetic option, though that may end up being counterproductive. Ultimately, then, assessment of the rights-based objection to a legal market in rhino horn depends on empirical questions about the prospects for alternative conservation options. If these options show any promise, then if animals have rights, it's probably wrong to establish a legal market in rhino horn.

We're simplifying here, as a lot turns on what it means for one of these options to "show any promise." Suppose that the probability that a legal rhino horn market will save rhino species is 50% and that the synthetic horn option has a 25% chance of success. Is the synthetic horn option promising enough that it would be wrong to commodify animals in the hope of saving them? Or would the synthetic horn option need to be at least as likely to succeed as the legal rhino horn market? It isn't clear what a rights theorist would say here.

One particular worry about a rights position that opposes a market in rhino horns concerns the formation of what's called a Baptist–Bootlegger coalition (Wiltshire 2019). This interprets a rhino horn market ban motivated by animal rights through the lens of Prohibition in the US, where alcohol markets were banned based on the views of Baptists. Bootleggers, however, made plenty of alcohol for which consumers had to pay high prices. No one liked Prohibition except the Baptist anti-alcohol lobby and the marketers of illegal alcohol. And, of course, plenty of alcohol was still drunk; it was just illegal to do so. The parallel worry then is clear: animal rights defenders get the ethical ban they want and poachers benefit because of the high price of illegal rhino horn; meanwhile individual rhinos suffer, rhino populations decline, and everyone who wants rhinos to continue to exist loses out.

10.7 Semiotics: What do Markets Communicate?

Animals are commodified when they are treated as mere means by market actors. However, even if animals aren't being treated as mere means, having a market in rhino horn might still communicate certain objectionable messages about rhinos. At least from the perspective of many conservationists, people ought to value species or the biodiversity they embody intrinsically (Chapter 2) or recognize that the species is morally considerable. On this view, rhinos shouldn't simply be conserved for the sake of their use value (for instance, for the ecosystem services they provide), but because the world is somehow better with rhino in it. Once it is legal to buy and sell rhino horn, however, someone might worry that this, in practice, communicates that the value of these animals can be represented by the (market) value of their horns – that is, their instrumental value (Chapter 2). If so, then the market would be sending the wrong message to the individuals whose views conservationists ultimately want to change. The market would also be legitimizing beliefs that make rhino horn desirable in the first place. It is not true that rhino horn is a good cure for hangovers, but that's what some consumers believe. In the case of dagger handles made from rhino horn in Yemen, there are no empirical misconceptions – they are just valued highly culturally because they have been used for this purpose historically and some people feel they look good. If a legal market in rhino horn just entrenches the kinds of beliefs that lead to conservation crises, then can it possibly be the right strategy?

This is sometimes called the "semiotic" objection to a market: namely, that whatever the effects of the market, it can be objectionable because of what it communicates about what's being sold – where what a market communicates to people depends, in part, on their beliefs.

Semiotic objections are very powerful when they show that a particular market would be counterproductive. If the goal is to conserve rhinos, and a market in rhino horn would actually result in their loss because it reinforces beliefs about the acceptability of the use of rhino and increases its value for those who participate in the market, then it's obvious that the market is a bad idea. However, semiotic objections are not so compelling when they are independent of concerns about effectiveness. If, in fact, rhino conservationists have no realistic alternative to markets in rhino horn, then the choice is between a future with rhinos and one without them – not between two futures with rhinos, one of which includes people having more rational beliefs about the effectiveness of traditional medicines. So, if the market really is conservationists' last hope, then the semiotic objection should probably be addressed by education campaigns, not by opposing the market.

10.8 How Important is Wildness?

Another moral objection to a legal market in rhino horn is that, while it might result in certain species being conserved, this strategy requires sacrificing what might be seen as an important good: namely, the *wildness* of rhinos.

As we discussed in Chapter 3, there are a number of relevant senses of wildness. First, animals can be wild in the sense of not being tame. Second, they can be wild in the sense of not being domesticated. Third, they can be wild in some sense of being "free to do their own thing," to express something like their own autonomy. And fourth, they could be wild in the sense of roaming in wild (or at least less managed) places. A legal rhino market might result in less wildness in at least some of these senses. For instance, rhinos would spend more time in the vicinity of people (including when having their horns regularly removed), and this could make them tamer. It's unlikely that they would be domesticated, but it certainly seems possible that there might be interventions to encourage breeding rhinos with larger horns. And the need for monitoring and harvesting would be likely to restrict rhino movements in various ways, resulting in rhinos living in environments that are at least partially managed by people. Since investors have a strong financial incentive to ensure that their product doesn't wander off or die, they will want to keep those horns close and well surveilled – which means the same for the rhinos attached to those horns.

So, there is likely to be some loss in rhino wildness, and perhaps in the wildness of the places in which they are found too. But perhaps, given the alternatives, this doesn't matter very much. Tighter surveillance and closer human contact are likely to exist without a market if serious attempts are made to keep poachers at bay. Furthermore, a successful market would keep more rhinos alive and located in their native landscapes – not existing only in captivity. Additionally, landscapes with native species like rhinos might be seen as in some sense wilder than those that have lost such species (see Chapters 3 and 18). In any case, it seems reasonable to argue that the goal of protecting rhinos' lives and conserving the species is important enough to outweigh the loss of some wildness.

10.9 The Wrong Beneficiaries?

Let's consider one final worry about a legal market in rhino horn. There is a long colonial history of local Africans being prevented from hunting in certain areas or from killing animals of certain species. Game preserves set up by European colonists in the nineteenth century frequently excluded local Africans from their traditional hunting grounds, an issue of environmental injustice (see Chapter 8). From the perspective of some current Africans, national parks and private rhino ranches are a continuation of the same colonial exclusion: poor local communities aren't allowed to make a living from the natural resources in their area – including rhinos – and the income from those resources go directly to the already wealthy (Spierenburg and Brooks 2014). Is it wrong to conserve species in a way that continues the history of economic and political exploitation and marginalization? (See also Chapter 13 for a more detailed exploration of this issue in relation to whaling.)

On one level, there appear to be some straightforward solutions to these problems. Governments could levy heavy taxes on the sale of rhino horn from private ranches and direct those funds, in the form of both cash transfers and social programs, to members of the impoverished communities surrounding those ranches. Tax incentives could encourage those who own rhinos to hire local people to work on their properties. And for rhino horn that's harvested from public land, governments could establish profit-sharing arrangements with local communities. These arrangements could both demonstrate the importance of the communities and, at the same time, make conservation more financially rewarding than poaching (especially given that profits on black market rhino horn are predominantly made by intermediaries, not those supplying it to the market).

Such inclusive ideas are not only theoretical; they are increasingly being applied in southern Africa. One example comes from a community program in southern

Mozambique, adjacent to South Africa's Kruger National Park, where a community ranger initiative has been developed to move toward a more inclusive and sustainable approach to anti-poaching and conservation (Massé et al. 2017).

It is, however, doubtful that this would actually happen if a rhino horn market was established. So, the question becomes whether it's wrong to conserve species in a way that may well perpetuate an unjust arrangement, at least from the perspective of many observers. Addressing this in detail is beyond the scope of this chapter. However, insofar as conservationists support a legal market in rhino horn, they should also propose and support remedies for the economic and political disparities that rhino ranching perpetuates and to which it contributes. "Supporting," of course, doesn't mean "delivering." But recognizing such environmental justice concerns are an important part of trying to deal fairly with the individuals who have reason to object to the status quo.

10.10 Conclusion

This chapter has explored ethical issues associated with a market-based solution to a particular conservation problem: the poaching of rhinos in southern Africa. In the case of rhino conservation, there are at least five ethical issues (a list that surely is not comprehensive), relating to animal welfare, commodification, semiotics, wildness, and the degree to which the market benefits the right human individuals.

Some of these issues can be navigated, at least if a market in rhino horn has the intended effect of saving rhinos. Even if animals have rights, commodification might be tolerable if it saves the lives of individual animals, and the semiotic objection can probably be sidestepped for the same reason. But if there's significant doubt that a market in rhino horn would save either individual rhinos or the species, then these objections, including worries about lost wildness, may provide good reasons not to experiment with one. The issue relating to the human beneficiaries of the market is harder, but it's also a problem for many other activities in areas with legacies of injustice. A shared problem is no less a problem, but it's a reminder that conservationists aren't doing anything more objectionable than, say, those who promote ecotourism in the same areas.

A great deal turns on the question of whether there are viable alternatives to a market in rhino horn, as well as the odds that markets can in fact save rhinos. The findings from empirical literature here are mixed. Many studies argue that markets can protect the rhino species – partly because, as we saw in the case of alligators, marketization has worked before. And it's certainly plausible that the welfare compromises involved in legally de-horning rhinos are substantially lower than the welfare compromises involved in poaching. If death is considered to be a welfare issue (see Chapter 5), it's safe to say that being shot is generally worse than being immobilized with anesthetics (Derkley et al. 2019). It's also likely that the strategy would come at some cost to the commodified animals' freedom – frequently harvested rhinos would live in conditions that more closely resemble managed livestock. Those who own rhinos will have a strong financial incentive to raise and protect the rhinos on their land (Taylor et al. 2021). But as we mentioned at the outset, the case for a legal market is not decisive; there are serious reasons to worry that it will fail to repress poaching and so thus will also fail to improve the plight of individual rhinos and rhino species in the long term.

References

Barrow, M.V. (2009). Dragons in distress: naturalists as bioactivists in the campaign to save the American alligator. *Journal of the History of Biology* 42 (2): 267–288.

Biggs, D., Courchamp, F., Martin, R., and Possingham, H.P. (2013). Legal trade of Africa's rhino horns. *Science* 339 (6123): 1038–1039.

Brown, A.A., Dean, A.J., Possingham, H., and Biggs, D. (2019). The role of animal welfare values in the rhino horn trade debate. *Conservation Science and Practice* 1 (11): e103.

Büscher, B., Dressler, W., and Fletcher, R. (2014). *NatureTM Inc.: Environmental Conservation in the Neoliberal Age*. Tucson, USA: University of Arizona Press.

Chapman, L.A. and White, P.C. (2020). The future of private rhino ownership in South Africa. *Wildlife Research* 47 (6): 441–447.

Chen, F. (2017). The economics of synthetic rhino horns. *Ecological Economics* 141: 180–189.

Derkley, T., Biggs, D., Holden, M., and Phillips, C. (2019). A framework to evaluate animal welfare implications of policies on rhino horn trade. *Biological Conservation* 235: 236–249.

Eikelboom, J.A., Nuijten, R.J., Wang, Y.X. et al. (2020). Will legal international rhino horn trade save wild rhino populations? *Global Ecology and Conservation* 23: e01145.

Fàbregas, M.C., Fosgate, G.T., Ganswindt, A. et al. (2021). Unforeseen consequences of conservation management practices: case study on herding rhino as an anti-poaching measure. *Animal Conservation* 24 (3): 412–423.

Hanley, N., Sheremet, O., Bozzola, M., and MacMillan, D.C. (2018). The allure of the illegal: choice modeling of rhino horn demand in Vietnam. *Conservation Letters* 11 (3): e12417.

Lunstrum, E. (2014). Green militarization: anti-poaching efforts and the spatial contours of Kruger National Park. *Annals of the Association of American Geographers* 104 (4): 816–832.

Massé, F., Gardiner, A., Lubilo, R., and Themba, M.N. (2017). Inclusive anti-poaching? Exploring the potential and challenges of community-based anti-poaching. *South African Crime Quarterly* 60: 19–27.

Penny, S.G., White, R.L., MacTavish, L. et al. (2020). Negligible hormonal response following dehorning in free-ranging white rhinoceros (*Ceratotherium simum*). *Conservation Physiology* 8 (1): coaa117.

Rice, K.G., Percival, H.F., Woodward, A.R., and Jennings, M.L. (1999). Effects of egg and hatchling harvest on American alligators in Florida. *Journal of Wildlife Management* 63 (4): 1193–1200.

Spierenburg, M. and Brooks, S. (2014). Private game farming and its social consequences in post-apartheid South Africa: contestations over wildlife, property and agrarian futures. *Journal of Contemporary African Studies* 32 (2): 151–172.

Taylor, A., Balfour, D., Brebner, D.K. et al. (2017). Sustainable rhino horn production at the pointy end of the rhino horn trade debate. *Biological Conservation* 216: 60–68.

Taylor, W.A., Child, M.F., Lindsey, P.A. et al. (2021). South Africa's private wildlife ranches protect globally significant populations of wild ungulates. *Biodiversity and Conservation* 30: 4111–4135.

Thorbjarnarson, J. (1999). Crocodile tears and skins: international trade, economic constraints, and limits to the sustainable use of crocodilians. *Conservation Biology* 13 (3): 465–470.

Trendler, K. (2014). Rhino horn: there is never the right way to do the wrong thing. In: *Assessing the Risks of Rhino Horn Trade: A Journal of Arguments Presented at the April 2014 CITES Conference in South Africa*, 60–65. Pretoria, South Africa: International Rhino Coalition.

USAID Wildlife Asia (2018). Research Study on Consumer Demand for Elephant, Pangolin, Rhino and Tiger Parts and Products in China. www.usaidrdw.org//resources/reports/inbox/final-20180612_infosheet-china-quantitative_8june2018_usaid.pdf

Wiltshire, J. (2019). The Rhinoceros Horn Trade Ban: Can Scenario Formulation Help Build Consensus amongst Highly Polarised South African Stakeholders? PhD thesis. Paris, France: International School of Management.

Woodward, A.R. and Elsey, R.M. (2019). American alligator: *Alligator mississippiensis*. In: *Crocodiles: Status Survey and Conservation Action Plan*, 3e (ed. S.C. Manolis and C. Stevenson), 1–6. Darwin, Australia: Crocodile Specialist Group.

11 Hyperabundant Native Species: Deer in the Suburbs

11.1 Introduction: White-Tailed Deer

In 2016, New York City launched an integrated deer impact management plan for the native white-tailed deer population on Staten Island. According to the City, the population of deer on Staten Island had grown so large that it was causing major negative impacts, including vehicle collisions, the spread of tick-borne diseases, damage to forests, and loss of biodiversity. Hunting, however, was not an option, since it's illegal to hunt or discharge a firearm within City limits. So, the plan to control deer populations focused on sterilizing bucks with surgical vasectomies (Figure 11.1). Updates to the plan, reported in September 2021, indicated some success: the total estimated population of deer on Staten Island had dropped by 21% and there was a 60% reduction in fawn births (City of New York 2021).

Staten Island isn't alone in attempting to reduce its white-tailed deer populations; many eastern US states are now doing the same. However, this hasn't always been the case. While historically abundant, deer numbers had declined significantly by the early twentieth century, mainly because of hunting for consumption and recreation. As important game animals, there were various population recovery efforts. White-tailed

Wildlife Ethics: The Ethics of Wildlife Management and Conservation, First Edition. Clare Palmer, Bob Fischer, Christian Gamborg, Jordan Hampton, and Peter Sandøe.

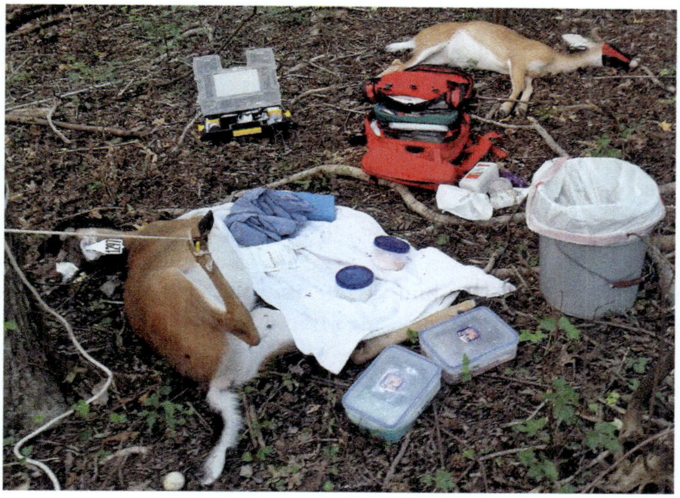

Figure 11.1 Surgical sterilization of hyperabundant white-tailed deer to achieve fertility control in peri-urban areas of Staten Island, New York State, USA. *Source:* Courtesy of Dave Kenny.

deer were reintroduced to some locations, maximum numbers of animals allowed to be killed (bag limits) were imposed on hunters, and habitat was managed by creating the kind of forest clearings within which deer thrive. However, as time passed, such land management became unnecessary; ideal habitat for white-tailed deer was being created without the need for deliberate design or intervention. As ecological generalists, deer settled comfortably into former agricultural lands, now partially reforested, and dined in the many gardens scattered throughout leafy suburbs. Not only did these landscapes provide plentiful resources but they also contained few predators, especially of adult deer. Consequently, white-tailed deer numbers increased significantly across much of eastern North America (Edelblutte et al. 2021), reaching densities many times higher than they ever had before.

When native species reach high population densities in urban, suburban, and rural environments – think, for instance, of kangaroos in Australia (discussed in Chapter 5), wild boar in parts of Europe, and elephants in some locations in southern Africa – they are often labeled "excess," "chronically abundant," "overabundant," or "hyperabundant." And as is the case with white-tailed deer in New York City, wildlife managers often attempt to reduce their numbers.

Such situations generate significant disagreements about what to do, both within and beyond affected human communities. These disagreements may primarily be of a technical or economic nature. Frequently, though, they concern conflicting worldviews, values, and ethical commitments. What *counts* as being overabundant or hyperabundant for a native species – hyperabundant for whom? Whose interests or values should be prioritized? How far should past humans' responsibility for creating such situations affect the way present humans respond? Can managing hyperabundant animals lead to injustice between people, or toward the animals? How should decision-makers weigh the many factors involved, such as human safety and wellbeing, human convenience and preferences, animal welfare, the wildness of animals and their environments, biodiversity, and ecosystem flourishing? In this chapter, we try to disentangle key values and ethical principles at stake in such questions.

11.2 What Is "Hyperabundance" and Why Does It Matter?

"Hyperabundant" is a term that's generally (though not exclusively) applied to herbivores, often in situations where predators are no longer active in regulating their population. Without predators or human intervention, populations are regulated primarily by the availability of food, increasing rapidly when food is plentiful and declining precipitously during food shortages or disease outbreaks (Forsyth and Caley 2006). In principle, the term "hyperabundant" could be used in a purely descriptive way, relative to some baseline population size, where it doesn't tell us anything about the (un)desirability of a particular level of abundance. However, "hyperabundant" is what philosophers call a "thick" term – it has both descriptive and evaluative content. In this case, the evaluative content is decidedly negative: "hyper" means *too many*. This immediately prompts the question: too many for what or for whom?

One possibility is that what's really meant by "hyperabundant" is "too many for *human societies* to tolerate." In the case of white-tailed deer, high populations can mean frequent vehicle/deer collisions, the widespread destruction of gardens and yards by voracious browsing, and an increase in cases of tick-borne infections such as Lyme disease (Levi et al. 2012). White-tailed deer are "hyperabundant," then, when their population size makes them of high instrumental *disvalue* to at least some of the humans who live around them (see Chapter 2). It's worth noting, however, that there's unlikely to be a consensus within a community about optimal white-tailed deer population size, since hunters, gardeners, and drivers (among others) are likely to have rather different perspectives. So, what counts as hyperabundance from a human perspective will most likely be contested.

This "anthropocentric disvalue" interpretation of hyperabundance isn't the only one. The term can also be used to mean something like "too many for *ecological resilience*," referring to factors such as very heavy browsing on native vegetation (Côté et al. 2004). Such heavy browsing can in turn have negative impacts on other wild herbivores that compete for the same land and resources, as well as smaller species that rely on intact understory vegetation for shelter, such as lizards (Howland et al. 2014). These impacts matter from an ecocentric perspective, when species diversity is seen as being jeopardized, or where there might be concerns about the continued successful provision of ecosystem services (see Chapters 2 and 3).

There could also be situations where hyperabundance is seen as problematic for the sake of the hyperabundant animals themselves – where there are "too many for the *animals' own good*." Due to a lack of predators, there could be so many white-tailed deer that they outstrip available environmental resources, leading to a likely decline in deer welfare and ultimately to deaths from malnutrition, starvation, and disease. This situation reflects the more traditional idea of a species exceeding so-called environmental carrying capacity (McShea et al. 1997).

All this means that different population levels may be called "hyperabundant" depending on whether the locus of concern is human health and convenience, ecological resilience, animal welfare, or some combination of all three. So, for instance, a white-tailed deer population may be labeled "hyperabundant" by local human residents whose gardens are being wrecked, even though the deer have good welfare and don't threaten native flora and fauna. However, another population of a similar size might be tolerated or cherished by local human communities while nonetheless causing significant ecological damage.

Whether, and in what ways, populations of animals such as white-tailed deer should be managed for size depends in part, then, on the context in which hyperabundance is understood. Some disagreements about management will flow from whether people believe the relevant population needs to be managed at all or could reasonably be left alone. In other situations, like the ones on which we'll focus here, there's broad agreement that management would be useful or is required, but there are uncertainties or disagreements about management *methods*.

Assessments of management methods depend on the values and ethical theories different individuals prioritize. So, for instance, from a wholly anthropocentric value perspective, if deer populations are seen as a nuisance (or worse) to humans, then their populations should be reduced by the method that best balances effectiveness, price, and other human interests (such as safety). From a utilitarian perspective, by contrast, what matters is the overall outcome in terms of positive and negative experiences, including the experiences of the animals involved; this could mean being critical of management strategies that look desirable from an anthropocentric perspective.

In any case, in the interest of taking a closer look at the ethics of controlling hyperabundant populations, we'll focus on cases like Staten Island where there's general agreement that deer populations require *some* management response, though there's disagreement about what that response should actually be.

11.3 Managing Hyperabundant White-Tailed Deer Populations

This brings us to the leading options for managing white-tailed deer populations.

1) Separation, discouragement, and coexistence
2) Lethal control by hunting and sharpshooting
3) Biocontrol (reintroduction of predators)
4) Surgical and chemical fertility control (sterilization of males or females)

We'll now consider some of the key ethical questions these options raise.

11.3.1 Separation, Discouragement, and Coexistence

This approach doesn't aim to reduce deer populations so much as to develop strategies for people to coexist with them. This is, in fact, part of the official policy of some US cities, such as Austin, Texas, the policy of which is to ". . . practice tolerance and co-existence with deer" (City of Austin, Texas 2013, p. 1). From such a perspective, there may be a moral presumption in favor of trying to resolve conflicts without reducing population size. However, this is unlikely to be the easiest or cheapest option for deer management, and it's unlikely to be adopted from a wholly anthropocentric perspective, where other options such as hunting or sharpshooting may be more attractive.

Attempts to coexist with deer might be underpinned by the conclusion that humans are ultimately primarily responsible for the "problems" for which deer are blamed, and so humans – not deer – should bear the cost of correcting them. After all, humans removed the predators that kept deer populations in check, humans decided to develop land that had previously been deer habitat, and humans created deer-friendly urban and suburban environments without much thought for the way deer would respond.

Trying to resolve conflicts without reducing population size may be possible via three basic methods: first, deer/human separation (in particular through deer fencing); second, discouraging deer from lingering in certain environments by making the environments less attractive to them (for instance, by creating gardens of deer-resistant and deer-repelling plants); third, increasing human tolerance for higher deer populations (including changing human behaviors that increase conflict or risk, especially on the road, reducing deliberate feeding of deer, or encouraging attitudinal changes). Such an approach would be very much in tune with the growing attitude to wildlife, namely, mutualism, explained in Chapter 8, with its focus on caring, sociable responses to wild animals and a striving toward coexistence (McCance et al. 2015). Based on this kind of attitude, white-tailed deer in the suburbs (Figure 11.2) may be viewed as an asset.

However, numerous studies have demonstrated that it's extremely difficult to implement such measures successfully. For example, even if deer fencing turns out to be effective, it may come at considerable esthetic, practical, and economic cost and may have unforeseen impacts on other animals that inhabit the same area. While it may sound appealing to increase human tolerance for cooperative living, such changes rarely occur on a large enough scale to reduce *perceptions* of conflict. Prior to the nineteenth century, people were used to living amid livestock and wild animals. Since that time, though, people have grown accustomed to the idea of the so-called "sanitary city," free of visible animal influences. Attempts to foster live-and-let-live mindsets challenge "the perception of cities and suburbs as human territories" (Connors and Short Gianotti 2021, p. 2).

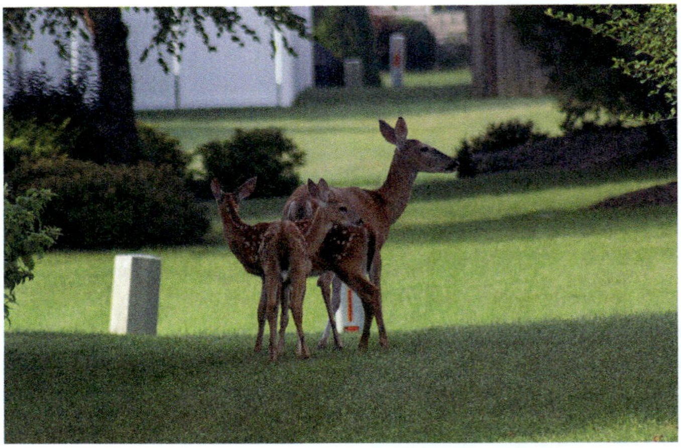

Figure 11.2 White-tailed deer in the suburbs of a US town. *Source:* Alvin Trusty/Flickr/CC BY-NC 2.0.

Finally, reducing human/deer conflict doesn't remove the *other* reasons why some people want to control deer populations, whether to reduce ecological damage or to make population boom and bust cycles less dramatic for the sake of the deer themselves. Some barrier methods can effectively keep deer out of areas designated for ecological protection, such as the construction of "slash walls" at the periphery of regenerating forest areas (Smallidge et al. 2021).

Unfortunately, though, the more effective the measures that restrict deer to particular locations, the more likely it is that the population will exceed its environmental resources, leading to animal welfare issues. So, measures that don't alter population size may solve one problem (conflict with human interests, ecosystem flourishing, or biodiversity) while not dealing with, or even exacerbating, another problem (deer welfare). As a result, other management options need to be considered.

11.3.2 Lethal Control by Hunting and Sharpshooting

White-tailed deer have been hunted for consumption and recreation in the US for centuries. Indeed, as we saw in Chapter 7, the North American Model of wildlife management is organized around the sustainable hunting of so-called game animals such as white-tailed deer. However, neither subsistence nor recreational hunting *necessarily* helps to manage hyperabundant populations. Indeed, recreational hunters have some motivation to prefer hyperabundant populations to make deer easier to find, sometimes feeding deer over the winter to keep their populations high. Recreational hunters may also target trophy animals, such as antlered bucks, which has a relatively small effect on population size. So, if recreational hunting is to be used to control white-tailed deer populations, there need to be regulations that encourage hunters to target does. However, as we noted in Chapters 7 and 8, recreational hunting is on the decline in the US and in any case, the deer populations people are most interested in managing are frequently in densely populated suburban areas where a concern for human safety would restrict such hunting. Indeed, in many US municipalities, it's illegal to discharge a hunting weapon within 100 yards of any residence, which effectively prohibits hunting within suburbia. So, in many contexts recreational hunting is not an option.

An alternative lethal approach is culling by professional sharpshooters (DeNicola and Williams 2008), which can indeed control white-tailed deer populations. Nevertheless, such culling may, like recreational hunting, be controversial, first because any form of shooting can cause *suffering* to individual deer and second, because any form of killing involves *taking deer's lives*.

Let's begin with suffering. In principle, hunting may not cause much suffering to a deer that's shot; if the shot is accurate, death could occur very quickly, perhaps in less than a minute. This degree of accuracy is more likely to be achieved by sharpshooters than recreational hunters (DeNicola and Williams 2008); the latter group may be more likely to cause injury without killing, requiring a (sometimes unsuccessful) search to dispatch the wounded animal. Not much data on this exists; one study found that 7% of red and roe deer shot by hunters in Britain were not killed outright (Aebischer et al. 2014). Another study in Australia found that this outcome occurred in 13% of cases for shooting of rusa deer by professional cullers (Hampton et al. 2022). Where deer are hunted with bows rather than guns, higher wounding rates are likely. This means that the amount of suffering caused by the killing of deer will vary depending upon the chosen method, expertise of the person responsible, and so on.

However, even if there's very little suffering, obviously the *goal* of lethal control is to kill animals. One effect of killing, of course, is to deprive the animals of the rest of their lives. As we saw in Chapter 5, from some perspectives, the loss of a good future can be a significant value concern. And since, after all, the reason why deer are hyperabundant is because they live in environments without many natural predators and with plentiful food, unless there are too many of them for their resources, the lives they would be deprived of by hunting may well have been good (see Chapter 5). Killing may be especially concerning when the animals are young and healthy, with more life ahead and prospects of good experiences to come. Regardless of whether deer have good futures of which they're deprived, there are of course ethical perspectives on which it's still wrong to kill them. According to animal rights views, for instance, killing any sentient animals, even quickly by sharpshooters, is inherently unacceptable, as they have a right to life that should never be violated (see Chapter 6).

However, killing could be seen as preferable to the status quo from other ethical perspectives. From a utilitarian point of view, killing would be the preferred option if aggregate welfare would thereby be increased. This can occur when the deer themselves (collectively) benefit from reduced competition for resources (Gary Varner [2011] calls this "therapeutic hunting") or where enough other sentient animals would benefit from fewer deer. Ecocentric views committed to values such as ecosystem stability, ecosystem flourishing, the protection of species, and biodiversity may also prefer hunting if it's the best or most practical way of protecting these values. Likewise, hunting and sharpshooting may also be seen as positive by those who value wildness or naturalness in deer populations, since both generally allow deer to live out relatively "natural" lives, compared, for instance, to using fertility treatment (taking a "natural life" here to mean something like being free from human control in terms of the ability to perform species-specific behaviors [Gamborg et al. 2020]).

On the other hand, some research has indicated public concern about hunting causing an "unnatural death" (Urbanek et al. 2015), leading people to prefer fertility treatment – despite the more obvious "unnaturalness" of fertility treatment, and despite the possibility that, at least in some forms, hunting could potentially mimic "natural" predation. What's more, neither utilitarianism nor ecocentrism *necessarily* favors hunting as the best alternative. Ecocentrism, for instance, may imply that the best choice would be predator reintroduction, with hunting being a suboptimal alternative.

11.3.3 Biocontrol: Lethal Control by Predators

Predator reintroduction programs either allow or encourage predators to repopulate areas from which they have been locally extirpated. This strategy is frequently proposed as part of rewilding and restoration projects, especially in North America and Europe, so it may have other motivations. Still, population control is often one of them (Allen et al. 2019).

Reintroductions of native predators such as gray wolves do appear to have significant effects. One recent study from the USA, for instance, set out to quantify the effects of restored wolf populations on human lives and property. The study showed that deer–vehicle collisions were reduced by 24% after wolf entry, yielding an economic benefit 63 times greater than the costs of verified wolf predation on livestock. The authors, interestingly, suggest that much of this reduction in deer–vehicle collisions was due to a behavioral response of deer to wolves: while there wasn't a significant decline in deer population from wolf predation, the predators create a "landscape of fear" that keeps deer in woods and out of open areas and roads, thereby reducing the number of vehicular accidents (Raynor et al. 2021). Given that predator reintroductions may help control some hyperabundant species, what can be said for and against such reintroductions ethically?

Some ethical frameworks seem more likely to support predator reintroductions than others. As noted above, ecocentric theories, such as the Land Ethic (see Chapter 6), seem to imply that predator reintroduction is the best solution of those considered here. As has been argued of wolf reintroduction in Yellowstone National Park in the US, reintroduced (apex) predators are likely to have positive impacts on ecosystem flourishing as a whole, with effects on deer populations (both behaviorally and in terms of population size) being only one manifestation (Wilson 1997). In addition, just reintroducing native predators that have been absent for some time increases native biodiversity. Presumably, the ecosystem and species impacts of reintroduced predators are also likely to help promote other forms of native biodiversity. What's more, their presence in an ecosystem could be interpreted as increasing its wildness value by returning to it at least part of the complement of species once present (even though humans are carrying out and monitoring the reintroduction). Finally, while the "landscape of fear" that predators allegedly introduce (Ripple and Beschta 2004) may be stressful for the deer concerned, this is the "natural" state of affairs, whatever value that may be thought to have.

There are also arguments for reintroducing predators over (say) sharpshooting, based on a broadly *contextual* ethical account of restitutive (or restorative) justice (Forsyth et al. 2021). The US Rewilding Institute, for instance, maintains that there's a "moral argument" that humans have a responsibility to other species to carry out predator restorations of this kind, as humans were responsible for predator elimination (and for its subsequent ecological effects) (US Rewilding Institute 2021). Although there are difficulties in arguing that humans have moral responsibilities *to whole species* (see Chapter 4), there are other possibilities. For instance, people could have restitutive duties to inhabitants of an area (e.g., Indigenous peoples who valued the precolonial configuration of the ecosystem), to future generations (which is one influential way of understanding the moral significance of acting sustainably), or to ecosystems (if they are thought to have moral status; see Chapter 3). So, there are plausible arguments that current humans have some kind of responsibility to repair past ecological harms insofar as possible.

However, other ethical perspectives are less favorable to predator reintroductions. In terms of human-centered impacts, the reintroduction of predators is controversial. Historically, recreational hunters have viewed predators as competing for valuable quarry, and where recreational hunting is still practiced, similar attitudes may persist today. Moreover, predators face long-standing hostility from farmers and ranchers due to real or perceived conflicts with livestock and, as noted in Chapter 9, this can be a deep-seated issue of identity. If that's so, then even if direct economic benefits of predator reintroductions outweigh the costs (as the Raynor et al. [2021] study suggests), this may not shift human opposition. Such opposition creates risks to the reintroduced predators themselves – they may be shot, as has recently been the case with gray wolves straying outside Yellowstone National Park – and the perceived threat of predators may be viewed as a human welfare loss (Wilson 1997).

There are also reasons to be concerned about predator reintroductions from the perspective of both animal rights and welfare. Let's begin with rights. At first sight, wolves preying on deer don't obviously violate the deer's rights. On most accounts, rights can only be held against those who can *recognize* rights holders; so, just as deer have no right not to be struck by a lightning bolt, so they also have no rights against wolves or other predators not to be hunted. However, it's possible that deer can have rights against *humans* not to reintroduce wolves, at least not if the intention of reintroducing wolves is to kill deer. Admittedly, reintroduced wolves are not like trained attack dogs acting on human commands, where it seems clear that the dogs are, essentially, extensions of human agency. Nonetheless, wolves could be thought of as being more like intentionally placed biological weapons that act with predictable effects (Allen et al. 2019).

Things also look problematic from a welfare perspective. First, the reintroduced predators may have had their welfare compromised during the process of capturing and transporting them to the release site. Second, the "landscape of fear" that predators create for prey such as white-tailed deer may negatively impact deer's lives, with growing evidence that prey animals display PTSD-like responses to near-predation events (Zanette and Clinchy 2020). On top of that, predators can restrict access to food resources as the deer range more narrowly through forest and brush (Ripple and Beschta 2004). And it's also plausible that being hunted and killed by a predator is, in welfare terms, worse than being killed by a sharpshooter (though probably not worse than being wounded by a recreational hunter). Because of the potential for negative experiences through predation and fear, at least some ethicists who prioritize wild animal welfare, such as Oscar Horta (2011), reject predator reintroduction as a way of managing herbivores considered to be hyperabundant, such as deer. However, there are also the animal welfare benefits received by ground-dwelling smaller wildlife species inhabiting the same environment who will have a higher likelihood of survival once deer abundance drops, grazing pressure is reduced, and canopy or understory structure improves (Howland et al. 2014).

Whatever one thinks about predator reintroduction, however, it's not a realistic option in suburban areas and parkland, such as Staten Island. While sharpshooters may be used in these locations, fertility control is another possibility; and although it is a relatively new approach, it is increasingly widely proposed.

11.3.4 Fertility Control

As the name suggests, fertility control attempts to limit populations by preventing new individuals from being born rather than by killing existing individuals. So, it avoids the ethical concerns about killing that swirl around hunting and, to a lesser extent, control by reintroduced predators. However, fertility control raises other ethical questions, as we'll see.

Two main forms of fertility control have been tried in deer: on a small scale, surgical sterilization of does and vasectomies of bucks (as on Staten Island; Figure 11.1); on a larger scale, communities have been adopting chemical sterilization. Chemical methods today mostly rely on what are called immunocontraceptive vaccines: injecting deer with agents that prevent reproduction. Immunocontraception in turn takes two main forms. *Zona pellucida* vaccines prevent egg fertilization in does without interfering with hormonal cycling. Other vaccines stop reproductive cycles from occurring altogether by targeting reproductive hormones. For example, GonaCon™ is a commercial immunocontraceptive vaccine that induces the body of injected deer to produce antibodies against their own gonadotropin-releasing hormone (GnRH) (Curtis et al. 2008). This second form of immunocontraception can render both does and bucks infertile but does so via markedly changed behavior, physiology, and development (Hampton et al. 2015).

These methods all pose practical and economic challenges (surgical sterilization of does is especially expensive) and require a significant degree of expertise (in the surgical cases, veterinary expertise; Figure 11.1) to be successfully applied. In addition, efficacy is best in populations without much immigration from outside, since otherwise new deer may move in to replace those not born (Gamborg et al. 2020). For consequentialists at least, these drawbacks may be enough to make other management options preferable in most cases.

One further possible reservation concerns the "naturalness" of fertility control, at least if that notion is understood in terms of animals being free from human control with respect to their behavioral choices. While human hunting is episodic, and a "landscape of fear" was present long before humans removed predators, fertility control is a pervasive human influence, affecting deer lives and behavior all the time. Of course, the deer in question are already living in human-structured (or at least human-influenced) environments, so the significance of this point can be debated. Still, some may believe that a deer population that's constantly managed by fertility control is more "unnatural" than a population that's intermittently, if heavily, lethally controlled or one into which predators have been reintroduced.

Nevertheless, because fertility control doesn't involve killing, it's often regarded as a more "humane" alternative for managing hyperabundant populations (although what is meant by the word 'humane' is not always clear; Hampton et al. 2020). Most obviously, fertility control doesn't violate the right to life, if animals have such a right. Some ethicists argue that sentient animals also have reproductive rights (Donaldson and Kymlicka 2011), which *would* be violated by fertility control. But even such rights theorists may still regard fertility control as the lesser evil, given that some interventionist management option is going to be pursued.

There are likely to be welfare impacts from fertility control, though many of them are difficult to measure and their magnitudes remain unclear. For instance, some welfare issues arise in the process of *applying* fertility control. Surgical interventions require deer to be captured, immobilized, and, in the case of surgery, anesthetized prior to an invasive procedure (Figure 11.1). Increasingly, chemical fertility control agents (e.g. GonaCon) are administered via darting without the need for capture or anesthesia, but darting wild animals comes with its own risks (Hampton et al. 2015). In the case of surgery, at least it's one-and-done, but current forms of chemical fertility control require repeat applications every 1–4 years. Presumably, these interventions are, to some degree, distressing to the animals concerned.

Fertility control has significant impacts on the lives of the animals *after* application, especially the female deer. Most obviously, they won't get pregnant and have offspring. However, it's unclear how much this affects their welfare. In the case of surgical tubal ligation or the use of *zona pellucida* immunocontraceptive vaccines in female deer, the animals continue to cycle and the male deer continue to mate with them. Since the female deer don't get pregnant, this extends the rutting season (Miller et al. 2008). The worry that such constant sexual activity may be problematic for deer welfare has often been advanced but has been difficult to substantiate (McShea et al. 1997).

Chemical fertility control modalities that target the reproductive hormones ("endocrine disruption"; Hampton et al. 2015) can cause marked changes to the physiology of treated animals. For example, when GonaCon is used on *male* deer, it appears to reduce libido and lead to abnormal antler development, though the evidence here is rather weak (Killian et al. 2005). Furthermore, treated males have significantly lower weight and higher levels of infectious and parasitic lesions than untreated male deer (Curtis et al. 2008). All these forms of sterilization also mean that no offspring are produced, which deprives female deer of positive parenting experiences – assuming that these experiences are positive. On the other hand, negative experiences are also averted – for instance, if there's no mating, rutting injuries are reduced; if there's no pregnancy, the risks from birth and lactation are avoided. After all, and as discussed in Chapter 5, what occurs naturally isn't *necessarily* good for welfare. Perhaps natural breeding cycles are bad for deer, at least if welfare is understood in terms of the balance of subjective experiences.

In any case, all these uncertainties make it very difficult to give an assessment of the net welfare impacts of fertility control. It doesn't seem clear, however, that this is the ethical silver bullet resolving the difficulties that hyperabundant deer populations can present.

11.4 Conclusion

There are numerous values at stake in the management of hyperabundant animal populations. Most prominently, there are concerns about human welfare, animal welfare, animal lives, and ecological values, including the value of ecosystems, species, and biodiversity. People may agree that these are all, to a greater or lesser degree, important. However, they tend to prioritize these values differently. Moreover, as we have seen, each approach for controlling deer populations has ethical advantages and shortcomings. Together, this generates conflict about how best to address the issues created by hyperabundant deer.

In addition, there are several complicating factors that we haven't had room to discuss in detail. For instance, different population management strategies have different price tags. All methods of population control (except recreational hunting, which isn't necessarily very effective and may not be feasible in all cases) are expensive, especially surgical sterilization and hiring sharpshooters. While cost itself isn't of direct ethical relevance, it clearly matters indirectly. Such considerations are particularly important in consequentialist ethical frameworks that aim to maximize good outcomes, whether those are measured in terms of welfare or ecological outcomes, since it's important to consider how best to marshal economic resources. Wildlife management is chronically underfunded, and unless those making management decisions can secure additional resources, what they spend on one objective can't be spent on others. What's allocated to hiring sharpshooters, for instance, might promote animal welfare or ecological values much more effectively if spent on a different project.

However, it does seem that given the value shift toward mutualism in many urban and suburban (human) populations (see Chapter 8), some options are likely to be seen as more promising than others. Recreational hunting is unlikely to play a major role in suburban population management, and because of deep concerns about killing, sharpshooting is likely to remain highly controversial. This leaves many managers with a suite of nonlethal options, no one of which is likely to be effective on its own but which may, in combination, address the practical objectives that managers face while respecting the ethical concerns that many raise.

At the end of the day, though, when choosing a management policy, the aim should be to find robust compromises (see Chapter 9). This requires a fine-grained understanding of the ethical attitudes of stakeholders and a systematic application of their ethical views to multiple policy options. In many such cases involving highly abundant native wildlife species, the values of the public do not align with those of "experts" or wildlife professionals. However, such professionals and decision makers can provide public communications and dialogue by highlighting, rather than ignoring, the divergent ethical perspectives of their audiences, making such perspectives central to the ongoing conversation about how to live alongside hyperabundant animals.

References

Aebischer, N.J., Wheatley, C.J., and Rose, H.R. (2014). Factors associated with shooting accuracy and wounding rate of four managed wild deer species in the UK, based on anonymous field records from deer stalkers. *PLoS ONE* 9 (10): e109698.

Allen, B.L., Allen, L.R., Ballard, G. et al. (2019). Animal welfare considerations for using large carnivores and guardian dogs as vertebrate biocontrol tools against other animals. *Biological Conservation* 232: 258–270.

City of Austin, Texas (2013). Deer Policy. www.austintexas.gov/edims/document.cfm?id=192077

City of New York (2021). Managing Deer Impacts on Staten Island. https://storymaps.arcgis.com/stories/bffd49bd10b24b379a6c4d701c586230

Connors, J.P. and Short Gianotti, A. (2021). Becoming killable: white-tailed deer management and the production of overabundance in the Blue Hills. *Urban Geography* 2021: 1–23.

Côté, S.D., Rooney, T.P., Tremblay, J.-P. et al. (2004). Ecological impacts of deer overabundance. *Annual Review of Ecology, Evolution, and Systematics* 35: 113–147.

Curtis, P.D., Richmond, M.E., Miller, L.A., and Quimby, F.W. (2008). Physiological effects of gonadotropin-releasing hormone immunocontraception on white-tailed deer. *Human–Wildlife Conflicts* 2: 68–79.

DeNicola, A.J. and Williams, S.C. (2008). Sharpshooting suburban white-tailed deer reduces deer–vehicle collisions. *Human–Wildlife Conflicts* 2: 28–33.

Donaldson, S. and Kymlicka, W. (2011). *Zoopolis: A Political Theory of Animal Rights*. New York, USA: Oxford University Press.

Edelblutte, É., Short Gianotti, A.G., and Connors, J.P.C. (2021). Perceptions, concerns, and management of white-tailed deer among municipal officials. *Human Dimensions of Wildlife* 2021: 1–21.

Forsyth, D.M. and Caley, P. (2006). Testing the irruptive paradigm of large-herbivore dynamics. *Ecology* 87: 297–303.

Forsyth, M., Cleland, D., Tepper, F. et al. (2021). A future agenda for environmental restorative justice? *International Journal of Restorative Justice* 4 (1): 17–40.

Gamborg, C., Sandøe, P., and Palmer, C. (2020). Ethical management of wildlife: lethal versus nonlethal control of white-tailed deer. *Conservation Science and Practice* 2: e171.

Hampton, J.O., Hyndman, T.H., Barnes, A., and Collins, T. (2015). Is wildlife fertility control always humane? *Animals* 5 (4): 1047–1071.

Hampton, J.O., Fisher, P.M., and Warburton, B. (2020). Reconsidering humaneness. *Conservation Biology* 34 (5): 1107–1113.

Hampton, J.O., MacKenzie, D.I., and Forsyth, D.M. (2022). Animal welfare outcomes of professional vehicle-based shooting of peri-urban Rusa Deer in Australia. *Wildlife Research, online early* www.publish.csiro.au/wr/pdf/WR21131.

Horta, O. (2011). The ethics of the ecology of fear against the nonspeciesist paradigm: a shift in the aims of intervention in nature. *Between the Species* 13 (10): 163–187.

Howland, B., Stojanovic, D., Gordon, I.J. et al. (2014). Eaten out of house and home: impacts of grazing on ground-dwelling reptiles in Australian grasslands and grassy woodlands. *PLoS ONE* 9: e105966.

Killian, G., Wagner, D., and Miller, L. (2005). Observations on the use of the GnRH vaccine GonaCon™ in male white-tailed deer (Odocoileus virginianus). *Proceedings of the Wildlife Damage Management Conference* 11: 256–263.

Levi, T., Kilpatrick, A.M., Mangel, M., and Wilmers, C.C. (2012). Deer, predators, and the emergence of Lyme disease. *Proceedings of the National Academy of Sciences* 109 (27): 10942–10947.

McCance, E.C., Campbell, M.M., and Baydack, R.K. (2015). Identifying how human behavior influences urban white-tailed deer movement patterns in a Canadian metropolitan area. *Human Dimensions of Wildlife* 20 (6): 471–483.

McShea, W.J., Monfort, S.L., Hakim, S. et al. (1997). The effect of immunocontraception on the behavior and reproduction of white-tailed deer. *Journal of Wildlife Management* 61 (2): 560–569.

Miller, L., Gionfriddo, J., Fagerstone, K. et al. (2008). The single-shot GnRH immunocontraceptive vaccine (GonaCon™) in white-tailed deer: comparison of several GnRH preparations. *American Journal of Reproductive Immunology* 60 (3): 214–223.

Raynor, J.L., Grainger, C.A., and Parker, D.P. (2021). Wolves make roadways safer, generating large economic returns to predator conservation. *Proceedings of the National Academy of Sciences* 118 (22): e2023251118.

Ripple, W.J. and Beschta, R.L. (2004). Wolves and the ecology of fear: can predation risk structure ecosystems? *BioScience* 54: 123–138.

Smallidge, P., Chedzoy, B., Curtis, P., and Sims, K. (2021). Evaluating the construction and effectiveness of slash walls at the perimeter of regeneration harvests to exclude deer. *Forest Ecology and Management* 497: 119529.

Urbanek, R.E., Nielsen, C.K., Davenport, M.A., and Woodson, B.D. (2015). Perceived and desired outcomes of suburban deer management methods. *Journal of Wildlife Management* 79 (4): 647–661.

US Rewilding Institute (2021). What is Rewilding? https://rewilding.org/what-is-rewilding

Varner, G. (2011). Environmental ethics, hunting, and the place of animals. In: *Oxford Handbook of Animal Ethics* (ed. T.L. Beauchamp and R.G. Frey), 855–876. New York, USA: Oxford University Press.

Wilson, M.A. (1997). The wolf in Yellowstone: science, symbol, or politics? Deconstructing the conflict between environmentalism and wise use. *Society and Natural Resources* 10 (5): 453–468.

Zanette, L.Y. and Clinchy, M. (2020). Ecology and neurobiology of fear in free-living wildlife. *Annual Review of Ecology, Evolution, and Systematics* 51 (1): 297–318.

"Invasive" Animals: Predator Free New Zealand

12

12.1 Introduction

In 2016, the then Prime Minister of New Zealand, John Key (the leader of the conservative National Party) announced what the *Washington Post* called an "audacious effort" to make New Zealand "predator free" by 2050. Key said, "Our ambition is that by 2050 every single part of New Zealand will be completely free of rats, stoats, and possums … This is the most ambitious conservation project attempted anywhere in the world, but we believe if we all work together as a country, we can achieve it" (Roy 2016). This undertaking became known as Predator Free New Zealand (PFNZ).

There are no mammalian predators native to New Zealand. (In fact, it lacks any native mammals except bats and marine species.) But the country now has several such "predators" – primarily, but not exclusively, stoats, common brushtail possums, and rats – that have been introduced by humans. (Brushtail possums and rats are omnivores, not carnivores, as the term "predator" suggests.) These mammals are preying on or otherwise outcompeting New Zealand's native species, especially native birds (Figure 12.1), sometimes driving them toward extinction. As the then New Zealand conservation minister Maggie Barry said in a 2016 government media release: "New Zealand's unique

Wildlife Ethics: The Ethics of Wildlife Management and Conservation, First Edition. Clare Palmer, Bob Fischer, Christian Gamborg, Jordan Hampton, and Peter Sandøe.

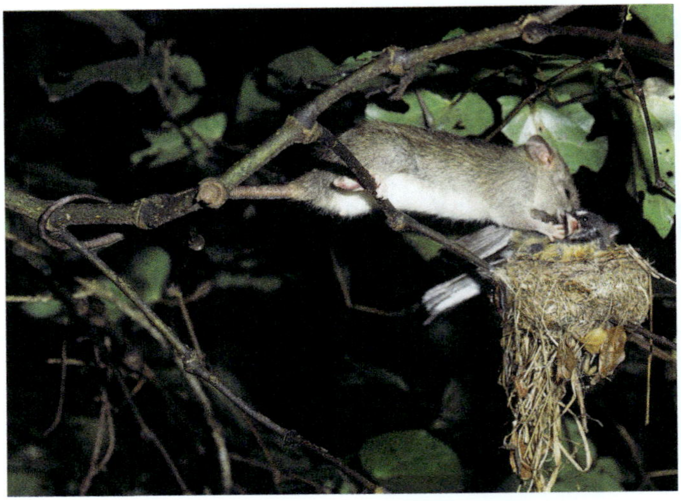

Figure 12.1 A ship rat attacking a fantail nest in a New Zealand forest. *Source:* Courtesy of David Mudge.

native creatures and plants are central to our national identity. They evolved for millions of years in a world without mammals and as a result are extremely vulnerable to introduced predators, which kill around 25 million native birds every year" (Office of the Minister of Conservation 2016).

A company – Predator Free 2050 Ltd. – was set up to launch PFNZ. The launch was largely welcomed by ecologists and conservationists worldwide, and, to a significant degree, by New Zealand's general public. Indeed, the initiative was geared to engage the citizenry generally and to involve New Zealand's Indigenous Māori peoples specifically; its vision was "[t]o connect and energise all New Zealanders toward a predator free New Zealand to enable our native species to thrive" (Predator Free New Zealand Trust n.d.). However, there were dissenting voices too. Some contested the *feasibility* of the project. No one has ever managed to eliminate multiple mammal species, including three species of rat, from islands the size of New Zealand, leading some biologists to claim that "the policy is flawed and risks diverting effort and resources from higher environmental priorities and better alternatives" (Linklater and Steer 2018, p. 1). Others questioned the *ethics* of the project; Morris (2020) for instance, argued that PFNZ is – among other things – an "unjust war" on sentient animals.

Moreover, the species targeted by PFNZ aren't the only undesired introduced predators in New Zealand, raising possible criticisms in terms of consistency and effectiveness. There are many domestic cats, owned and feral, whose negative ecological impacts on birds, reptiles, and amphibians gave rise to extensive culling in neighboring Australia. However, a decision was made to exclude free-roaming domestic cats from the scope of PFNZ, presumably because cats are a companion species for whom the general public has a high degree of empathy. Other introduced species are managed as valuable game animals if they are the target of recreational hunting (e.g., red deer) despite profoundly negative ecological impacts (Wardle et al. 2001).

In this chapter, we'll consider PFNZ more closely, as it raises common and contentious ethical issues in wildlife management. Worries about the impacts of undesired introduced animal species on native fauna and flora aren't unique to New Zealand; they exist almost everywhere. Concerns about such species also form an important part of the "pest management" approach to wildlife management, discussed in Chapter 7. But whether – and if so, how – to manage these species is increasingly contested. To tackle this issue, we'll begin with the idea of invasiveness itself. Then we'll focus on PFNZ, considering the merits – and limits – of the ethical arguments used to justify the interventions for which PFNZ is calling. We'll conclude by discussing a set of international principles that may be helpful in formulating policies around the control of undesired introduced species.

12.2 Invasive Species

What, exactly, is an "invasive species"? This question has no straightforward answer because the term is used in multiple ways in ecological literature (Pereya 2016). Indeed, it's worth pointing out that generally the term is not used to refer to a *species* at all, but rather to a *population*; other populations of the same species may well not be invasive. For instance, though stoats are regarded as an invasive species in New Zealand, they are native predators in the UK, just as common brushtail possums are native omnivores in Australia. Sometimes "invasive" is used just to mean a population that's been introduced by humans (either deliberately or by accident) to a place where it is not native. More commonly, however, invasive means more than that.

According to the International Union for Conservation of Nature (IUCN n.d.), "An alien species is a species introduced outside its natural past or present distribution; if this species becomes problematic, it is termed an invasive alien species." Developing this idea, Patricio J. Pereya (2016) identifies three key elements, any one or combination of which may lead a population to be described as invasive: *spread* (beyond parent populations into a new location); *dominance* over native species in the area; and *impact* on native species. But "invasive" (like "hyperabundant"; see Chapter 11) is what is called in philosophy a "thick concept" – the term is not merely descriptive but includes an evaluative component. And in this case, that evaluative component is decidedly negative. Calling a species' population "invasive," a term that implies something threatening and intrusive, is generally taken to convey the sense that there's something *bad* about the population and its members, an unwelcome intrusion into another's domain and (very often) that something should be done to suppress, control, or remove it (though such interventions may be regarded as more or less urgent, depending on the species and on the impacts it is having).

For those conservation biologists (see Chapter 7) who take the integrity or coherence of ecological communities to depend on their being composed only of native organisms adapted to one another over time, the mere *spread* of nonnative organisms among native organisms may be enough for them to be described as "invasive" in this negative sense (Larson 2011). More commonly, though, there needs to be significant negative *impact* on native species or biodiversity before a population is described as "invasive," with the implication that the population should be controlled.

This use of the term "invasive" has recently been widely challenged as unhelpfully negative and militaristic, almost suggesting that the organisms concerned are acting deliberately (Abbate and Fischer 2019). A study by Young and Larson (2011) indicated that many biologists who work with species labeled "invasive" themselves prefer the less value-laden terms "nonnative" or "introduced." Some authors have even coined the term "nativism" to describe discrimination against nonnative wildlife species (Wallach et al. 2018). PFNZ has been implicated in this context, with opponents highlighting rat-trapping and possum-killing competitions for school children in New Zealand as evidence that programs such as PFNZ reinforce a discriminatory norm (Wallach et al. 2018). So, in an effort to avoid imputing negative values to these populations before exploring the relevant issues, we'll use this more neutral terminology from now on.

That said, the discourse of PFNZ is saturated with the language of invasiveness. One of the organizations working to achieve its goals, for instance, is called Zero Invasive Predators, abbreviated to ZIP (Zero Invasive Predators, n.d.). And it's certainly true that the main animals at issue – stoats, rats, and brushtail possums – all count as "invasive" on *any* of the interpretations discussed above. All were introduced by humans. Two of the three were introduced deliberately: brushtail possums for fur production in 1837 and stoats to control populations of rabbits and hares (also introduced by European settlers) in 1884. Rats were probably introduced accidentally, with different species introduced at different times: the Polynesian ancestors of the Māori people likely introduced Polynesian rats (*kiore*) to New Zealand around 1250 CE; the black ("ship") and brown ("Norway") rats especially targeted in PFNZ were introduced by Europeans more recently. Stoats, possums, and rats are fast-breeding, adaptable animals that have spread all over New Zealand. And all have well-documented negative impacts on native wildlife, not adapted to terrestrial mammal competitors and predators.

Among a long list of impacts on native fauna, stoats and rats eat the eggs and chicks of ground-, tree-, and hole-nesting birds. Stoats also prey on full-grown birds (as do rats if the bird is small enough), while rats are good climbers and raid birds' nests in trees. Rats also eat native reptiles (e.g., hatchlings of the unique tuatara), amphibians, and invertebrates. Black rats seem to carry significant responsibility for the extinction of the bush wren, the greater short-tailed bat, and the South Island snipe, among other native species. Possums eat the berries and nectar preferred by native birds, making resources harder for native species to access. In addition, possums cause enormous browsing damage to native forests (Nugent et al. 2001) and – although this is not an impact on native wildlife – they also contribute to spreading bovine tuberculosis (TB), a costly infectious disease for the New Zealand cattle industry.

Such concerns explain why many New Zealanders support the PFNZ program. But what are the ethical arguments in its favor? How could an intervention to eradicate these species in New Zealand be ethically justified?

12.3 Ethical Arguments for Predator Free New Zealand

There are several arguments for pursuing PFNZ, including ones based on the protection or promotion of cultural, esthetic, and ecological values, where the last category includes both ecosystem services to people and ecocentric values related to ecosystems, species, and wildness. We'll consider these arguments in turn.

12.3.1 Protection of Nonuse Values

Predator Free New Zealand aims to protect a wide range of nonuse values including cultural, esthetic, and existence values (see Chapters 2 and 4) associated with threats to species and biodiversity. New Zealand has a high number of endemic birds and reptiles that, if lost in New Zealand, are lost to everyone everywhere, probably forever. For example, consider the small, forest-dwelling, orange-fronted parakeet (Māori: *kākāriki karaka*), a few hundred of which remain in three alpine beech valleys in Canterbury, on the South Island. Historically, orange-fronted parakeet populations were reduced by deforestation and by farmers protecting their crops and fruit from hungry birds. Now, however, the main threat is predation from rats and stoats. Without the removal of rats and stoats from the parakeets' habitat, it's likely that this species will go extinct (O'Donnell 1996).

The orange-fronted parakeet has *existence* value for many people; they want the orange-fronted parakeet to survive, even if they never personally see a member of the species and get no economic benefits from it. Native species, like the orange-fronted parakeet, also have *esthetic* value (see Chapter 4). Some are beautiful; others are fascinating and strange; some have melodious or intriguing songs that are already being missed. The significance of the "beautiful, thundering" sound of the birds in New Zealand forests in past decades has been recounted in interviews with Māori people. The loss of such species diminishes the esthetic value available both to residents and visitors to New Zealand, with potential knock-on economic effects due to lost tourism. And the loss is not only to people in New Zealand or to those currently alive. These species have value to people all over the world. And if they are lost, *future* people will never get the opportunity to see or hear orange-fronted parakeets, except in photos and films.

Native species in New Zealand also have significant *cultural* value, especially to Māori peoples. Some now threatened and protected species were central to Māori hunting and to related cultural traditions. In their study of the values of the Tuawhenua Māori, for instance, Lyver et al. (2017, p. 99) comment that even where some nonnative species can provide a provisioning service for many Māori communities, "they generally do not have cultural heritage values such as *whakapapa*, *wairua*, *te reo* (language), and *tūākiritanga-a-iwi* (cultural identity) associated with them, nor the *kōrero tawhito* (history of land and people including knowledge of sacred harvest sites) and customary protocols reserved for native *taonga* (treasured species) like the *kererū*, and therefore are not wholly substitutable." While Māori peoples do now hunt some of the nonnative species for food, these animals do not have anything like the same cultural significance as the native species.

This outlines just some of the nonuse values that are threatened by the activities of nonnative species, providing grounds to support an intervention such as PFNZ. However, they aren't the only values at stake; we now turn to ecological values.

12.3.2 Protection of Ecological Values

New Zealand is internationally renowned for its distinctive species and biodiversity, its flourishing ecosystems, and its magnificent wild landscapes. And as we have already seen, there's little doubt that rats, possums, and stoats threaten populations of native species. Those losses may not just be direct ones related to the potential loss of populations or entire species of native wildlife. Recall Bryan Norton's argument about the contributory value of species to ecosystems (Chapter 4). Norton argues that the loss of species can lead to the unraveling of ecological relationships, making other species, in turn, more vulnerable and potentially leading to cascading extinctions (Norton 1988). Seen from this perspective, rats, possums, and stoats spread risk through ecosystems much more widely than just the species that they directly threaten.

Such losses also matter for ecosystems, or ecological communities, certainly in terms of ecosystem services but especially if such communities are thought to be morally important. Recall the Leopoldian Land Ethic (Chapter 6), for instance: "A thing is right as it tends to preserve the integrity, stability, and beauty of the biotic community. It is wrong as it tends otherwise" (Leopold 1949, p. 242). The activities of the undesired introduced animals *do* seem worrying by this standard. They are undermining the integrity of New Zealand ecosystems, especially if "integrity" here is interpreted to mean something like "containing the full range of native species" (as discussed in Chapter 3). In addition, the reduction in these species' populations may also be reducing the beauty of their biotic communities.

Such worries may be behind the idea – broadly in line with contextual approaches to ethics – that in cases of ecosystem and species loss from introduced species, humans (or, at least, some humans) have special moral responsibilities to try to remove these particular species, since humans are the ones who caused the problem in the first place. For instance, the NGO Island Conservation states:

> Considering that human activities initially caused the problem of invasive species, humans have an obligation to restore the conditions for life wherever possible. Conservation intervention is an act of taking responsibility. Doing nothing would be culpable negligence.
>
> (Howald 2017)

In terms of the responsibility at stake, this seems a slightly odd way of putting it. After all, there's clearly *life* in these situations, it is just not the *desired* kind of life. But if "life" here is taken to mean "native species" or "traditional ecosystems," then this is an argument for intervention. Not only are valuable populations, species, and ecosystem functions lost, but humans are responsible for that loss; so, not acting would be blameworthy (provided, that is, that intervention has sufficient chance of success – a point to which we return below).

What about wildness values? Wildness is often taken to characterize the New Zealand landscape; a 2016 documentary series on New Zealand was (predictably) called "Wild New Zealand," emphasizing that New Zealand has been untouched since the "dawn of time" (Morgenstern et al. 2016). Leaving aside cinematic exaggeration, New Zealand was indeed colonized by people relatively recently. In fact, this was the last large habitable island to be discovered by humans. The Polynesian ancestors of the Māori peoples arrived around 800 years ago, as opposed, for instance, to the arrival of Indigenous Australians on the neighboring island between 50 000 and 65 000 years ago. This shorter human history, together with New Zealand's inhospitable mountainous landscapes, unpredictable geological activity, unique ecosystems, and (until recently at least) comparatively low levels of human influence, has led to the islands being labeled, and valued, as "wild."

Does the introduction and rapid growth of nonnative species on New Zealand, then, compromise this wildness value? Probably, at least to some degree. This wildness loss may not be so visible in the sweep of New Zealand's landscapes, though browsing brushtail possums can cause observable wide-scale tree canopy defoliation and mortality (Owen and Norton 1995). But populations of possums, rats, and stoats are now found across most of New Zealand. Since humans brought them to the island, they are, in a sense, an extension of human influence almost everywhere and their presence means that the *composition* of species in New Zealand ecosystems also reflects human activity. In these ways at least, the wildness value of New Zealand's environment is diminished by the spread of nonnative species.

Loss of species value, ecological value (including wildness value), and human cultural, esthetic, and economic values all seem to support an intervention like PFNZ. However, there has also been ethical criticism of the proposal. Let us consider some of these challenges.

12.4 Ethical Challenges to Predator Free New Zealand

Four main ethical worries have been expressed about PFNZ. The first concerns the challenge of thinking about introduced animals in the context of *anthropogenically* changing ecosystems. The second is that the proposal is difficult to justify in terms of the harms it causes to *individual animals*. The third is a more specific set of ethical concerns about the welfare impacts of the *specific methods* currently used for control of introduced species. The fourth maintains that the program's *overambitious goals* lack robust scientific support, and may therefore result in a high degree of animal suffering over time without achieving lasting benefits.

12.4.1 The Challenge of Anthropogenic Change

A first worry about PFNZ is, essentially, that introduced species are serving as scapegoats: they are being blamed for changes that are inevitable given more general trends for which humans are responsible. After all, introduced animals are hardly the only anthropogenic challenge to New Zealand's ecosystems. European settlers cleared about three-quarters of indigenous forest (Ewers et al. 2006), drained wetlands, and dedicated a huge acreage of former native wildlife habitat to agriculture (predominantly beef, dairy, and sheep farming). Most recently, there have been detectable impacts of anthropogenic climate change, such as rising temperatures. New Zealand has a large proportion of endemic species with small population and range sizes (Keegan et al. 2022) – factors that make species particularly vulnerable to climate change. All this means that introduced populations are just one of the many challenges native species are facing.

What's more, the growing human impact on New Zealand's ecosystems raises broader questions about whether interventions to try to restore anything like precolonial environments are worthwhile, especially where doing so raises other ethical issues. Even if targeted introduced species could be eliminated by 2050, other human impacts, in particular climate change, will also have intensified. Even now, there are cases where introduced populations have been eliminated but native ones are still struggling; many populations of native stitchbird (*hihi*), for instance, only do well when offered supplementary feed, despite now being in predator-free environments (Hare et al. 2019).

Given all this, some think that rather than trying to destroy introduced animal populations altogether, it would be better to be tolerant – at least in places – of the kind of "new nature" that's being created in New Zealand (for a defense of such a view, see Morris (2020)). New Zealand is now composed of many *novel ecosystems* – that is, mixtures of plant and animal species with no historical precedent, but which are nonetheless self-sustaining (Hobbs et al. 2013). So, a future of novel ecosystems seems inevitable. On this view, what's needed is a "significant revision of conservation and restoration norms and practices away from the traditional place-based focus on existing or historical assemblages" (Hobbs et al. 2009,p. 599) and an acceptance of a new kind of environment in which human-introduced species have their own role. (What that role might be, of course, is another matter.) However, since these arguments essentially involve, to a greater or lesser degree, giving up traditional conservation goals of protecting species and historical ecosystems, it's unsurprising that such arguments are highly controversial, not least within conservation biology (see Chapter 7). As long as most people adhere to such traditional views, these arguments are unlikely to be widely persuasive. However, given a growing concern for animal welfare, the following arguments may gain more popular traction.

12.4.2 Harming Sentient Individual Animals

Both the second and third concerns here relate to individual animals. In this section, we'll discuss the idea of harming and killing individual introduced animals to protect species and ecosystems in general sense. In the next section, we'll focus on specific current and projected *methods* of managing introduced animals, in particular the use of toxins and the ethical concerns they raise.

In this chapter thus far, we have focused on populations, species, and systems. Nevertheless, the welfare and lives of sentient animals are also at stake, as managing introduced populations at present generally means killing them. Having said this, wild animal lives are at stake *whatever* policy New Zealanders adopt. PFNZ certainly kills and causes suffering to stoats, possums, and rats. But then, the stoats, possums, and rats *themselves* kill and cause suffering to individual native animals. In some cases, the harm is largely indirect; the introduced animals outcompete native animals for resources (or needed resources are damaged, in the case of possums). In other cases, the harm is direct: rats and stoats prey on eggs, chicks, and sometimes adult native birds, as well as native reptiles and amphibians. So, there is no harm-free option available; whatever the adopted policy, some animals will be harmed or killed – the question is really about *which* animals will be harmed, by *whom*, and *how*.

One possible ethical approach to help settle this question would be broadly utilitarian: adding up all and only the positive and negative experiences of sentient individuals and looking for the net best outcome. The outcome of this kind of calculation will depend on how different harms are considered and over what time scale. If the calculus is restricted to intentional anthropogenic effects, a likely conclusion is that PFNZ is ethically *un*justified, given the large numbers of sentient, nonnative animals harmed. However, if the calculation includes *all* consequences (the utilitarian default), including the effects of nonnative animals on native animals, the animals killed by the policy need to be balanced against the native animals saved from predation.

Admittedly, these calculations are enormously complex, even in theory. First, many native animals killed by introduced predators will actually be unhatched embryos in eggs that aren't generally considered to meet the criteria for sentience – although they will still be deprived of possible future good lives (see Chapter 5). Second, even if native prey animals are saved from predation, they will ultimately still die from another, likely painful, cause (starvation, infectious diseases, etc.), though they are likely to have longer lives before doing so. Third, time scales matter. In the short term, the number of prey animals saved from predation will probably be more than predators killed, assuming that a creature like a stoat would typically kill multiple native birds (including their eggs) in a week. However, if the calculations are expanded to the long term, a larger disparity will likely develop between a relatively small number of predators killed and a relatively large number of native animals saved from predation, especially if eradication is successful (Warburton et al. 2012) (though, as discussed below, this calculation may shift depending on the killing method adopted). So, a lot more information would be needed to come to conclusions about how a utilitarian calculation would turn out.

A rights theory would adopt a different approach, suggesting that there are real worries about PFNZ. If animals have rights, then if humans kill introduced sentient animals, these animals' rights are violated. And it's difficult to argue that rights are violated whatever we do – that is, that the introduced animals are violating the rights of the native ones (though see Milburn 2022). The introduced animals aren't moral agents, able to make reasoned ethical judgments and recognize that others have rights; on most accounts, this means that they cannot violate rights (and some of the problem is due to eating eggs, which have not generally been argued to be rights holders). In addition, most of the non-native animals were not intentionally introduced to carry out population control on our behalf (unlike the reintroduced predators we discussed in the context of hyperabundant native species in Chapter 11). On this analysis, then, many rights approaches are unlikely to accept that PFNZ is ethically justified.

One individual-oriented ethical account that at least appears friendly to interventionist arguments is a contextual approach. Such an approach takes stock of how the introduced species issue arose and who's responsible for it. In outline, this would be rather like the argument from the NGO Island Conservation, quoted above, but here it would be applied from an individualistic perspective. Roughly, the idea would be that humans are causally responsible for introducing stoats, brushtail possums, and rats to New Zealand; without humans, these animals would not be on the islands, causing suffering and death to native animals (Doherty and Russell 2019). It may be true that no one *intended* that all these introduced animals would outcompete or prey on native species. Nonetheless, possums and other introduced species *do* cause harms that are, if somewhat indirectly, anthropogenic (Allen et al. 2019). And for that reason, since humans are responsible for causing these harms, they have a special responsibility to alleviate the harms that introduced species cause to individual native animals.

This argument suggests that even those concerned about harm to individuals should consider interventionist policies such as PFNZ to be ethically justified, because these policies aim to right a wrong, thus providing a kind of restitutive justice to individual native animals by protecting them from fatal anthropogenic threats.

The difficulty is that this argument also seems to work for the introduced animals themselves. It is not as though rats, stoats, and brushtail possums brought themselves to New Zealand; humans are also responsible for *their* situation. If humans' *past* activities create special responsibilities to animals *now*, those responsibilities seem just as strong to descendants of the translocated animals as to the native animals. And this certainly suggests that an argument to harm introduced animals based on special obligations to individual native animals because of human responsibility for their plight is not going to work here – it would be objectionably arbitrary to accept only responsibilities to the native animals while ignoring responsibilities to introduced ones.

To conclude this set of points, then, ethical positions that focus on animals' rights are likely to oppose PFNZ. However, viewed from a contextual position, the matter is much less clear and for utilitarians, much will depend on the methods used, as we'll now discuss.

12.4.3 Methods of Wildlife Control

In the previous section, we considered various "in-principle" ethical challenges to PFNZ. However, there's also an "in-practice" discussion to be had about wildlife control *methods*. The framework for "vertebrate pest control" discussed in Chapter 7 outlined methods that start from deterrence, move through trapping and relocating, and end at lethal management. With the exception of fenced reserves, deterrence plays a relatively minor role in PFNZ. Such "pest-free" fences can be very effective for protecting native species from introduced mammals (though less so against introduced mice). But these fences cannot be separated from lethal management, as a key part of the process of creating fenced reserves is to remove all the introduced mammals on the protected side of the fence – where "removal" means lethal management, as trapping and relocation are rare in New Zealand. After all, there's no location on the islands to which these animals can be relocated, as they aren't native anywhere in the country and shipping them overseas is both impractical (which country would take a few million rats?) and would anyway raise its own set of welfare issues.

So, PFNZ is largely focused on two major forms of lethal control: trapping and poisoning. Two kinds of traps are used: kill-traps, designed to crush the skulls or necks of captured animals (Figure 12.2), and nonlethal traps, whereby animals are captured

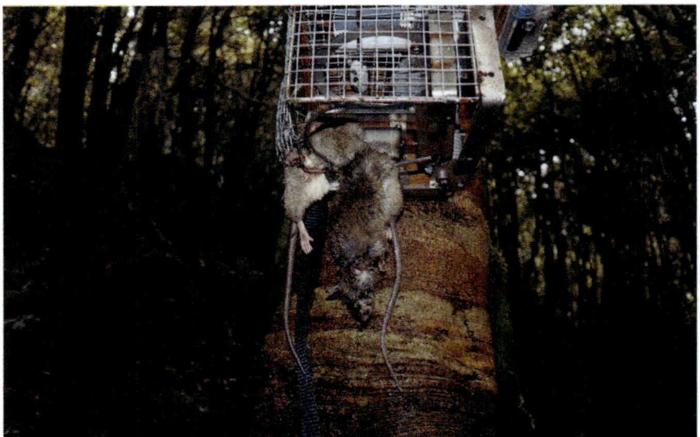

Figure 12.2 Rats killed by a kill-trap in a New Zealand forest. *Source:* Courtesy of Jeff Benson.

and must then be killed by another means. Many kill-traps have passed the standards of the National Animal Welfare Advisory Committee of New Zealand; to do so, traps must render 10/10 test animals irreversibly unconscious within three minutes (Morriss and Warburton 2014). So, there are relatively few welfare issues here. The main concerns are that killing animals deprives them of the good of their future lives and that the trap itself may cause acute suffering for a brief period.

Nonlethal traps may generate more welfare issues (Beausoleil et al. 2016). By law, they are to be checked daily; captured animals are then killed by blunt force trauma. While some traps have been modified to reduce the risk of injury, such as leg-hold traps for possums, injuries still occur (Cowan and Warburton 2011). And traps sometimes capture nontarget species, including native animals. One advantage of nonlethal traps, however, is that these animals can then be released (if they have not been severely injured).

Ethical assessments of trapping to kill vary widely. Practices that kill sentient animals to achieve some other end – here, the protection of native species – are unacceptable from a rights perspective, even if they cause very little suffering. Indeed, this is exactly the kind of practice that the animal rights philosopher Tom Regan (1983) called "ecofascism" – taking the life of a sentient being to protect a species (which he saw as an insentient collective that could not therefore have rights). However, from a utilitarian perspective, trapping might be justified, as discussed above, especially if only certified kill-traps are used and the animals being trapped inflict a good deal of suffering on their native prey. But the *justification* would be that trapping improved aggregate welfare overall; a utilitarian would not be concerned about protecting whole species as such. For a Leopold-type ecocentrist, however, there's no difficulty justifying the trapping as long as there's some likelihood that it will be effective in protecting and promoting native species and ecosystem flourishing.

While lethal traps (Figure 12.2) have been getting increasingly efficient, with some models self-resetting to allow multiple kills, they normally cannot, by themselves, get anywhere near eradicating whole populations of introduced animals, especially in more remote areas (Carter et al. 2016). This explains the popularity of poison baits which can be aerially broadcast in rough and rugged country. Most commonly, these poisons are fluoroacetate (usually referred to by its catalog number, "1080") or second-generation anticoagulants such as brodifacoum and bromadiolone. But these poisons raise significant animal welfare concerns. 1080 is a relatively fast-acting poison (relative to anticoagulants) that kills via neuroexcitation; several hours typically pass from ingestion to death and it's likely that animals feel significant distress and pain during parts of this period (Sherley 2007). Anticoagulants cause eventual loss of consciousness, but this can take much longer (typically days); what's more, the process is likely to cause distress and paralysis due to both external bleeding and internal hemorrhaging, especially into the skull. In humans, similar symptoms cause moderate to severe pain (Fisher et al. 2019).

In addition, baits dropped from an aircraft across a landscape are obviously available to any wild (or domestic) animal who encounters them. While New Zealand has no native terrestrial mammals other than bats, 1080-baiting programs targeting possums have been shown to kill large numbers of deer (Nugent and Yockney 2004), which aren't native but also aren't being targeted for eradication, being highly valued for recreational hunting. (In response, effective deer repellents have been developed for baits.) Even threatened native animals that are conservation targets themselves can consume baits and die; native *kea* (a species of parrot) have been killed in this way during 1080 drops (Weser and Ross 2013). There may also be secondary poisoning, if birds of prey eat poisoned small mammals, although these risks are much higher with the use of anticoagulants than 1080 (Fisher et al. 2019).

There are much stronger ethical objections to the use of 1080 and anticoagulant poisons than to trapping. Obviously, animal rights theorists will object to these poisons. But the suffering these poisons cause can be compared to whatever suffering the introduced animals bring about by competing with and preying on native animals – which will matter from a utilitarian perspective. Even from an ecocentric perspective, such poisons are ethically problematic: nontarget native animals may be affected, residues may remain in the landscape and waters (albeit only briefly) and the widespread scattering of poison bait could be argued to compromise wildness value.

However, from an ecocentric perspective, it still seems as though traps and poisons can be justified in fenced areas where there's a realistic possibility both of completely eliminating introduced populations and of preventing their return, thus ensuring that the use of poison has a clear end-date. This would allow for the establishment of something more like the ecosystem prior to the arrival of the introduced species, even though such ecosystems would still be encountering climate change (Keegan et al. 2022) and other anthropogenic changes.

12.4.4 Overambitious Goals?

A final ethical concern about PFNZ is that the goals seem to be highly ambitious, in terms of achieving complete eradication of multiple introduced populations across both main islands by 2050. This has led critics to argue that the program is not evidence-based, having inadequately dealt with scientific uncertainty or achievability (Linklater and Steer 2018). In addition, the *ad hoc* nature of PFNZ (with much control work being undertaken by volunteers, local councils, and even school children) means that little knowledge may be gained along the way. In this sense, PFNZ does not align well with the idea of a "knowledge-based ethic": careful monitoring of outcomes to reduce scientific uncertainty and maximize learnings from any failures (Warburton and Norton 2009).

This achievability worry also has implications for animal welfare over time. If it is not possible to *eradicate* these species over the land area targeted and with the tools available – and it is not clear that it is – then the only realistic goal is population *suppression*. But this means that trapping and poisoning will have to continue indefinitely; any let-up and the numbers will increase again. While such an ongoing suppression program may be adequate to protect some native species, the cumulative impact will be especially costly in terms of animal welfare (Warburton et al. 2012).

An indefinitely extended killing program that causes significant suffering to thousands of mammals seems to be in tension with aspects of the growing public attitude of "wildlife mutualism" across much of the world (Chapter 8) – a view that emphasizes caring, sociable attitudes to wild animals and striving toward coexistence. It also runs counter to compassionate conservation, with its "first do no harm" principle and its commitment to "treating individuals with respect and concern for their wellbeing"

(Wallach et al. 2018,p. 1260). Even if some compassionate conservationists aren't opposed to all killing (there might be occasions when certified kill-traps would be acceptable, for instance), it seems they would be unlikely to accept the indefinite use of poisons with such significant welfare impacts.

12.5 Technological Possibilities: The Future of Predator Free New Zealand?

Traditional technologies – traps and poisons – have allowed introduced populations to be eradicated on a number of small islands. However, as discussed above, PFNZ faces logistical challenges, given the size of New Zealand's main islands, and ethical concerns associated with traditional technologies. So, there is increasing interest in new technologies that can address all these problems. The relevant technologies include fertility control, gene editing, and the development of a *gene drive* – all potentially "silver bullet" technologies that aim to eliminate entire populations by preventing the population from generating new members, rather than by killing already existing individuals. (We will say more about changing technologies in wildlife management in Chapter 19.)

Gene drives are perhaps the most promising technology here. Gene drives are "systems of biased inheritance that enhance the likelihood a sequence of DNA passes between generations through sexual reproduction" (Collins 2018). Researchers are currently working to create gene drives that could push desirable characteristics quickly through populations. Mice are particularly good candidates for this research and are a key focus of what's called the GBIRd (Genetic Biocontrol of Invasive Rodents) program (Campbell et al. 2019); researchers are currently manipulating a natural gene drive found in mice to create "daughterless" mice. The goal is to get to a situation where "all offspring are phenotypically male, eventually creating a population that is not reproductively viable" (Leitschuh et al. 2018,p. S121). This could theoretically eradicate a mouse population on an island over a few years (Birand et al. 2022).

However, the implementation of such technology for the target species of PFNZ is still far away. First, rats, stoats, and possums are all more complicated biologically than mice. Second, not only does the technology have to work, there has to be a confinement mechanism (so that, for instance, a gene drive designed to eliminate all New Zealand brushtail possums does not spread to Australia, resulting in the loss of brushtail possums even in areas where they are native). Third, hundreds of modified animals would have to be bred to release, raising the typical concerns associated with keeping wild animals in captivity. Gene drives, of course, also raise a whole range of other ethical problems that we cannot explore here, including humans' role in nature (De Graeff et al. 2021).

However, assuming such technology could be developed both to function effectively on New Zealand and also to remain confined to it, this could both make achieving PFNZ's goals easier and significantly reduce ethical objections to it. The rights of animals that do not come into existence cannot be violated, and even if the impacts on experimental animals in developing the technology are included, the elimination of introduced mammals over several generations would cause much less suffering than the ongoing "rolling toll" of killing, especially through poison.

12.6 Concluding Thoughts: Principles of Ethical Wildlife Control

Human-influenced ecosystems, or so-called hybrid landscapes, are here to stay; even if it were possible, it certainly is not politically feasible to completely recreate New Zealand's ecosystems as they were prior to the arrival of humans. Still, there are good reasons to try to protect at least some of New Zealand's threatened species from some introduced animals. At the same time, it also seems ethically problematic to protect (parts of) nature by endlessly and painfully poisoning thousands upon thousands of sentient animals, some of whom aren't even the target of the poison. Indeed, from a rights perspective, doing so is morally wrong. And while the other ethical approaches we have considered aren't necessarily incompatible with all killing, they would all recommend reducing the harms that PFNZ causes.

In 2015, a group from academia, industry, and nongovernmental organizations met to develop the first international principles for so-called ethical wildlife control (Dubois et al. 2017). Their approach was broadly *consequentialist* – allowing for the "weighing of outcomes of control actions" (Dubois et al. 2017,p. 258) – but it was also *pluralist* in terms of the values recognized as being important. This group came up with seven principles:

1) modify human practices when possible
2) justify the need for control
3) have clear and achievable outcome-based objectives
4) cause the least harm to animals
5) consider community values and scientific information
6) include long-term systematic management, and
7) base control on specifics of the situation (Dubois et al. 2017).

These principles can help stakeholders think through the New Zealand case. The first principle, for instance, usefully turns attention to *human* environmental practices (for instance, agricultural and other development), not just the activities of introduced animals. Setting aside arguments for accepting novel ecosystems, PFNZ can satisfy the second principle based on evidence of impacts on native species. We've already noted difficulties with the third principle (see above); the eradication objectives look virtually impossible to meet by 2050. One possible way of responding to this would be to recalibrate the objectives, perhaps following the suggestion of Dubois et al. (2017) that species protection policies are better focused on specific increases in endangered species populations rather than on reducing or eliminating the target (introduced) animals (Clayton and Cowan 2010). As our discussion has indicated, it's controversial whether the fourth principle has been addressed in the case of PFNZ, especially in terms of the use of poisons. In any case, there's clearly room for improvement; for brushtail possums at least, cyanide – which kills much more quickly – would seem to be preferable to more convenient poisons such as 1080. The fifth principle insists on community involvement in policy making about wildlife control (which does appear to have played a role in the creation of PFNZ). Principles six and seven also appear to have been addressed by PFNZ, with the program having a multi-decade timeline and having been designed specifically for contemporary New Zealand.

The ethical wildlife control principles of Dubois et al. (2017) will not eliminate difficult choices. But that is not their aim. Instead, these principles can help to structure conversations among stakeholders about the trade-offs that different policies make. In so doing, they can feed into processes of deliberative democracy such as deliberative mini-publics, town halls, or community forums (see Chapter 9). Most stakeholders value both the protection of New Zealand's unique species and the aim of not causing suffering or killing – values that are in tension when decision-makers must either lose native species or kill the members of an introduced species by painful means. The seven principles of Dubois et al. (2017) make values and priorities explicit both in their content and in the way they are ordered. By structuring policy debates around such principles, stakeholders can be more explicit about what they value, why they value it, and where those values rank relative to others. This is a first step toward adjudicating some disagreements and deciding how to negotiate when disagreements are ineliminable.

References

Abbate, C. and Fischer, B. (2019). Don't demean "invasives": conservation and wrongful species discrimination. *Animals* 9 (11): 871.

Allen, B.L., Allen, L.R., Ballard, G. et al. (2019). Animal welfare considerations for using large carnivores and guardian dogs as vertebrate biocontrol tools against other animals. *Biological Conservation* 232: 258–270.

Beausoleil, N., Fisher, P., Littin, K. et al. (2016). A systematic approach to evaluating and ranking the relative animal welfare impacts of wildlife control methods: poisons used for lethal control of brushtail possums (*Trichosurus vulpecula*) in New Zealand. *Wildlife Research* 43 (7): 553–565.

Birand, A., Cassey, P., Ross, J.V. et al. (2022). Gene drives for vertebrate pest control: realistic spatial modelling of eradication probabilities and times for island mouse populations. *Molecular Ecology* 31 (6): 1907–1923.

Campbell, K.J., Saah, J.R., Brown, P.R. et al. (2019). A potential new tool for the toolbox: assessing gene drives for eradicating invasive rodent populations. In: *Island Invasives: Scaling up to Meet the Challenge* (ed. C.R. Veitch, M.N. Clout, A.R. Martin, et al.), 6–14. Gland, Switzerland: IUCN.

Carter, A., Barr, S., Bond, C. et al. (2016). Controlling sympatric pest mammal populations in New Zealand with self-resetting, toxicant-free traps: a promising tool for invasive species management. *Biological Invasions* 18 (6): 1723–1736.

Clayton, R. and Cowan, P. (2010). Management of animal and plant pests in New Zealand – patterns of control and monitoring by regional agencies. *Wildlife Research* 37 (5): 360–371.

Collins, J.P. (2018). Gene drives in our future: challenges of and opportunities for using a self-sustaining technology in pest and vector management. *BMC Proceedings* 12 (8): 9.

Cowan, P. and Warburton, B. (2011). Animal welfare and ethical issues in island pest eradication. In: *Island Invasives: Eradication and Management* (ed. C.R. Veitch, M.N. Clout, and D.R. Towns), 418–421. Gland, Switzerland: IUCN.

De Graeff, N., Jongsma, K.R., and Bredenoord, A.L. (2021). Experts' moral views on gene drive technologies: a qualitative interview study. *BMC Medical Ethics* 22 (1): 1–15.

Doherty, T.S. and Russell, J.C. (2019). Ethical dimensions of invasive animal management. In: *The Routledge Handbook of Animal Ethics* (ed. B. Fischer), 420–431. Oxford, UK: Routledge.

Dubois, S., Fenwick, N., Ryan, E.A. et al. (2017). International consensus principles for ethical wildlife control. *Conservation Biology* 31 (4): 753–760.

Ewers, R.M., Kliskey, A.D., Walker, S. et al. (2006). Past and future trajectories of forest loss in New Zealand. *Biological Conservation* 133 (3): 312–325.

Fisher, P., Campbell, K.J., Howald, G.R., and Warburton, B. (2019). Anticoagulant rodenticides, islands, and animal welfare accountancy. *Animals* 9 (11): 919.

Hare, K.M., Borrelle, S.B., Buckley, H.L. et al. (2019). Intractable: species in New Zealand that continue to decline despite conservation efforts. *Journal of the Royal Society of New Zealand* 49 (3): 301–319.

Hobbs, R.J., Higgs, E.S., and Harris, J.A. (2009). Novel ecosystems: implications for conservation and restoration. *Trends in Ecology & Evolution* 24 (11): 599–605.

Hobbs, R.J., Higgs, E.S., and Hall, C. (2013). *Novel Ecosystems: Intervening in the New Ecological World Order*. Oxford, UK: Wiley-Blackwell.

Howald, G. (2017). Embracing the ethics of conservation. www.islandconservation.org/embracing-ethics-conservation

International Union for the Conservation of Nature (IUCN) (n.d.). Invasive alien species. www.iucn.org/our-work/topic/invasive-alien-species

Keegan, L.J., White, R.S., and Macinnis-Ng, C. (2022). Current knowledge and potential impacts of climate change on New Zealand's biological heritage. *New Zealand Journal of Ecology* 46 (1): 3467.

Larson, B. (2011). *Metaphors for Environmental Sustainability: Redefining our Relationship with Nature*. New Haven, USA: Yale University Press.

Leitschuh, C.M., Kanavy, D., Backus, G.A. et al. (2018). Developing gene drive technologies to eradicate invasive rodents from islands. *Journal of Responsible Innovation* 5 (1): S121–S138.

Leopold, A. (1949). *A Sand County Almanac*. Oxford, UK: Oxford University Press.

Linklater, W. and Steer, J. (2018). Predator Free 2050: a flawed conservation policy displaces higher priorities and better, evidence-based alternatives. *Conservation Letters* 11 (6): e12593.

Lyver, P.O'.B., Timoti, P., Gormley, A.M. et al. (2017). Key Māori values strengthen the mapping of forest ecosystem services. *Ecosystem Services* 27 (A): 92–102.

Milburn, J. (2022). *Just Fodder: The Ethics of Feeding Animals*. Montreal, Canada: McGill-Queens University Press.

Morgenstern, R., Flowers, M., and Easton, N. (2016). *New Zealand: Earth's Mythical Islands*. London, UK: BBC.

Morris, M.C. (2020). Predator Free New Zealand and the 'war' on pests: is it a just war? *Journal of Agricultural and Environmental Ethics* 33: 93–110.

Morriss, G.A. and Warburton, B. (2014). Modifying the Victor® Easy Set® rat trap to improve the animal welfare of stoats and ship rats trapped in New Zealand. *PLoS One* 9 (2): e86760.

Norton, B. (1988). *Why Preserve Natural Variety?* Princeton, USA: Princeton University Press.

Nugent, G. and Yockney, I. (2004). Fallow deer deaths during aerial-1080 poisoning of possums in the Blue Mountains, Otago, New Zealand. *New Zealand Journal of Zoology* 31 (2): 185–192.

Nugent, G., Fraser, W., and Sweetapple, P. (2001). Top down or bottom up? Comparing the impacts of introduced arboreal possums and 'terrestrial' ruminants on native forests in New Zealand. *Biological Conservation* 99 (1): 65–79.

O'Donnell, C.F. (1996). Predators and the decline of New Zealand forest birds: an introduction to the hole-nesting bird and predator programme. *New Zealand Journal of Zoology* 23: 213–219.

Office of the Minister of Conservation (2016). Predator Free New Zealand 2050 to be a massive team effort. www.doc.govt.nz/news/media-releases/2016/predator-free-nz-2050-to-be-a-massive-team-effort

Owen, H.J. and Norton, D.A. (1995). The diet of introduced brushtail possums *Trichosurus vulpecula* in a low-diversity New Zealand *Nothofagus* forest and possible implications for conservation management. *Biological Conservation* 71 (3): 339–345.

Pereyra, P.J. (2016). Revisiting the use of the invasive species concept: an empirical approach. *Austral Ecology* 41 (5): 519–528.

Predator Free New Zealand (n.d.). https://predatorfreenz.org/about-us/

Regan, T. (1983). *The Case for Animal Rights*. Berkeley, USA: University of California Press.

Roy, E.A. (2016). No more rats: New Zealand to exterminate all introduced predators. www.theguardian.com/world/2016/jul/25/no-more-rats-new-zealand-to-exterminate-all-introduced-predators

Sherley, M. (2007). Is sodium fluoroacetate (1080) a humane poison? *Animal Welfare* 16: 449–458.

Wallach, A.D., Bekoff, M., Batavia, C. et al. (2018). Summoning compassion to address the challenges of conservation. *Conservation Biology* 32 (6): 1255–1265.

Warburton, B. and Norton, B.G. (2009). Towards a knowledge-based ethic for lethal control of nuisance wildlife. *Journal of Wildlife Management* 73 (1): 158–164.

Warburton, B., Tompkins, D.M., Choquenot, D., and Cowan, P. (2012). Minimising number killed in long-term vertebrate pest management programmes, and associated economic incentives. *Animal Welfare* 21 (1): 141–149.

Wardle, D.A., Barker, G.M., Yeates, G.W. et al. (2001). Introduced browsing mammals in New Zealand natural forests: aboveground and belowground consequences. *Ecological Monographs* 71 (4): 587–614.

Weser, C. and Ross, J.G. (2013). The effect of colour on bait consumption of kea (*Nestor notabilis*): implications for deterring birds from toxic baits. *New Zealand Journal of Zoology* 40 (2): 137–144.

Young, A.M. and Larson, B.M. (2011). Clarifying debates in invasion biology: a survey of invasion biologists. *Environmental Research* 111 (7): 893–898.

Zero Invasive Predators (n.d.). The big challenge. https://zip.org.nz/about

Indigenous Wildlife Use: Whaling and the Makah People

13

13.1 Introduction

On May 17, 1999, for the first time in over 70 years, members of the Makah Tribe hunted and killed a gray whale (*Eschrichtius robustus*). The Makah are a North American Indigenous tribe with about 2600 members, some 1200 of whom live on a 121 square kilometer reservation that surrounds the Neah Bay in Washington state, in the northwestern corner of the US mainland. On that day in 1999, the Makah whalers were greeted on the shore by celebrating tribespeople, delighted to see their traditional cultural practices revitalized (Coté 2017).

Others, however, were protesting. Hundreds of anti-whaling activists, prompted by groups such as the Sea Shepherd Conservation Society and the Animal Welfare Institute, flocked to Neah Bay before the hunt. Tensions were high between anti-whaling protesters and the Makah at several points, both on land and on water. When the Makah hunters returned to shore with the whale, protestors blared loud horns over the Makah celebrations (Martello 2004). The Makah also received bomb threats and were subject to derogatory chants and roadblocks in the weeks leading up to the hunt. These protests extended to locations around North America.

Wildlife Ethics: The Ethics of Wildlife Management and Conservation, First Edition. Clare Palmer, Bob Fischer, Christian Gamborg, Jordan Hampton, and Peter Sandøe.

In the years since, activists have fought a series of legal battles against the Makah in attempts to prevent further whaling. Those efforts have been largely successful thus far. Apart from one illegal hunt in 2007, which was condemned both by the Makah tribe and US authorities, the Makah have not had a successful hunt since 1999. However, as described in the next section, that may change.

This controversy is one example of the tensions that can arise when Indigenous peoples' traditional wildlife use practices conflict with the values that other people associate with wildlife (Daoust 2021) – which in this case include species and biodiversity (Chapter 4) and the protection of the welfare, lives, and rights of individual animals (Chapter 5). It's also an example of the tensions that can arise between commitments to environmental justice (Chapter 8) – which include valuing self-determination, sustaining traditional cultures, respecting treaty agreements, and the rectification of historical wrongs – and more general political commitments to equal treatment and consistent policy. Here, we map out some of these ethical tensions in the context of the Makah's resumption of traditional whaling.

13.2 The History of Makah Whaling

The Makah are the only Wakashan-speaking people in the US. Their name in their native language is "qwidiččaʔa·tx̌" (pronounced *Kwih-dich-chuh-ahtx*), which means "people who live by the rocks and sea gulls." The name "Makah" was given to them by a neighboring tribe and means "generous with food." It became their formally recognized name after the US government used it in its 1855 treaty with the tribe (Coté 2017). In that treaty – the Treaty of Neah Bay – the Makah gave up 1214 square kilometers of territory. In exchange, they received educational and health services, cash payment dispersed over the next 20 years, and "[t]he right of taking fish and of whaling or sealing at usual and accustomed grounds" (Article 4, which does not specify an expiry date). It's the only treaty between the US government and an Indigenous tribe that includes the right to hunt whales (Beldo 2019a).

Archaeological evidence suggests that whaling played a significant cultural, subsistence, and economic role for the Makah for at least 1500 years. Whale hunts were ceremonial events and Makah social structures were shaped by the roles people played in them. Whale-derived products were important to the community and also provided commodities that the Makah traded both with nearby tribes and, starting in the 1800s, with European settlers. These practices continued until the beginning of the twentieth century (Figure 13.1).

But by the 1920s, commercial whalers had all but eliminated the gray whale population in the northeastern part of the Pacific Ocean. This led to various tribal, national, and international efforts to save the gray whale species so that whales remained available for future hunters. The Makah themselves voluntarily stopped hunting gray whales to prevent further depletion of the population. In 1946, the International Whaling Commission (IWC) was formed to "provide for the proper conservation of whale stocks and thus make possible the orderly development of the whaling industry" (IWC n.d.). The goal of the IWC in the 1940s was sustainable use (see Chapter 7): the idea that conservation of whale species at a global scale would allow for hunting to continue or resume later.

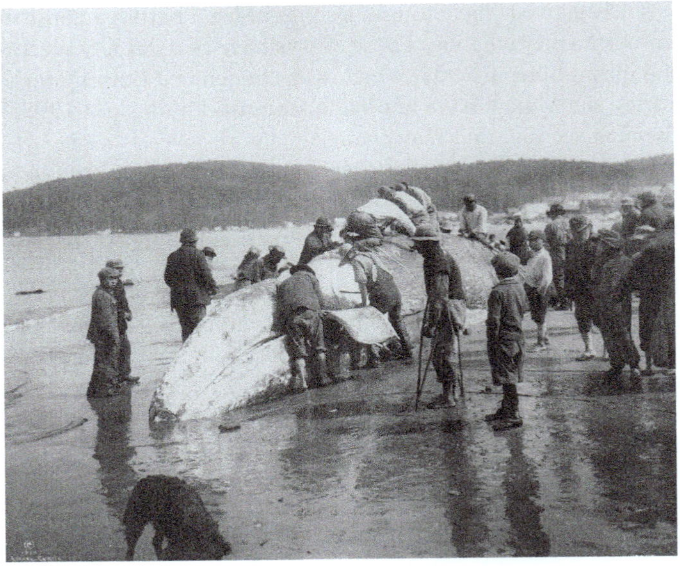

Figure 13.1 Indigenous whaling by the Makah tribe in the Pacific Northwest of the USA in 1910. *Source:* University of Washington Libraries, Special Collections, A. Curtis 18752, reproduced with permission.

However, the treatment of whales as "stocks" became increasingly controversial in the United States over the next few decades, with a shift toward the idea of preserving whale species to protect the whales as such, rather than conserving them for later use in hunting. In 1972, the Marine Mammal Protection Act became law in the US, forbidding the "hunting, killing, capture, and/or harassment of any marine mammal" in US waters. In 1973, the Endangered Species Act became law, and the gray whale was placed on the list of protected species. And in 1982, the IWC itself decided there should be a moratorium on commercial whaling, implemented in 1985–1986 and still in force (Harrop 2003). This moratorium, however, had some exceptions for noncommercial whaling, including what the IWC calls "aboriginal subsistence whaling" (IWC n.d.)

By the early 1990s, gray whale populations displayed a healthy annual growth rate and were considered recovered. So, the whale was removed from the Endangered Species List in 1994. Shortly thereafter, the Marine Mammal Protection Act was amended to allow for subsistence hunting by Indigenous groups and, in 1995, the Makah applied to the IWC for a waiver to resume their hunts. The National Oceanic and Atmospheric Administration (NOAA) entered into an agreement with the tribe in October 1997 to pursue this goal, issuing an environmental assessment (under the Environmental Policy Act) finding that the Makah's request would have no significant impact on the gray whale population. The IWC set a total catch limit of 620 gray whales for 1998–2002. This was split between the Russian Federation (acting on behalf of the Chukotkan people), which was allocated 600 whales, and the US (acting on behalf of the Makah), which was allocated 20 whales, or five per year. In 1998, the NOAA officially allocated the 20-whale quota to the Makah (Beldo 2019a).

The chaotic scenes described at the beginning of this chapter occurred in the year that the Makah (briefly) resumed whaling. Subsequently, in 2000, after a failed whale hunt in May, a legal decision paused whaling until a new environmental assessment was made. This precipitated various hearings, rulings, and appeals: in brief, the Makah continued to submit whaling requests, the NOAA continued to attempt to grant them, but various objecting groups, including the Humane Society of the United States, continued to raise environmental challenges. Perhaps most notably, some researchers identified a much smaller subset of the eastern North Pacific gray whale population, composed of some 200 individuals, which is now known as the Pacific Coast Feeding Group. The legal battle has come to focus on this group, which could be further threatened if the Makah are allowed to resume hunting. In 2021, however, a US administrative law judge recommended that the Makah be allowed to resume hunting as long as the tribe takes precautions to avoid killing members of the Pacific Coast Feeding Group (Mark 2021). Assuming a favorable decision from the NOAA, this means that the Makah will be allowed to resume hunting whales.

It should be noted that the Makah are not unanimously in favor of whaling, nor is there a supportive consensus among other tribes in the area (Kim 2015, p. 142). Some members of the tribe favor making money via whale *watching* and other forms of whale-based tourism (Figure 13.2) instead of hunting, which is the way other Indigenous peoples in the region have adapted to the whaling ban. However, it still seems to be the case that the majority of Makah consider whaling to be important affirmation of tribal rights as enshrined in the Treaty of Neah Bay (Kim 2015).

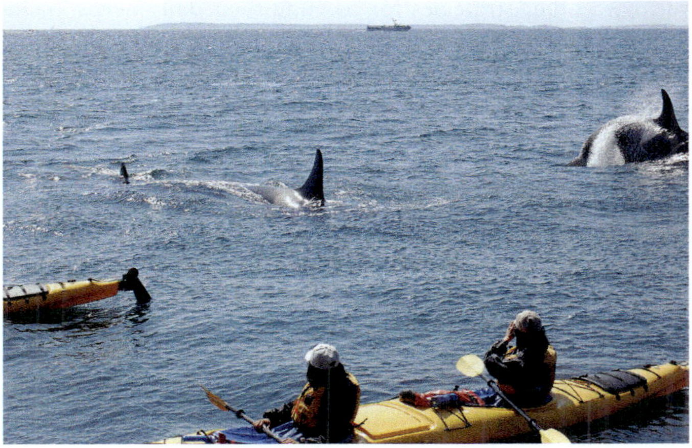

Figure 13.2 Modern tourism centered on viewing gray whales in the Pacific Northwest of the USA. *Source:* JC Winkler/Flickr/CC BY 2.0.

13.3 Two Sides of the Controversy

As a first pass, we can think of this controversy as having two sides – those who do and those who do not think that the Makah should be permitted to hunt whales. What concerns motivate these positions? What ethical concerns *could* be used to motivate them? We'll consider these two sides in turn.

13.3.1 The Pro-Makah Whaling Side

On the side favoring a right to whaling, there are, of course, the Makah themselves. The tribe's own website describes their position this way:

> Whaling and whales are central to Makah culture. The event of a whale hunt requires rituals and ceremonies which are deeply spiritual. Makah whaling is the subject and inspiration of Tribal songs, dances, designs, and basketry. For the Makah Tribe, whale hunting provides a purpose and a discipline which benefits their entire community. It is so important to the Makah, that in 1855 when the Makah ceded thousands of acres of land to the government of the United States, they explicitly reserved their right to whale within the Treaty of Neah Bay. Makah whaling tradition provides oil, meat, bone, sinew and gut for storage containers: useful products, though gained at a high cost in time and goods.
>
> (Makah Tribal Council 2019)

There are four obvious concerns here: cultural, religious, legal, and practical. Let us begin with the last of them.

The tribe clearly acknowledges the practical value of whale products, but it also downplays them by describing them as "gained at a high cost in time and goods." This is not completely surprising, as the Makah have been living without whaling for many years and have found other strategies for meeting their daily needs, including buying products from ordinary retailers and grocery stores. That being said, at least as of this writing, the Makah reservation has one grocery store and one convenience store, each of which is stocked once per week. In the winter, road closures on the highway that connects the reservation to the nearest town (120 km away) often prevent restocking. So, the Makah rely on their own reserves of food, especially meats from hunting and fishing – which whaling would greatly increase. So, while practical concerns aren't preeminent in the case for whaling, they aren't entirely negligible either.

The other three concerns are somewhat difficult to disentangle. Consider the legal argument for a right to whale, based on the Treaty of Neah Bay. Based on Article Six of the US Constitution, such treaties are considered "contracts among nations" and "the supreme law of the land," providing the foundation for federal Indian law (which specifies the rights and responsibilities of Native American tribes and the US government). It seems plausible, then, that rights guaranteed by such treaties could not be abrogated by subsequent legislation, though this has not always been respected in the US courts. More specifically, in a 2002 case, a US court reached the conclusion that the Makah should follow the Marine Mammal Protection Act, even though this was in conflict with respecting their treaty rights. This has shifted the focus of the argument to the Makah's application for an exception to the Marine Mammal Protection

Act, which rests largely on the cultural and religious significance of whaling. It's also an exception that, as we noted earlier, it seems likely that the Makah will ultimately receive.

While much more could be said concerning complicated legal debates about religious and cultural accommodation in US law and the controversial history of US treaties with Native American tribes, here, we are more concerned with the relevant ethical considerations. What could be the best ethical case for the Makah having a right to whale?

Thinking more generally about the bases for exceptions to otherwise justified laws, there is little debate that people have rights to religious and cultural expression; these are widely recognized and have been enshrined in the United Nations' Universal Declaration of Human Rights. Instead, the debate is about the *extent* of those rights. One argument for a fairly generous interpretation was proposed by Will Kymlicka (1995). Kymlicka argued that if individual rights should be protected, then the claims of minority cultures need to be protected (to include minority religious traditions). The basic idea is that individual rights exist to protect, insofar as possible, the pursuit of the good life as individuals understand that notion. However, individuals' conceptions of the good life are often tied to their culture. So, if rights are going to do the work they are supposed to do, they need to protect the culturally specific ways of life that are important to particular groups of people. Invariably, though, a dominant culture sets standards that privilege one way of life – with its attendant system of values – over other, minority cultures. Working with the assumption that someone's starting point in life should not result in systematic disadvantages, Kymlicka argues that the law should do its best to accommodate the interests of minority cultures, since doing so protects the basic rights of the members of those cultures.

That sort of argument indeed implies that the Makah ought to be permitted to hunt whales, at least given the assumption that no human rights would be violated by whaling. Of course, if animals have rights, then the *whales'* rights would be violated by whaling – an idea to which Kymlicka returns in a later piece on animals and multiculturalism (Kymlicka 2017). We'll come back to this below.

But whatever the merits of this argumentative strategy, there are plausibly also some important additional historical considerations. Native American tribes, like many Indigenous people more generally, were the victims of genocide, land grabs, cultural erasure, and any number of other injustices. As a result, the interests of such people groups might be seen to deserve special consideration in policy settings, aside from their status as minority cultures.

Kyle Powys Whyte, a scholar of Indigenous environmental justice, offers one influential way of thinking about the significance of such historical injustices via the concept of "settler colonialism":

> As an injustice, settler colonialism refers to complex social processes in which at least one society seeks to move permanently onto the terrestrial, aquatic, and aerial places lived in by one or more other societies who already derive economic vitality, cultural flourishing, and political self-determination from the relationships they have established with the plants, animals, physical entities, and ecosystems of those places
> (Whyte 2017, p. 158)

The "social processes" mentioned here are diverse, including the physical occupation of land and associated waters, the reconfiguration and repurposing of that land and associated waters, the replacement of the original legal and political order, and the forced assimilation of the members of the original culture into the new one. Jointly, these and other processes contribute to the *erasure* of the prior society – which is not just its destruction but also the attempt to eliminate any trace of it.

On this view, the efforts to prevent the Makah from partaking in the practice of whaling are a continuation of the legacy of settler colonialism and the erasure of Indigenous peoples. The Makah's whaling rights were guaranteed by the Treaty of Neah Bay, but that treaty is not being honored (Van Ginkel 2004). In denying the Makah their treaty rights, the US government is continuing its legacy of erasing their culture, which does not simply disregard the right to self-determination – it disregards their right to exist. From this perspective, then, the Makah should be allowed to hunt whales not just because whaling is culturally and religiously important, but because permitting hunting is a way of beginning to rectify the wrongs of colonialism. Promises that were broken need to be kept. Rights to sovereignty and self-determination need to be respected and protected. Identities that have been erased need to be recovered and cultivated, in hopes of preserving the continuity of the community.

Strikingly, this historical way of framing the situation makes the discussion of whether whaling is necessary (or needed) for the Makah people irrelevant. Instead, what matters is that Makah people have the right *not* to have a specific identity erased – namely, the one that bans on whaling (among other things) effectively undermined.

So, general considerations that favor accommodating important minority group cultural and religious practices, justice-oriented responses to affirm tribal rights against settler colonialism provide significant support for letting the Makah resume whaling.

13.3.2 Against the Resumption of Makah Whaling

What about the arguments on the other side? Essentially, there are two kinds of arguments against the Makah being permitted to whale, both of which correspond closely to arguments we considered in the first half of this book. The first is a broadly ecocentric argument, maintaining that whaling may risk reducing biodiversity and may have other broader negative ecological consequences apart from the fact that it undermines the aim of species preservation. The second argument focuses on the impacts of whaling on individual whales.

The ecocentric argument begins with the observation that whale populations have declined significantly due to whaling. From 1890 to 2001, there was an estimated 64% reduction in the global number of "great" whales and an 81% reduction in their biomass. Gray whales specifically were nearly driven to extinction in the mid-1800s, when an estimated minimum population size of 4000–5000 was reached (Christensen 2006). The population size for gray whales is now estimated at over 20 000 but progress has not been linear, as there have been periodic "unusual mortality events." Most recently, the population peaked at nearly 27 000 in 2016 and then suffered a 24% decline between then and 2021, suggesting that gray whale populations are still vulnerable (Stewart and Weller 2021). Insofar as the gray whale species and the biodiversity it embodies and promotes are valuable, this seems to provide some reason to restrict whaling.

This argument, however, does not seem to go all the way to a conclusive objection to Makah whaling. True, it provides a reason to *restrict* hunting gray whales, but not to eliminate whaling entirely. As mentioned above, the IWC explicitly makes exceptions from its moratorium on commercial whaling for Indigenous groups:

> From the outset, the IWC recognised that Indigenous or aboriginal subsistence whaling is not the same as commercial whaling. Aboriginal whaling does not seek to maximise catches or profit. It is categorised differently by the IWC and is not subject to the moratorium. The IWC recognises that its regulations have the potential to impact significantly on traditional cultures, and great care must be taken in discharging this responsibility.
>
> (IWC n.d.)

In 1994, as noted above, the gray whale was removed from the US Endangered Species List, which allowed the Makah to apply to hunt whales in the first place. Moreover, environmental assessments consistently found that whaling at the rate that the Makah propose – no more than five whales per year – should not have any impact on the health of the gray whale population. So, the species protection and biological diversity argument provides only a weak reason to prevent the Makah from whaling. While all hunting may be less than optimal for the species, such low catch rates do not pose any real threat to it.

There is, however, a second kind of argument against permitting whaling by the Makah: that there's something objectionable about the impact of whaling on *individual* whales, quite apart from any concerns about the species (Daoust 2021). Those sympathetic to this idea, however, disagree about what, exactly, is objectionable here. Proponents of animal rights, of course, object to all consumptive use of sentient animals, which would preclude killing whales for any reason, except in the most desperate life and death circumstances. Defenders of animal rights will also object to the way that so much of the discourse about the Makah focuses on the health of the gray whale *population* (i.e., on sustainability), instead of focusing on individual gray whales. That framing, they argue, makes individuals seem expendable so long as the population overall is not harmed (Donaldson and Kymlicka 2011). Given that the state should not permit people to violate the rights of others – whether human or nonhuman – proponents of animal rights are likely to insist that the state should not give the Makah permission to hunt whales.

For those who do not have a categorical objection to consumptive use, the case depends on the welfare impacts of whaling. First, there are the welfare impacts of the method of killing. In their 1999 hunt, the Makah whalers used hand-held harpoons to catch the whale, followed by shooting with a 0.50 caliber rifle to kill the whale more quickly (Van Ginkel 2004). Identifying a lethal spot on a large animal that may be moving fast, with much of their body submerged, in potentially inhospitable ocean conditions, is notoriously challenging. The failure to achieve immediate death has been used to criticize other forms of whaling on animal welfare grounds, e.g., Japanese "scientific" whaling (Gales et al. 2008). And then there are those whales that are chased but not harpooned, and those that are harpooned but not killed; these escaping animals are known as "struck and lost" in marine mammal hunting. This type of outcome comes with risks of longer-term suffering but it is unknown how frequently this occurs in the context of hunting practices like those of the Makah. Finally, there is the suffering imposed on surviving members of a pod when a cohort animal is removed.

Clearly, hunting gray whales causes those individuals suffering, and, as we note in Chapter 5, on some accounts of welfare, deprives them of the good of the rest of their lives. On the face of it, the method used for killing gray whales seems no worse than animal welfare issues that many people accept or defend in other wildlife contexts, such as bow hunting for white-tailed deer (see Chapter 11) or using kill-traps for brushtail possums (see Chapter 12). However, gray whales are pursued *before* being harpooned, so there are the effects of fear and exhaustion from pursuit (Allen et al. 2019) to be considered in addition to pain from killing. But then there is the question of quantity – thousands of deer and possums are killed in these ways each year, but after all, the Makah only want to hunt five whales per year. Of course, it may be argued that these other hunting and culling practices aren't justified either, on the grounds that the relevant human interests do not outweigh the animals' interest in avoiding pain.

However, there is also a perhaps surprising *animal welfare*-oriented argument in favor of permitting the Makah to whale. In brief, consider what the Makah will eat if they *do not* whale – namely, some combination of locally caught fish and conventional meats from grocery stores. So, they will be directly harming – or supporting an industry that harms – many more sentient animals per pound of meat, simply because of the enormous difference in size between whales, the fish the Makah catch, and the animals raised on farms. The pounds-of-meat-per-animal-harmed ratio is far better for whales than the members of these other species. Hunting of large animals that produce a lot of food may also cause less net suffering than agricultural food production methods that require land clearing, fencing, irrigation, etc. and thereby have profound negative effects on many individual local wild animals (Hampton et al. 2021). If the aim is to minimize harm relative to the realistic options available, then this seems to be an additional consideration in favor of allowing the Makah to whale.

Furthermore, the reasons the Makah have for resuming whaling seem particularly substantial and serious, given both the political rights at stake and the importance of their religious and cultural interests in whaling. Consistency here would appear to demand that if the Makah should not whale, many majority population practices that involve killing animals for much less serious reasons should also be stopped. And this in turn raises the uncomfortable question Kymlicka (2017, p. 297) puts this way: "The question is not whether minorities have a moral waiver to maintain their cultural traditions, but rather whether majorities apply demands for moral accountability in culturally biased ways, holding minorities accountable while exempting themselves."

Therefore, those who are opposed to Makah whaling but who are willing to tolerate other, majority-culture practices that involve harming animals for human benefits will have to make the case that there is something *particularly* objectionable about Makah whaling. Some might be inclined to argue that it's particularly objectionable because it affects *whales*; after all, one recent (mostly US) study found that nearly 87% of respondents were opposed to whaling (Naylor and Parsons 2018). But since animals' popularity is not relevant to their welfare, this just pushes the question back. What makes whales morally special? This question is akin to the one we posed relating to native versus introduced species in Chapter 12.

One answer goes as follows. Even if all sentient beings deserve equal moral consideration, they might not have equally strong interests. It may turn out, for instance, that animals with more sophisticated cognitive capacities can be harmed more severely than simpler creatures – perhaps the lowest welfare low for a dolphin is worse than the lowest welfare low for a shrimp. If that's true, then it may be important to avoid causing more cognitively sophisticated animals to suffer, as their suffering may be worse. So, on this view, if gray whales are more cognitively sophisticated than white-tailed deer, and all other things being equal, whaling with harpoons would be a more significant welfare issue than, say, bow hunting deer.

However, the first problem with this answer is that it is not clear whether there are such differences in how severely animals can be harmed; it remains an open question whether cognitive capacities are related to welfare in this way. The second problem is that very little is known about the cognitive capacities of gray whales, and it's unclear that they are as sophisticated as other cetaceans (such as dolphins and orcas), which are well studied and have demonstrated impressive abilities (Marino et al. 2007).

A different answer is indirect. Instead of saying that there is something special about the gray whales themselves – where they *intrinsically* deserve greater protections than the members of other species – the claim is that there is something special about the whales *because of human attitudes toward them*. This idea is familiar from the related notion of "flagship species" that has been used to promote conservation causes (Thomas-Walters and Raihani 2017); for instance, the giant panda logo which became the logo for the World Wildlife Fund; see Chapter 14 in 1961. The thought here is that animal advocates are able to drum up more public support for whales than for other animal welfare causes – and so, presumably, can be more effective in their campaigns against whaling relative to other causes. This type of impact has been empirically demonstrated for conservation charities, whereby people have been found to donate more to the campaigns of charities featuring flagship species than to appeals featuring non-flagship species (Thomas-Walters and Raihani 2017).

But whatever the merits of this approach in conservation circles – which have been contested – it is not clear that it makes much sense in this context. Even if it's more likely that advocates can make a difference for whales, the return on investment is very small. Yes, whales experience pain when harpooned and shot, but few animals are affected. Other practices, such as concentrated livestock rearing operations, have dramatically larger impacts on animal welfare by impacting millions of animals for much longer durations per animal. If the goal of such advocacy is to maximize expected impact on animal suffering, then it is difficult to see how it could make sense to focus on the Makah's whaling.

How strong, then, is the case against the Makah being allowed to whale? If the worry is either from a perspective concerned with species extinction and biodiversity loss, or a modest concern about animal welfare, it's rather weak. The argument against whaling is much stronger, though, assuming that animals have rights or taking on a very demanding view of when it's permissible to cause harm. But then these stronger positions will have implications for a whole swathe of common animal uses, not just Makah whaling.

13.4 Making Decisions across Deep Disagreements

As we have seen, there are plausible arguments both for and against the Makah being permitted to whale. This is one of many circumstances where it's effectively impossible to achieve consensus about a specific practical question. In those cases, a procedural approach to disagreement is needed – one whereby people are willing to accept the outcome because they respect the process that led to it (see Chapter 9). That procedure, however, cannot be a simple one like voting, since that ignores considerations – such as a history of historical injustices – that count in favor of giving special latitude to certain minority groups. In the US and many other contemporary democracies, the courts play this role: the citizens delegate the work of adjudicating the scope of reasonable accommodations to judges and juries.

Unsurprisingly, US courts are fairly anthropocentric, reflecting the laws in place governing human–animal relations, which in this case biases them toward the Makah. This seems reasonable, given what the courts otherwise permit. After all, while there are some legitimate concerns about what the Makah want to do, the US readily allows practices known to have negative effects on whale populations, including commercial shipping (resulting in ship strikes and noise pollution), commercial fishing (where whales are bycatch), and oil and gas extraction (which can result in habitat degradation and loss). The provocatively titled article "How we all kill whales" (Moore 2014) provides an insight into the extent of these unintentional impacts. If the US tolerates preventable harm to whales that's a foreseeable byproduct of these activities, it's unclear why it should draw a hard line when the interests of the Makah are at stake. However, from some ethical perspectives, there is an important ethical distinction between *intentional* and *unintentional* actions (here, killing) and we discuss the implications of these different types of "harms" (Fraser and MacRae 2011) in Chapter 17.

One byproduct of this institutional anthropocentrism – however reasonable it may be – is that some views are essentially marginalized. Proponents of animal rights cannot make their case in court the way they'd like; instead, they have resorted to defending *individual* gray whales by making arguments about whaling's impact on populations, which makes their position seem relatively weak. That's why, as discussed earlier, many anti-whaling advocates must ignore their belief in the wrongness of killing *any* whales in order to argue for the wrongness of killing *specific* whales – namely, the members of the Pacific Coast Feeding Group. Although the identification of this subset was an effective legal tool to delay the decision to either allow or prohibit the Makah's whaling practices, it did not morally condemn whaling as wrong on the basis of violating the rights of sentient beings. As one animal rights advocate put it, "Morally speaking, there is a world of difference between a blanket moral prohibition on killing whales and a harvest quota of zero" (Beldo 2019b, p. 52). Procedural approaches to disagreement are bound to be limited in various ways; they are imperfect solutions to the problem of deep disagreement. Still, they are often the best solutions available.

13.5 Conclusion

In this chapter, we have considered a challenge that crops up around the world: namely, navigating tensions between the values of dominant and minority cultures. This challenge is especially complex when the minority culture has been subjected to past injustices (as discussed in Chapter 9).

There is considerable global momentum behind movements to strengthen the participation of Indigenous and traditional peoples in the management of the lands and oceans (see Chapter 8). However, enabling that participation may create conflict with other values. From the above discussion of the Makah, we can see that special consideration may be given to values that involve the livelihoods and cultural continuity of formerly colonized and disadvantaged Indigenous peoples. These are unique cases in which only certain people are permitted to act in ways that the dominant legal regime forbids. This seeming divergence from an egalitarian approach to access to wildlife arises from what are, in effect, attempts to achieve equity relating to historical injustices or in the interests of keeping alive threatened cultural practices. As emerging paradigms such as environmental justice become more influential in wildlife management, it is likely that the dilemmas arising in the case of the Makah will become more widespread, especially as more conservation estate is returned to Indigenous peoples.

References

Allen, B.L., Allen, L.R., Ballard, G. et al. (2019). Animal welfare considerations for using large carnivores and guardian dogs as vertebrate biocontrol tools against other animals. *Biological Conservation* 232: 258–270.

Beldo, L. (2019a). *Contesting Leviathan: Activists, Hunters, and State Power in the Makah Whaling Conflict*. Chicago, USA: University of Chicago Press.

Beldo, L. (2019b). Stock morality: whalers, activists, and the power of the state in the Makah whaling conflict. *American Ethnologist* 46 (1): 47–60.

Christensen, L.B. (2006). Marine mammal populations: reconstructing historical abundances at the global scale. https://open.library.ubc.ca/collections/52383/52383/items/1.0074757

Coté, C. (2017). *Spirits of our Whaling Ancestors: Revitalizing Makah and Nuu-Chah-Nulth Traditions*. Seattle, USA: University of Washington Press.

Daoust, P.Y. (2021). Navigating social norms and animal welfare in hunted animals. In: *Animals, Health, and Society* (ed. C. Stephen), 255–262. Boca Raton, USA: CRC Press.

Donaldson, S. and Kymlicka, W. (2011). *Zoopolis: A Political Theory of Animal Rights*. New York, USA: Oxford University Press.

Fraser, D. and MacRae, A.M. (2011). Four types of activities that affect animals: implications for animal welfare science and animal ethics philosophy. *Animal Welfare* 20 (4): 581–590.

Gales, N., Leaper, R., and Papastavrou, V. (2008). Is Japan's whaling humane? *Marine Policy* 32 (3): 408–412.

Hampton, J.O., Hyndman, T.H., Allen, B.L., and Fischer, B. (2021). Animal harms and food production: informing ethical choices. *Animals* 11 (5): 1225.

Harrop, S.R. (2003). From cartel to conservation and on to compassion: animal welfare and the international whaling commission. *Journal of International Wildlife Law and Policy* 6 (1–2): 79–104.

International Whaling Commission (n.d.). The International Whaling Commission – IWC. https://iwc.int/en

Kim, C.J. (2015). *Dangerous Crossings: Race, Species and Nature in a Multicultural Age*. Cambridge, UK: Cambridge University Press.

Kymlicka, W. (1995). *Multicultural Citizenship: A Liberal Theory of Minority Rights*. Oxford, UK: Clarendon Press.

Kymlicka, W. (2017). Realigning multiculturalism and animal rights. In: *Animals, Race and Multiculturalism* (ed. L. Cordeiro-Roderigues and L. Mitchell), 295–304. Cham, Switzerland: Palgrave Macmillan.

Makah Tribal Council (2019). The Makah whaling tradition. https://makah.com/makah-tribal-info/whaling

Marino, L., Connor, R.C., Fordyce, R.E. et al. (2007). Cetaceans have complex brains for complex cognition. *PLoS Biology* 5 (5): e139.

Mark, J. (2021). A tribe has not hunted whales in decades. Now, it might have a chance – and animal rights groups aren't happy. www.washingtonpost.com/nation/2021/09/29/makah-whaling-judge-recommendation

Martello, M.L. (2004). Negotiating global nature and local culture: the case of Makah whaling. In: *Earthly Politics: Local Global in Environmental Governance* (ed. S. Jasanoff and M.L. Martello), 263–284. Cambridge, USA: MIT Press.

Moore, M.J. (2014). How we all kill whales. *ICES Journal of Marine Science* 71 (4): 760–763.

Naylor, W. and Parsons, E.C.M. (2018). An online survey of public knowledge, attitudes, and perceptions toward whales and dolphins, and their conservation. *Frontiers in Marine Science* 5: 153.

Stewart, J.D. and Weller, D.W. (2021). Abundance of eastern North Pacific gray whales 2019/2020. https://repository.library.noaa.gov/view/noaa/27928

Thomas-Walters, L. and Raihani, N.J. (2017). Supporting conservation: the roles of flagship species and identifiable victims. *Conservation Letters* 10 (5): 581–587.

Van Ginkel, R. (2004). The Makah whale hunt and Leviathan's death: reinventing tradition and disputing authenticity in the age of modernity. *Etnofoor* 17 (1–2): 58–89.

Whyte, K.P. (2017). The Dakota access pipeline, environmental injustice, and US colonialism. *Red Ink* 19 (1): 154–169.

Ex situ Conservation: The Giant Panda

14

14.1 Introduction

In Spring 2021, a controversy broke out about two giant pandas housed in Edinburgh Zoo in Scotland, a female called Tian and a male called Yang Guang (Stewart 2021). As with all giant pandas in zoos outside China, they were leased from the Chinese government. Typically, zoos pay around $1 million per year per panda couple, money that's earmarked for panda conservation in China. These two pandas had arrived in Edinburgh in 2011 with a 10-year lease. Their 10 years being up, they were due to fly back to China in December 2021 where, like other retired zoo pandas, they would live in a breeding facility until their natural deaths.

However, Edinburgh Zoo wanted to extend its panda lease and, via the Scottish government, opened negotiations to do so (Stewart 2021). The zoo made the request because the two pandas – the only ones on display in the UK in 2021 – were important for attracting visitors. Before the pandas arrived in 2011, the zoo reported a deficit of around $1.6 million; during the pandas' first year, this became a surplus of $3.5 million. A pattern of financial surpluses continued until 2020, when COVID-19 restrictions for visitors created predictable financial difficulties. Given the influence of the pandas on visitor numbers, the zoo likely considered them important for its economic recovery.

Wildlife Ethics: The Ethics of Wildlife Management and Conservation, First Edition. Clare Palmer, Bob Fischer, Christian Gamborg, Jordan Hampton, and Peter Sandøe.

To the delight of zoo management, the negotiations were successful: the Chinese government agreed to let the pandas stay for two more years. David Field, the chief executive of the Royal Zoological Society, Scotland – which owns Edinburgh Zoo – commented that "Yang Guang and Tian have helped millions of people connect with nature, so it is fantastic that they will be with us a little longer before we say goodbye ..." (BBC 2021).

While the two giant pandas have been economically valuable to the Edinburgh Zoo, they have disappointed in another respect: despite many attempts to get them to mate naturally, they failed to produce a cub. Tian was artificially inseminated eight times, using semen from both Yang Guang and another captive panda, and although she did get pregnant several times, none of the pregnancies went to term (Brocklehurst 2021). Even in failure, however, David Field claimed that the attempts had nonetheless still been useful, as they contributed directly to panda breeding research and indirectly to panda conservation (BBC 2021).

However, this positive view wasn't universally shared. The animal rights organization People for the Ethical Treatment of Animals (PETA), for instance, maintained: "Pandas are not breeding machines but individuals, and they should not be sexually assaulted to produce babies for human amusement and display. Young animals are destined to spend the rest of their miserable lives imprisoned between four walls – all so zoos can turn a profit. The only real hope for pandas lies in protecting their rapidly disappearing natural habitat" (Stewart 2021).

This response takes us to the key questions in this chapter. Does captive breeding and display in zoos meaningfully contribute – via reintroduction, funding, or in other significant ways – to wild panda conservation or to the conservation of other species? And even if breeding and displaying pandas does contribute to conservation, would that justify such practices? In other words, do the conservation ends justify the captive means? We'll begin investigating these questions by outlining some relevant history about this particular case.

14.2 The History of Giant Panda Conservation

Fossil records suggest that giant pandas have existed for some 7 million years (Lindburg and Baragona 2004) and were widely distributed throughout eastern Asia for about 2.5 million of them. Over the last 3000 years, however, due primarily to habitat destruction but also to hunting, the land occupied by pandas has been reduced to less than 1% of its original size (Loucks et al. 2001). The animals now live in a partly interconnected habitat in mountainous parts of southwest China (IUCN 2016) and have been pushed to the brink of extinction.

Efforts to protect wild giant pandas began in the 1960s, when the Chinese government banned hunting and established four panda reserves (WWF 2004). Further *in situ* conservation work was initiated by an agreement signed in 1979 between the multinational NGO, WWF (the Worldwide Fund for Nature, still officially known as the World Wildlife Fund in the US and Canada), and the Chinese authorities. This work redoubled in the mid-1980s with the discovery that, despite this agreement, giant panda habitat had more than halved in the previous decade. So, there was an increased focus on protecting and planting bamboo (pandas' only food) and stopping timber production in panda habitat. However, a scientific study published in 2017 concluded "that panda habitat covered less area and was more fragmented in 2013 than in 1988 when the species was listed as endangered" (Xu et al. 2017, p. 1635), suggesting that at least some land clearing or timber production had continued. Nonetheless, surveys showed that panda numbers were slowly increasing over this time period. It may be the case, then, that much of the progress in wild panda abundance should be attributed to strict enforcement of an existing ban on hunting pandas.

Early phases of panda conservation efforts were founded on a limited understanding of panda biology and behavior. For example, during the 1980s, many panda cubs were taken from the wild into captivity based on the false belief that they had been abandoned by their mothers. However, later studies revealed that mothers would leave cubs for up to 50 hours at a time to forage (Schaller 1994). An important element in ongoing panda conservation was, therefore, improving understanding of behavior, diet, and reproduction. Research in the 1980s found that, despite being a relative of the otherwise omnivorous bear family, the giant panda is nearly 100% herbivorous, needing access to at least two different species of bamboo (Schaller 1985). This highlighted new problems: large stretches of the same species of bamboo were found to flower and die simultaneously. Such periods of bamboo death seemed to be a major threat unless pandas could migrate to other areas where different species of bamboo were not in flower. This, in turn, reemphasized the need for pandas to have large or at least connected areas of habitat, allowing them freedom to travel to access seasonal food resources.

Researchers also studied pandas using radiotelemetry to examine home ranges, how the pandas spend their time, and other aspects of panda behavior. Among other things, they found that the animals spend most of the time they are awake feeding (Schaller 1985); indeed, each panda eats massive amounts of bamboo, which has low caloric density – a staggering 12–38 kg per day (Nicholls 2010).

From the 1970s onwards, panda populations were surveyed once a decade. In the first two decades, the estimated number of giant pandas living in the wild more than halved from 2459 to 1216 individuals (excluding dependent cubs), leading the IUCN to classify giant pandas as "Endangered" in 1990. The 2014 count, however, identified 1864 individuals (IUCN 2016). Of course, this was less than their estimated abundance in the 1970s; moreover, developments in counting methods make the estimates difficult to compare. Nonetheless, there seems to have been considerable recent success in reversing the decline of the species. In 2016, IUCN assessors were convinced that sufficient progress had been made to warrant an upgrade of the panda's conservation status from "Endangered" to "Vulnerable." At the same time, however, the report stressed that "the giant panda will remain a conservation-dependent species for the foreseeable future" (IUCN 2016).

In parallel to *in situ* conservation work, the 1950s saw the launch of *ex situ* captive breeding programs in specialist centers in China. The first success came in 1963 when a female panda cub was born in the Beijing Zoo (Zhang et al. 2006). However, panda breeding turned out to be much more difficult than initially imagined; for decades, the population of captive pandas had to be continuously supplemented from the wild. The obstacles to captive breeding were significant, including a very narrow annual fertility window for female pandas (just a few days per year) and the need for both pandas to be able and willing to mate.

So, artificial insemination techniques were developed to try to improve the breeding rate. This led to some progress, but the main breakthrough came by a combination of two additional approaches. Every other time a panda gives birth, she produces two cubs, but only one normally survives. (In the wild, the panda mother will leave the weaker cub to die and choose to raise the stronger one. She does not have enough milk or energy to care for two cubs.) However, scientists discovered that both cubs could be kept alive if they were, from birth, rotated between incubator and mother, later being separated from their mothers entirely and raised in groups in panda "nurseries" (Figure 14.1) (Nicholls 2010). Second, more effort was put into adjusting natural mating to the behavioral needs and choices of the animals. Pandas that are mating prospects are now first introduced to one another via olfactory stimuli prior to the actual event. In addition, the Chinese breeding centers tried to give the animals their choice of mating partners; this improved both copulation and birth rates (Martin-Wintle et al. 2015).

Combined with efforts to improve care generally and feeding specifically, these initiatives improved pandas' survival to adulthood and led to a sustainable captive population that no longer required supplementing with wild-caught pandas. By the end of 2020, the global captive population consisted of 633 individuals (Xinhua News Agency 2021). That is, one in four living pandas was a captive animal – a few of whom, like the two pandas from Edinburgh, were rented out to zoos across the globe.

At present, then, the project of protecting the giant panda species seems to be having some success. Wild populations are slowly recovering and captive populations are growing. Since there's general ethical agreement about the value of protecting species like the giant panda (see Chapter 4), this seems like a good thing. Indeed, the panda in the wild is especially important because it also serves as an *umbrella species*: protecting its habitat could also protect a large number of other species living in the same ecosystem

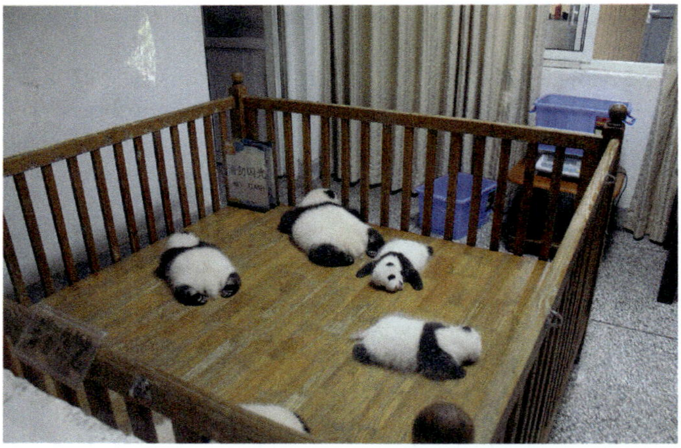

Figure 14.1 Captive giant panda pups, separated from their mothers, and being raised in a "nursery" within a captive breeding center in Chengdu, China. *Source:* Melissa Borquet/Dreamstime LLC.

(Li and Pimm 2016). Granted, some worry that conserving pandas and other so-called "flagship" species skews the allocation of conservation resources, resulting in the neglect of more needy but less charismatic species and/or other habitats that are important for biodiversity (as discussed in Chapter 13; see also Thomas-Walters and Raihani 2017). But we will not pursue this argument here. Instead, our focus will be on the ethics of *ex situ* conservation – particularly captive breeding of large populations of giant pandas and their display in zoos across the world.

14.3 Should Large Populations of Giant Pandas Be Captive Bred?

14.3.1 Captive Breeding and Wild Populations

Almost all panda breeding takes place in Chinese breeding facilities. The goal of creating these facilities was to help preserve the species not just in captivity but also in the wild. As discussed above, this seems, in itself, to be a valuable goal, especially from the ecocentric ethical perspectives we considered in Chapter 6. But how, in practice, could captive panda breeding contribute to conservation of pandas in the wild? There are at least three possibilities. First, captive-bred pandas might be reintroduced into wild populations and thereby boost numbers and genetic diversity, especially for more isolated populations in fragmented areas. Second, captive-bred pandas might provide an "insurance population" (Hogg et al. 2017) in case a disaster struck their wild kin. Third, captive-bred pandas might provide knowledge that could help protect populations of wild pandas.

Do China's captive panda populations contribute to wild populations in any of these ways? Let's begin with reintroduction to the wild. Captive-bred panda populations became sustainable around the turn of the millennium. At that time, the Chinese government initiated the Captive Giant Panda Project (Hong et al. 2019), the aim of which was to introduce genetic diversity from captive populations to small, isolated wild panda subpopulations that faced local extinction partly due to threats from inbreeding (Shan et al. 2014). Accordingly, 14 pandas were released into the wild between 2005 and 2018, 12 of whom were born in captivity. According to a 2019 paper, three pandas died soon after release (Hong et al. 2019). Based on these low numbers, the release of captive-born pandas seems to have played "at best a supportive role" in panda conservation (Lindburg and Baragona 2004, p. 274).

According to Zhang Hemin, one of the scientists in charge of the breeding program, there is some chance that, in time, the ability to release captive-bred pandas into the wild will improve (Holland 2016). However, it's widely recognized that the main problem facing wild pandas is a limited amount of suitable habitat; what's most needed is habitat expansion and better connections between habitats. Without this, reintroducing new captive-bred pandas to the wild is unlikely to make much difference.

What about the second possible contribution that captive-bred pandas could make: keeping a so-called insurance population? Suppose, for example, that the population size of wild pandas drops significantly due to an infectious disease or natural disaster – so-called stochastic factors that make small populations highly susceptible to extinction.

If a well-managed population of captive wild pandas could be reintroduced after the threat has passed, it might be possible to rebuild the population.

Given the patchy record of panda reintroduction so far, there's no guarantee that such a reintroduction would be a success. But it's certainly a strategy that *might* be important, and it has been used in other conservation cases. For instance, a sustainable captive population became a central plank of the conservation strategy for the Tasmanian devil in Australia when an unusual infectious disease nearly caused the species' extinction (Hogg et al. 2017) – though so far, large-scale releases of these animals have not been needed. So, while not guaranteed to succeed, the idea is plausible enough and does provide a conservation reason for keeping a sufficient number of captive pandas as back-ups for their wild counterparts.

The third contribution captive-bred pandas could make to conserving wild pandas concerns scientific research. Many of the findings regarding nutritional needs, reproduction, and behavioral biology of pandas originated – either entirely or in part – from studies conducted on captive-bred animals. Moreover, if the wild panda population became challenged by, say, an infectious disease, then a population of captive pandas may be an important target for research about how to prevent or alleviate such a problem.

So, if the conservation of the panda species in the wild is a good thing, then insofar as captive-breeding pandas contributes to the success of that goal, there's an ethical reason to breed them. However, this may not be sufficient ethical justification overall; there are also ethical concerns about breeding pandas in *captivity*. These reasons concern the welfare, and perhaps the rights, of individual pandas. Ecocentric views that focus primarily on the value of species and/or ecosystems are likely to be willing to trade off pandas' welfare for significant conservation gains, assuming these gains are forthcoming. However, from other ethical perspectives, panda welfare is a primary concern.

14.3.2 Panda Welfare and Rights in Captivity

As we saw in Chapter 5, "welfare" is a complex term that can be understood in different ways. On a narrow definition of animal welfare – one that focuses primarily on avoiding physical suffering and fulfilling basic physiological needs – captive-bred pandas probably have reasonable welfare, since they have adequate food and water and some space for movement.

However, as with most wild animals kept in captivity, the amount of space available for adult species members is significantly less than it would be in the wild. Furthermore, social relationships may not follow natural patterns. Panda cubs, for instance, are typically kept in groups due to the breeding schemes described above, even though they are generally solitary animals. In the wild, female pandas remain with their cub for at least 18 months and raise a cub about once every four years; in the breeding centers, by contrast, females are bred each spring and cubs are taken from them much younger than they would separate in the wild (Loeffler 2015). These practices may give rise to questions about panda welfare. Furthermore, some of the problems generated by the inability of male captive pandas to engage in natural mating may be linked to the way the animals are raised in captivity.

So, where *positive* welfare or welfare as the expression of natural behavior is emphasized, captive pandas may not do so well. Some of the problems here may be solved by changing the ways pandas are raised in the breeding centers. For example, keeping panda cubs with their mothers may improve welfare and the ability to breed naturally, though at the cost of breeding efficiency, and at the expense of the attractiveness to tourists of the display of groups of panda cubs at some breeding centers in China (Holland 2016). The breeding process itself also clearly raises some potential welfare issues. Stereotypic behavior, for instance, is especially expressed by male pandas in the form of pacing and head-tossing during mating season; researchers at Chinese panda breeding facilities concluded that "the pattern of increasing stereotypies during the mating season in males is largely the result of frustrated motivation by males to access neighboring females" (Martin et al. 2020).

What are the ethical implications of all this? From anthropocentric ethical perspectives that only consider human interests, there's nothing inherently wrong with breeding and keeping pandas in captivity. Similarly, if pandas turn out to have good welfare overall, then keeping them in captivity may be morally justified from a utilitarian perspective. However, if current forms of captivity impose welfare costs (as they seem to), then for captive breeding to be ethically acceptable, utilitarianism would require either improving panda welfare or (if this is not feasible) identifying the welfare benefits to humans, wild pandas, and/or other species that outweigh the costs imposed. So, for instance, if panda breeding had a substantial positive welfare impact on *wild* pandas by introducing diverse genetic material that improved wild panda health, the captive breeding program could perhaps be justified. But as we have seen, there's little evidence that this benefit has materialized so far.

From an animal rights perspective, it's difficult for captive breeding to be justified at all, even if the captive pandas have good welfare and contribute to the welfare of wild populations. They are, after all, being created as a mere means to protect the species to which they belong, whether through reintroduction, research or being held as an insurance population. For many rights views (e.g., Regan 1983), this would be ethically unacceptable. It might be argued, in response, that captive-bred pandas need not be understood *merely* as means. If someone selects a human embryo to serve as a "savior sibling" (see Sheldon and Wilkinson 2004) to provide matching bone marrow for a sick brother or sister, the savior sibling need not *only* be treated as a means to helping their sibling, even if the parents would not otherwise have had another child. So, there may be a window for arguing that captive breeding for the purpose of helping current or future wild pandas does not *in itself* mean that the captive-bred pandas have purely instrumental value. However, given the whole context of being kept in captivity, used in research, and being subject to reproductive technologies, most defenders of animal rights will judge panda breeding to be rights violating.

While animal rights defenders would object in almost any case, consequentialist approaches – whether their concern is maximizing welfare or the flourishing of ecosystems and species – are likely to permit trade-offs between the welfare of individual captive pandas and the flourishing of the wild population, either in terms of the welfare of wild pandas or the protection of the species and ecosystems to which they belong. The final answer, then, depends on how these trade-offs balance out in practice.

However, our concern here is not just with captive breeding centers in China. As we saw earlier in the chapter, some captive-bred pandas end up being distributed to zoos internationally. Do these displays contribute in any way to wild panda conservation? And is this an ethically acceptable way of treating pandas?

14.4 Is It Ethically Acceptable to Put Pandas on Display in Zoos around the World?

Pandas seem to have been displayed in China as far back as the second century CE. At that time, the species was treasured and people ascribed it healing powers (Catton 1990). However, it wasn't until the twentieth century that a panda was displayed in a zoo outside China; that first occurred in the USA in the mid-1930s. The popularity of the attraction led to a series of pandas being imported for zoo display.

However, access to pandas depended on foreign policy relationships with the Chinese government. From the late 1950s, the Communist government gifted giant pandas as "goodwill ambassadors," first for Communist allies and later for others; in particular, Chairman Mao presented US President Richard Nixon and UK Prime Minister Edward Heath with pairs of pandas following their state visits to China in 1972 and 1974, respectively (Buckingham et al. 2013).

In the mid-1980s, the practice of leasing pandas to zoos on a commercial (and often short-term) contract began. Initially, the pandas leased this way were taken from the wild, causing widespread objections in terms of CITES restrictions on trade in endangered species (Buckingham et al. 2013). However, around the turn of the millennium, the Chinese government switched to the current leasing model (the kind adopted by the Edinburgh Zoo). But the link between panda leasing and foreign policy seems to have been retained (which, though we will not discuss this here, may present ethical dilemmas for organizations and countries receiving pandas, in terms of discouraging critical responses to human rights violations in China).

Two changes to these leasing arrangements are of direct concern to our questions in this chapter. First, the rent for pandas is now earmarked for the panda conservation program (where it was used, for instance, to rebuild research and breeding facilities after a devastating earthquake in 2008). Second, the leased pandas are captive bred, not wild caught. These two changes mean that the display of zoo rental pandas no longer comes at the expense of the wild panda population; moreover, zoo pandas are contributing to panda conservation in China through their rental fee. Together with other reasons given for the benefits of zoos, could these considerations be used to justify pandas' display, despite the existence of ethical objections to zoos?

We'll start with the latter point. In-principle ethical objections are often raised against the display of *any* animals in zoos. These are generally based on the idea that captivity instrumentalizes animals (Regan 1995) or violates their rights to liberty (Rachels 1989). But other ethical theories are relevant here, too. Dale Jamieson (1985, p. 117) maintains that displaying animals in zoos is wrong for broadly virtue-ethical reasons. Zoos, he argues, present animals as separate from and inferior to humans, suggesting that animals can be used for our pleasure and our purposes. Accordingly, zoos teach us "a false sense of our place in the natural order." In so doing, visiting zoos may encourage a loss of humility or an inappropriate sense of human self-importance.

However, we will not consider these arguments further here. Rather, we'll assume for the sake of argument that zoos are not, in principle, ethically impermissible or problematic, but that to justify any welfare compromises for their animals, zoos ought, through their collections, to make significant practical contributions to promoting conservation.

And the more that good welfare is compromised, the stronger the conservation justification should be (Palmer et al. 2020).

A good place to start here, then, is with panda welfare in zoos. As in the Chinese breeding centers, the question is not whether minimal requirements are met: the pandas get to eat fresh bamboo and they normally live in reasonably accommodating enclosures. Still, there are significant restrictions on free movement and much of the rest of the behavioral repertoire of the wild-living panda is missing, in particular free mating and care of cubs for the females. So, there is reason for concern about panda welfare, especially in terms of positive welfare and the ability to perform natural behavior.

In addition, some of the specific arrangements in place with China are potentially welfare compromising. In particular, it does not seem to be in the best interest of the pandas placed in zoos overseas to have to return to China after a set number of years. There are considerable animal welfare costs associated with long-distance transport and very likely costs in having to adapt to a new environment in old age. These policies could of course be changed to allow pandas to stay in the zoo environment to which they have adapted (Yan et al. 2020).

While zoo panda welfare could be much worse, there are enough worries here to suggest that a plausible conservation justification is needed for the practice of putting pandas on display in zoos. Such a conservation justification, however, is not going to be *direct*, in the sense that these pandas are themselves candidates for wild reintroduction; and zoo pandas make next to no contribution to panda breeding, which is, after all, amply supplied by the Chinese breeding centers from which they were acquired. Rather, the pandas displayed in zoos seem to be a kind of "surplus" animal that is being *used* by being leased.

So, if there's a positive impact on conservation from displaying pandas in zoos, it must be *indirect* – and indeed, the arguments made in favor of having pandas in zoos typically refer to such indirect effects. As we saw earlier, the chief executive of the Royal Zoological Society, Scotland, claimed that the pandas in the Edinburgh Zoo helped to connect people to nature (BBC 2021). Perhaps those who see pandas in zoos become more aware of the need for wildlife conservation and more supportive of conservation efforts. And if pandas draw people to zoos who would not otherwise come, might there not be both conservation education benefits with respect to those visitors *and* financial benefits for conservation, since part of the revenue from the visit funds panda conservation?

Maybe. However, the jury is still out concerning the effects of zoos on visitor attitudes to wildlife conservation (let alone effects on visitors' subsequent behavior). Some studies seem to show positive changes in attitudes. One study, for instance, concluded that a zoo/aquarium visit "has a measurable impact on the conservation attitudes and understanding of adult visitors" (Falk et al. 2007, p. 9), strengthening attitudes and values regarding conservation and connection to nature. However, the conclusions of studies that show positive changes in attitudes have also been questioned. A 2018 qualitative metaanalysis of 31 papers studying empirical visitor research concluded that: "The overall evidence that the visitors learn about conservation and biodiversity, and even more importantly, that this learning results in behavioral changes, remains quite weak" (Nygren and Ojalammi 2017, p. 64). Another recent review concluded that "repeat visitors are more likely to engage in conservation efforts," but adds that little is known about whether people become more engaged because they visit zoos or whether they visit zoos because they are more engaged in the first place (Godinez and Fernandez 2019). So, there may be a correlation of sorts between visiting zoos and a positive attitude to conservation, but it is not clear that visiting zoos *causes* a change in attitude among visitors.

There may also be concerns raised by the ways zoos market pandas to attract visitors. For example, *personalizing* pandas by giving them names may detract from the issue of protecting the wild living panda *population* – this is why some zoos, including the Copenhagen Zoo (Mads Frost Bertelsen, personal communication), have a policy of not giving their animals names. Similarly, activities like celebrating the birthday of a panda in a zoo (Figure 14.2), while appealing to visitors, certainly does not contribute to conservation education of zoo visitors. And it seems unlikely that seeing a panda would in itself increase visitor conservation concern or commitment more than seeing other zoo animals. However, because they are highly charismatic, pandas do draw more people into zoos in the first place, so if there is a positive effect of zoos on public attitudes or behaviors, it's plausible that pandas displayed in zoos can amplify it.

A more tangible and seemingly obvious way in which pandas in zoos may have an indirect effect on conservation is, as mentioned above, through the significant amount of money channeled back to conservation work in China via the rental schemes. Leaving aside the conservation effectiveness of these schemes, however, even this ostensible benefit is somewhat complicated. The cost of the panda lease is very high and pandas' bamboo diet is very expensive to maintain. As an example, the director of Copenhagen Zoo estimates that the feeding costs for the zoo's two pandas equals half the cost of feeding all the other animals in the zoo (Mads Frost Bertelsen, personal communication). So, while pandas may bring in more visitor revenue, they are also a drain on resources. In fact (although this does not seem to have been the case for the Edinburgh Zoo) some studies have found that having pandas in zoos can end up generating a

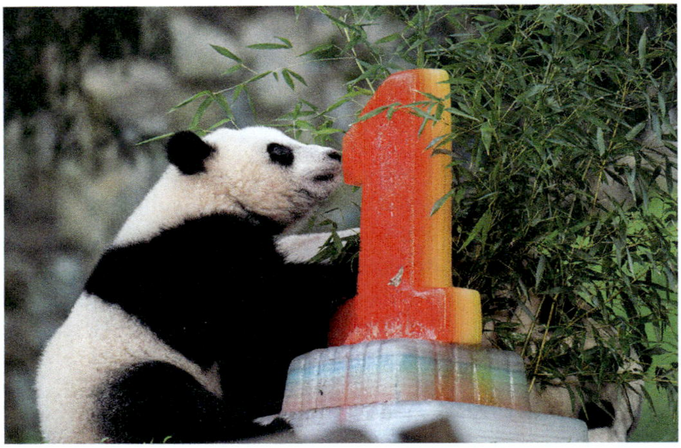

Figure 14.2 The first birthday of a captive giant panda is celebrated at Smithsonian's National Zoo, Washington, DC, USA. *Source:* Angela N/Flickr/CC BY 2.0.

financial deficit, thereby potentially diverting funds from conservation work to which the zoos might otherwise contribute (Driml et al. 2017). In terms of conservation funding, then, it's unclear whether the display of pandas is a net benefit.

Here's one final argument that could be made in favor of having pandas in zoos: it may help to build up relevant expertise for giant panda conservation. There's no doubt that when research in panda conservation took off, experts from San Diego Zoo and other zoos with experience of giant pandas played a key role. However, with the huge build-up of expertise in China, this kind of effect is bound to be of less importance in the future.

14.5 Conclusion

In this chapter, our focus has been on captive breeding and display in zoos of wild animals, taking the giant panda as a case. On animal rights views, both captive breeding and display of pandas are normally unacceptable. On other influential ethical views, however, where trade-offs are permissible, we have claimed that such breeding could be justified if it were to make meaningful contributions to the flourishing of the wild panda population and/or the ecosystems in which wild pandas live. To reach this goal, however, there may be good ethical reasons *not* to continue the expansion of the already large captive-bred panda population and instead to focus on improving, connecting, and expanding wild panda habitat.

With respect to the display of pandas in zoos, there's no positive effect in terms of *direct* panda conservation (by reintroducing to the wild, for instance). Given the various welfare compromises it involves, any defense of this practice must go by way of *indirect* positive effects on panda conservation (though such justifications will not work for animal rights defenders who reject zoos in principle). It's very difficult, however, to document the positive effect of seeing pandas (and other zoo animals) on the conservation attitudes of visitors. (That said, lack of proof of an effect is not the same as a proof of lack of effect.) There is a stronger argument in favor of saying that zoo pandas contribute via leases to panda conservation efforts in China but at the same time, costly pandas may detract from more pressing conservation efforts in which zoos may otherwise engage.

Overall, then, it seems that the conservation ends may justify the captive means for breeding limited numbers of pandas in captivity in China. However, even assuming zoos are acceptable in principle, given their welfare costs, there's at present little evidence that displaying leased pandas in zoos can be ethically justified in terms of their benefits to wild panda populations and ecosystems.

References

BBC (2021). Edinburgh Zoo's giant pandas to stay another two years. www.bbc.com/news/uk-scotland-edinburgh-east-fife-59562362

Brocklehurst, S. (2021). "Rock star" pandas – not exactly a love story. www.bbc.com/news/uk-scotland-23856890

Buckingham, K.C., David, J.N.W., and Jepson, P. (2013). Environmental reviews and case studies: diplomats and refugees: panda diplomacy, soft "cuddly" power, and the new trajectory in panda conservation. *Environmental Practice* 15 (3): 262–270.

Catton, C. (1990). *Pandas*. London, UK: Christopher Helm.

Driml, S., Ballantyne, R., and Packer, J. (2017). How long does an economic impact last? Tracking the impact of a new giant panda attraction at an Australian zoo. *Journal of Travel Research* 56 (5): 613–624.

Falk, J., Reinhard, E., Vernon, C. et al. (2007). *Why Zoos & Aquariums Matter: Assessing the Impact of a Visit to a Zoo or Aquarium*. Silver Spring, USA: Association of Zoos and Aquariums.

Godinez, A.M. and Fernandez, E.J. (2019). What is the zoo experience? How zoos impact a visitor's behaviors, perceptions, and conservation efforts. *Frontiers in Psychology* 10: 1746.

Hogg, C.J., Lee, A.V., Srb, C., and Hibbard, C. (2017). Metapopulation management of an endangered species with limited genetic diversity in the presence of disease: the Tasmanian devil *Sarcophilus harrisii*. *International Zoo Yearbook* 51 (1): 137–153.

Holland, J.S. (2016). Pandas get to know their wild side. www.nationalgeographic.com/magazine/article/giant-pandas-wild-animals-national-parks#:~:text=Like%20many%20endangered%20species%2C%20giant,was%20labeled%20endangered%20in%201990

Hong, M., Wei, W., Zhou, H. et al. (2019). Creative conservation in China: releasing captive giant pandas into the wild. *Environmental Science and Pollution Research* 26: 31548–31549.

International Union for Conservation of Nature (2016). IUCN Red List of Threatened Species. www.iucnredlist.org/

Jamieson, D. (1985). Against zoos. In: *In Defense of Animals* (ed. P. Singer), 108–117. New York, USA: Wiley-Blackwell.

Li, B.V. and Pimm, S.L. (2016). China's endemic vertebrates sheltering under the protective umbrella of the giant panda: China's protected areas and biodiversity. *Conservation Biology* 30 (2): 329–339.

Lindburg, D.G. and Baragona, K. (ed.) (2004). *Giant Pandas: Biology and Conservation*. Berkeley, USA: University of California Press.

Loeffler, K. (2015). Panda chronicles: a veterinarian's firsthand perspective on the health and welfare of giant pandas in China's breeding industry. www.hsvma.org/panda_chronicles_1

Loucks, C.J., Lü, Z., Dinerstein, E. et al. (2001). Giant pandas in a changing landscape. *Science* 294: 1465–1465.

Martin, M.S., Owen, M., Wintle, N.J.P. et al. (2020). Stereotypic behaviour predicts reproductive performance and litter sex ratio in giant pandas. *Scientific Reports* 10: 7263.

Martin-Wintle, M.S., Shepherdson, D., Zhang, G. et al. (2015). Free mate choice enhances conservation breeding in the endangered giant panda. *Nature Communications* 6: 10125.

Nicholls, H. (2010). *The Way of the Panda: The Curious History of China's Political Animal*. London, UK: Profile Books.

Nygren, N.V. and Ojalammi, S. (2017). Conservation education in zoos: a literature review. *Finnish Journal for Human-Animal Studies* 4: 62–76.

Palmer, C., Morrin, H., and Sandøe, P. (2020). Defensible zoos and aquariums. In: *The Routledge Handbook of Animal Ethics* (ed. B. Fischer), 394–406. New York, USA: Routledge.

Rachels, J. (1989). Why animals have a right to liberty. In: *Animal Rights and Human Obligations* (ed. T. Regan and P. Singer), 122–131. Englewood Cliffs, USA: Prentice Hall.

Regan, T. (1983). *The Case for Animal Rights*. Berkeley, USA: University of California Press.

Regan, T. (1995). Are zoos morally defensible? In: *Ethics on the Ark: Zoos, Animal Welfare and Wildlife Conservation* (ed. B.G. Norton, M. Hutchins, E. Stevens, and T. Maple), 38–51. Washington, D.C., USA: Smithsonian Institution Press.

Schaller, G.B. (ed.) (1985). *The Giant Pandas of Wolong*. Chicago, USA: University of Chicago Press.

Schaller, G.B. (1994). *The Last Panda*. Chicago, USA: University of Chicago Press.

Shan, L., Hu, Y., Zhu, L. et al. (2014). Large-scale genetic survey provides insights into the captive management and reintroduction of giant pandas. *Molecular Biology and Evolution* 31: 2663–2671.

Sheldon, S. and Wilkinson, S. (2004). Should selecting saviour siblings be banned? *Journal of Medical Ethics* 30: 533–537.

Stewart, K. (2021). Anger as Edinburgh zoo aims to keep hold of pandas. www.thetimes.co.uk/article/anger-as-edinburgh-zoo-aims-to-keep-hold-of-pandas-f3bq6g772#:~:text=Plans%20to%20extend%20Edinburgh%20Zoo's,of%20putting%20profit%20over%20welfare

Thomas-Walters, L. and Raihani, N.J. (2017). Supporting conservation: the roles of flagship species and identifiable victims. *Conservation Letters* 10 (5): 581–587.

World Wildlife Fund (2004). History of the giant panda. https://wwf.panda.org/wwf_news/?13588/History-of-the-Giant-Panda

Xinhua News Agency (2021). World's captive panda population hits 633. www.xinhuanet.com/english/2021-01/03/c_139637991.htm

Xu, W., Viña, A., Kong, L. et al. (2017). Reassessing the conservation status of the giant panda using remote sensing. *Nature Ecology & Evolution* 1: 1635–1638.

Yan, Q., Hu, Y., and Ye, H.B. (2020). Time to update China's panda loan terms. *Science* 367: 373–373.

Zhang, Z., Zhang, A., Hou, R. et al. (2006). Historical perspective of breeding giant pandas ex situ in China and high priorities for the future. In: *Giant Pandas* (ed. D.E. Wildt, A. Zhang, H. Zhang, et al.), 455–468. Cambridge, UK: Cambridge University Press.

Wildlife Research: Toe-Clipping

15

15.1 Introduction

In 2004, the journal *Science* published an article called "Do not touch my toes." The topic? Toe-clipping, the dominant method by which wildlife researchers mark amphibians, reptiles, and other small wild animals for subsequent reidentification. As the name suggests, toe-clipping involves cutting unique combinations of digits, or parts of digits, from the animal in question (Figure 15.1). First described in the 1940s, toe-clipping is a cheap, quick, long-lasting, and easily taught method; as a result, it has long been considered the standard marking technique for many species of amphibians and reptiles (and occasionally mammals). Here, we'll focus on the toe-clipping of frogs.

No vertebrates are more threatened than wild amphibians, with their staggering rate of species loss now known as the "amphibian extinction crisis" (Wake and Vredenburg 2008). So, it's particularly important to be able to reidentify individuals to track trends in diminishing wild populations. Toe-clipping has mostly been used in "mark-recapture" studies that allow researchers to estimate population sizes and survival rates of individual animals. Tissue clipped from toes can also be used to estimate the age of captured animals, for genetic analysis, and to diagnose infectious diseases.

Wildlife Ethics: The Ethics of Wildlife Management and Conservation, First Edition. Clare Palmer, Bob Fischer, Christian Gamborg, Jordan Hampton, and Peter Sandøe.

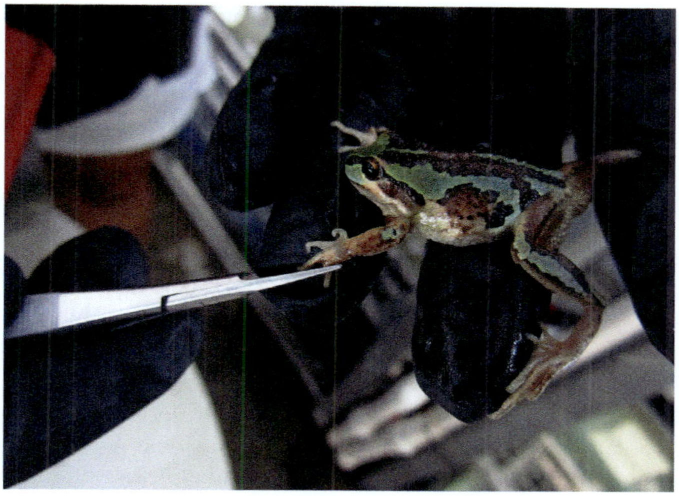

Figure 15.1 Toe-clipping of a digit of the left forelimb of a threatened Australian alpine tree frog during ecological research. *Source:* Courtesy of Laura Brannelly.

Together, this information can help provide a detailed understanding of an animal's natural history (Phillott et al. 2007).

The specific occasion for the 2004 *Science* article was a publication by two Australian ecologists, Michael McCarthy and Kirsten Parris, who used advanced statistical methods to reexamine data derived from studies on frogs and toads by means of toe-clipping (McCarthy and Parris 2004). In brief, they assessed the correlation between the number of toes removed and the likelihood of ever seeing that animal again; they found that the more toes clipped, the lower the chances that the animal would be rediscovered (the likelihood of recatching a frog diminished by 4–11% for each toe removed after the first). This study alone could not itself provide an explanation for the finding. The disappearance of the frog or toad might have been because the animals were more likely to die after toe-clipping (perhaps due to increased predation risk associated with decreased mobility). Alternatively, as a consequence of the treatment, the animals may have fled the area. But if either explanation is correct, the finding seems to cast doubt on the legitimacy of toe-clipping as a research tool, since it introduces biases into the data that researchers collect. If animals with clipped toes do not behave like animals without clipped toes, data collected from their movement or survival may not be reflective of what's happening to the wild population. This limits the value of knowledge gained from such research.

Questions about toe-clipping do not stop there: the practice raises ethical as well as further scientific concerns. Most obviously, toe-clipping is an invasive and likely to be a painful procedure for the individual animal; in addition, it may have long-term effects on animals' fitness, such as compromising climbing or "clinging" ability in geckoes (Bloch and Irschick 2005). And these animal welfare concerns aren't unrelated to the scientific concerns, as some loss of locomotion may be a contributor to mortality – which might explain the lower recapture rate.

But even if these worries about toe-clipping are legitimate, the practice could still be justified. If the practice helps to protect whole species from extinction, might it be a price worth paying? In this chapter, we'll think through some of the ethical questions raised by invasive practices like toe-clipping for the purpose of wildlife research.

15.2 Background: Animal Research Regulatory Frameworks

We'll begin by considering the context in which the debate about toe-clipping occurs. Research on wild animals is normally governed by the same regulations or guidelines as research with typical laboratory animals such as rabbits, mice, and rats. So, to understand the shape of the controversy over toe-clipping, we need to take a brief look at core principles of animal research ethics.

The use of animals in research has been controversial since the nineteenth century. At least in part because of its controversial nature, permission is required to use animals for research in almost all postindustrial countries (unlike the use of animals for most other purposes). To obtain permission, the researcher in charge must submit a proposal describing the project and its goals to a committee, typically an institutional animal use committee at university or research institute level (in North America and Australasia) or a committee formed by the state (in much of Europe). Similar processes are increasingly being established in other countries, where national guidelines for animal research ethics are being developed and research institutions are increasingly creating animal use committees (Retnam et al. 2016). These committees are usually formed from animal research scientists, but they also often contain ethicists and sometimes representatives of the general public or animal advocacy groups (Olsson et al. 2016). Research proposals are assessed in the context of widely accepted ethical principles, though different jurisdictions apply the principles more or less stringently, and some only work with the first of the three principles mentioned below.

The first principle requires minimizing harm to research animals. This is typically expressed using the so-called 3Rs: *Replace*, as far as possible, experiments using live animals with alternative methods; *Reduce* the number of animals used to the minimum necessary for scientific validity; and *Refine* procedures for the remaining experiments so as to minimize animal suffering (see section 13.6 below).

The second principle is that committees should ensure a proper balance between harm imposed on animals and expected benefits from the experiments. While it's fair to say that almost all countries with regulations on animal experimentation implement the 3Rs, this idea of a harm–benefit assessment, while widely accepted, is not universally practiced (Brønstad et al. 2016).

The third principle – which has so far really only been implemented in the European Union (Olsson et al. 2019) – is to put an absolute cap on the suffering that animals may endure as part of research. Experiments should not be allowed if they involve *severe* suffering. Of course, this requirement could be seen as a special case of the requirement to refine procedures, but whereas the requirement to refine is always relative to what is possible without sacrificing the goal of the research, the requirement to avoid severe suffering is more or less absolute (in the EU, some countries have so-called "safeguard clauses" allowing exceptions to the principle in special cases).

A wide variety of more detailed guideline documents have been developed in recent years to address these principles, including the PREPARE (Smith et al. 2018), ASAB (Bee et al. 2020), and ARRIVE (Du Sert et al. 2020) guidelines. The focus of these guidelines has largely been laboratory and domestic animals, but many of these principles also apply to wildlife studies and increasingly it is a requirement made by international journals, funders, universities, and other academic institutions that such guidelines are complied with.

15.3 Ethical Underpinning of Research Regulations

There's no simple one-to-one correlation between research regulations and the ethical theories discussed in Chapter 6, but we can see how these regulations might relate to different theoretical views. The fundamental idea of the 3Rs seems to be that all research benefiting humans is permissible, provided that suffering is minimized to the degree compatible with the research taking place at all. This appears at least weakly anthropocentric: since minimizing suffering matters, animals clearly count for something, but human interests always trump animal interests. If, however, the second principle is added, a genuine effort is required to achieve a balance between the harm imposed on animals and the expected benefits from the experiments. This makes the regulatory framework broadly utilitarian. It can also be defended within virtue ethics where contextualized practical wisdom – using reason and emotions to inform a context sensitive judgment – can be seen as key to achieving such a balance (Hursthouse 2011, pp. 134–138).

Finally, if the third principle is included, absolute limits are set to the suffering that animals may endure as part of the research. This could reflect several different ethical approaches: a consequentialist framework that prioritizes animal welfare (Hampton et al. 2019), the idea that human virtue does not permit causing certain levels of harm, or the idea that causing severe pain is incompatible with showing some minimal respect for sentient life. It might even be argued that this aspect of regulation, in absolutely forbidding some practices, reflects parts of rights theory (Beauchamp and Morton 2015). That being said, the absolute-limit view is not equivalent to a commitment to animal rights. One central idea of leading forms of animal rights is that animals should not be used merely as means or tools for the sake of others (even if those others are members of the same species). It's very difficult to reconcile a thoroughgoing animal rights view with animal research at all, with the exception of research from which the research subjects themselves stand to benefit (sometimes called "therapeutic" research).

This is, in part, because of the problem of *consent*. It's widely agreed that it's unethical to do research on humans without their free, prior, and informed consent (and some of the biggest scandals in medical research history were occasions when consent wasn't sought). Since animals cannot consent, they are, in this respect, like human infants, and the only people entitled to consent on their behalf are their guardians. Infants' guardians would not consent to potentially harmful experimental work that would not benefit the infants so, presumably, animals' guardians would not either, as that would not be in the best interests of the animals as individuals. So, while it's likely that at least some animal research can be justified from other ethical perspectives, only research that has no significant overall negative effects on the affected animals can be justified if animals have rights.

For the sake of understanding the debate about toe-clipping within the research community, then, we'll largely set aside rights theory and focus on the three ethical principles of animal research ethics mentioned above, and their associated moral frameworks.

15.4 Distinctive Features of Wildlife Research: Animal Identification

Wildlife research frequently has at least two features that distinguish it from (say) animal research to test human vaccines or experimental drugs. First, much wildlife research is undertaken either to gain knowledge about the biology and ecological relationships of wild organisms or, more frequently, with management and conservation goals in mind. So, the purposes and justifications for wildlife research often differ from those in medical research on animals, which has goals related to *human* health and welfare. (Of course, some wildlife research is also ultimately about human welfare, especially that related to zoonotic disease; see Chapter 16.) Second, while some wildlife research happens in captivity (with zoos, captive breeding, or wild-caught animals), the majority is carried out *in situ*, in field studies. These studies take very different forms, including merely observing animals (in person or through camera traps), habituating them to human presence, tracking their movements and populations, altering their environments, removing some of them, and relocating some of them. All these practices raise questions about potential harm to the animals, but the set of ethical issues we'll discuss here focuses on *identifying* animals.

Obviously, animals in the field are not contained and controlled in the ways in which lab animals are. Checking the whereabouts and welfare of any particular animal requires being able to *find* it. This means the animal has to be tracked or marked. The technology here has been dynamic. Many older practices are now ethically controversial, including banding the flippers of penguins, due to negative impacts on survival rates, reproduction or body condition of marked animals. Other marking methods have additionally become controversial for esthetic reasons, e.g., placing radio collars on tigers and branding pinnipeds (seals, sea lions, and walruses) (Figure 15.2). However, the debate surrounding toe-clipping captures most of the central ethical issues relevant to wildlife marking contexts, so we'll focus on that.

While there's a general consensus to the effect that toe-clipping should only be used "when necessary," there does not appear to be much consensus about when that is. The Australian Society of Herpetologists (2007), for instance, begins its position statement on toe-clipping by insisting that it "is the only practical and reliable long-term technique for marking some taxa." The US-based Association of Reptilian and Amphibian Veterinarians (2009), by contrast, "recommends that, when possible, toe-clipping be avoided," and is much more positive about alternative marking strategies. As of this writing, toe-clipping remains a common practice in amphibian and reptile wildlife research, and this leads us to the question of how it might fit with the research principles discussed above. To what degree is it ethically defensible?

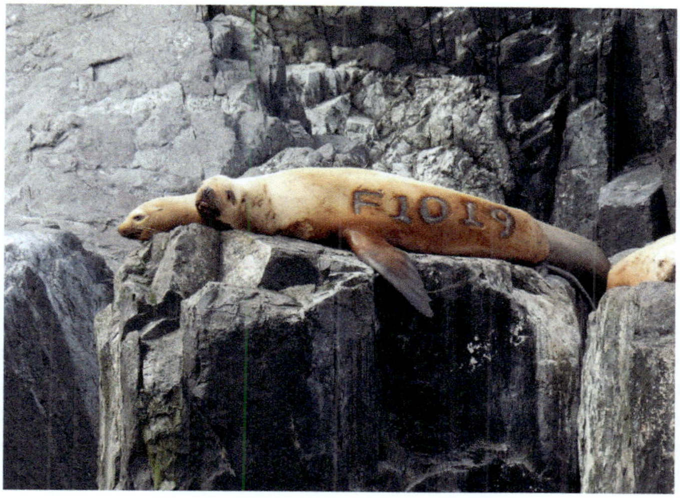

Figure 15.2 Freeze-branding of a Steller sea lion for ecological research, near Haida Gwaii, Canada. *Source:* Courtesy of Michael Jackson.

15.5 Toe-Clipping and Welfare

Before moving on to the research principles more specifically, the first thing we need to establish is what toe-clipping might mean for frogs. How does it affect their welfare – especially if they are going to be released into the wild after the clipping? Does it cause them significant pain? As discussed in Chapter 5, animals' subjective experience of pain cannot be measured directly, so various "proxy" measures are relied on. In this case, urinary stress hormone concentrations did indicate marked stress responses after toe-clipping (Narayan et al. 2011) (we'll return to these stress-measuring experiments below). This does at least *suggest* that toe-clipping causes pain (although as we noted in Chapter 5, cortisol may not always be a reliable measure of negative stresses).

Some researchers try to qualify this conclusion. For instance, one paper defending toe-clipping argues:

> While invasive procedures should not be applied without due consideration of the pain and stress caused to the animal, it must be remembered that mammals have a greater capacity to perceive pain than do other vertebrates. Toe-tipping/clipping amphibians cannot be considered as causing the equivalent distress and pain as digit amputation in a human or other mammal… In addition the Herpetological Animal Care and Use Committee (2004) regards pain as an adaptive response that reduces the use of an injured limb during recovery, and describes the use of anesthetics in procedures such as toe-clipping as undesirable. This reduces handling time and allows post-operative, field-released animals to adapt their activity to compensate for the affected limb/s
>
> (Phillott et al. 2007, p. 307)

There are three claims made here to defend toe-clipping. The first is that the *capacity* for pain experience is less in amphibians than mammals. This claim appears to be contested (for example, Machin [1999] claims that "pain perception in amphibians is likely analogous to that in mammals"; p. 2). But in any case, even if it were true, having a *lesser* capacity to perceive pain is compatible with having a capacity to perceive *significant amounts* of pain. So, even if animals are not anthropomorphized, by assuming that toe-clipping harms them as much as it would harm humans, care should be taken not to make an error in the other direction, assuming that if amphibians and reptiles have a reduced capacity to perceive pain, then toe-clipping is trivial to them.

The second claim is that in this case, pain is *useful*, since it means that the animals protect the damaged limb and learn more quickly how to move without the lost digits. (This claim seems to be at least in tension with the first, as it implies that post-toe-clipping pain is sufficiently bad that the animal will avoid using the limb.) The third claim is that the animals' *welfare* is improved by not using anesthesia for the procedure, since that means the animals can be released more quickly after the toe-clipping. The second and third claims together certainly create an argument that would be strange in human or veterinary practice. Imagine a finger amputation where the doctor said: "Better to do it without anesthetic, so that you quickly learn to protect your injured hand more carefully, and thus adapt to the lost finger more quickly." Admittedly, the frogs are being released into a threatening wild but as the McCarthy and Parris (2004) study may suggest, in this respect they would likely be better off with all their digits.

In sum, it seems reasonable to conclude that toe-clipping is experientially unpleasant for the frogs involved, and that it's also likely to affect their ability to perform some natural behaviors. So, it is not welfare neutral. This is important when we apply the research principles to the case. In the next few sections, we consider the implications of the 3Rs, the relative costs and benefits of toe-clipping, and the idea of a cap on suffering to our assessment of toe-clipping.

15.6 The 3Rs: Replace, Reduce, Refine

Strictly speaking, it's not possible to apply the 3Rs to toe-clipping without considering all the alternatives, which space does not allow. Still, a rough sense of what might be expected is within reach here. Let's consider each "R" in turn.

15.6.1 Replacement

Replacement requires using nonanimal models when possible. When studying wildlife, especially in the context of wildlife management and conservation, this is very rarely possible; there's no cell culture, for instance, that could help a researcher to understand how frogs behave in an ecosystem. A small number of wildlife research projects may be able to "replace" the use of living animals by obtaining genetic fingerprints from fecal samples or tufts of fallen fur. But in most cases, there are no relevant nonanimal models that could replace basic research on wild animals, particularly not in reintroduction projects, where there are no preexisting wild populations that can be studied. Refraining from causing suffering in frogs by substituting a nonanimal model is not going to work. So, this "R" does not count against toe-clipping.

15.6.2 Reduction

Reduction requires using the minimum number of animals necessary to achieve valid results. The number of frogs who need to be reidentified will depend in part on what the researchers want to learn. Are they measuring population size, favored habitat, how far individual frogs have traveled, or something else? Whatever the answer, reduction only dictates that researchers not clip the toes of any frogs unnecessarily; it does not count against toe-clipping in itself. Indeed, reduction may actually count in *favor* of toe-clipping via indirect benefits of the practice. If, for instance, toe-clipping provides tissue samples that can be used for other purposes, it could result in a reduction of the total number of animals captured, since fewer animals would be needed just for the purpose of tissue sampling.

15.6.3 Refinement

The third "R" – refinement – requires employing methods that minimize the harm caused to animals. The question refinement poses here is whether technique refinements are possible, either to toe-clipping or its alternatives, that reduce the harm to frogs.

There are possible refinements of toe-clipping itself. For instance, researchers can minimize the amount of each digit amputated (toe-"tipping" rather than "clipping"; Phillott et al. 2007). Alongside this, they can minimize the number of digits clipped, be careful not to clip any digits that are especially important for mating or climbing, and properly clean and disinfect all wounds.

However, refinement is as much about method choice as it is about improving any particular method, and there are many alternatives available, such as passive integrated transponder tags (which involves injecting a device under the skin that can be read by a scanner), visible implant elastomer tags (which involves injecting a liquid under the skin that turns into a pliable, brightly colored solid), and pattern mapping (where researchers identify animals based on distinctive natural patterns on the skin; Heard et al. 2009). Is toe-clipping worse for frog welfare than these alternatives?

That question is, at one level, easy to answer: pattern mapping is obviously better for frog welfare than toe-clipping. The problem is that it is practically impossible to reliably reidentify many species based on skin patterns, as they have no distinct markings. If pattern mapping was required for animal welfare reasons, some research (on those species without distinct markings) could not proceed. This may be the right result, but it is certainly not the approach that's accepted by most people who review research protocols. Instead, the standard approach is to assume that refinement requires using the least harmful method *that can deliver the desired results.*

So, this rules out pattern mapping for some frog species. What about other methods? Although microchips intuitively sound less painful than amputation, the tiny size of many conserved frog species (Figure 15.1) means that implants like microchips are relatively massive and their implantation can create relatively massive holes in the skin of the animal. It's difficult to make comparative judgments here, because the empirical data are ambiguous and depend on what animal welfare measures are prioritized. Langkilde and Shine (2006), for instance, used blood cortisol as a measure of stress; on this measure, toe-clipping appeared less stressful than microchip implantation in a lizard species; they also found that toe-clipping was less stressful than superficially trivial manipulations such as housing the animal in an unfamiliar enclosure. On the other hand, Narayan et al. (2011) (mentioned earlier) used urinary cortisol as a measure of stress and found toe-clipping to be more stressful than capture and handling alone in a toad species.

Another question here requires thinking some more about the "can" as in "can deliver the desired results." Is this a point about what's feasible given practical constraints? Or about what could be done in principle, given appropriate funding? The materials required for toe-clipping are cheap; they can all be secured for less than $100. As of this writing, a visible implant elastomer tagging kit, by contrast, costs over $1000 and a passive integrated transponder kit can be $5000 or more. If economic feasibility is allowed to enter calculations, then it means essentially pricing animal welfare. Depending on ethical perspective, this will be more or less problematic. If research committees are pragmatic, funding will be accepted as a critical constraint on what wildlife research is conducted and how it is done. This will tip calculations toward allowing toe-clipping, perhaps especially in the Global South where funding may be most limited (but amphibian species are most threatened; Wake and Vredenburg 2008). If, by contrast, economic feasibility is not allowed to enter the calculations, then it will be rare for toe-clipping to be justified, since there are usually alternatives available that, though more costly, have fewer negative consequences for the animals' welfare.

15.7 Balancing Harms and Benefits

The second animal research principle discussed above concerns the balance of harms and benefits. On this principle, animals should not be harmed for "trivial" reasons; there should be sufficiently weighty reasons to justify harmful research. Since toe-clipping does appear to harm frogs, there need to be significant gains from harming them.

Answering this question requires more thought about the kinds of knowledge that can be gained from research. In Chapter 2, we distinguished between intrinsic and instrumental values. The same kind of distinction applies here: knowledge might be valued intrinsically, in its own right, regardless of whether it can be put into practice. When science is pursued for these reasons, it's often referred to as *pure* or *basic* research. Or – or in addition – knowledge might be valued instrumentally. In that case, the value of knowledge would be because it allows us to advance certain other interests: in conservation, for instance, or in developing new medicines or technologies. When science is pursued for these reasons, it's often referred to as *applied* research.

Admittedly, this division may be oversimplified. One complication is that the results of a good deal of applied research aren't actually put into practice, so it does not end up having much instrumental value. For instance, much applied ecological research does not lead to conservation actions that follow the recommendations the authors offer. As a result, there is a vigorous debate about the capacity of conservation biology, as a scientific discipline, to effectively contribute to actions that preserve and restore biodiversity (Arlettaz et al. 2010), partly because many of the processes threatening rare species may not be reversible – such as climate change (see Chapter 18).

Where does the toe-clipping case fit here? The majority of published studies that use toe-clipping seek a specific kind of instrumental knowledge: they are applied studies aiming to improve the conservation of their chosen species, for example the threatened Australian alpine tree frog (Figure 15.1) (Brannelly 2014). No one expects this research to lead, say, to the discovery of chemical compounds that could have pharmaceutical applications; moreover, very few are projects seeking knowledge that people value intrinsically regardless of its application, such as information about amphibian anatomy or behavior. Given this, the argument for research involving toe-clipping needs to show that it does, in fact, have significant value to the relevant conservation objectives. Here again, though, we need to note the disconnect between conservation research and implementation (Arlettaz et al. 2010). For example, even if such a research project established conclusively that an infectious fungal pathogen is causing a rapid decline in the population size of an alpine frog species, there is no guarantee that this knowledge will enable the species to be saved from extinction.

So, this answer does not clearly settle the issue. In the case of toe-clipping, most published research has a conservation goal: it's aimed at finding out more about the conservation status of particular species, and whether strategies to protect or to reintroduce these species are working. It's worth noting that this goal needn't be anthropocentric; it might be ecocentric, concerned with protecting valuable species and ecosystems in their own right. In cases where research succeeds in helping to fulfill conservation goals – especially where species are highly endangered and, where if toe-clipping is not used, the research will not happen at all – then the research may be justifiable on this harm–benefit measure. The balancing of harms and benefits is going to have to be taken on a case-by-case basis.

15.8 The Severe Suffering Limit

The third principle, which is, as mentioned above, currently only part of animal research policy in the EU, is the severe suffering limit: there is some threshold beyond which harm to animals should not be permitted, however valuable the knowledge (either intrinsically or instrumentally) that could be gained from the experiment. In other words, there are some harms that no benefits could justify. In practice, many people now accept this. For instance, Harry Harlow's famous maternal deprivation studies from the 1930s–1950s, where infant monkeys were taken away from their mothers and placed alone in cages with surrogate "mothers" made of metal wire (Harlow et al. 1965), would not be approved by any committee in charge of assessing animal research today. (Though outside Europe where this principle applies, this may in part be due to the involvement of monkeys in the experiments; similar experiments might be permissible on rats and other so-called uncharismatic species – a factor that may also affect wildlife research.)

However, this principle does not seem immediately applicable to the toe-clipping case. Even though toe-clipping is likely to cause pain and possibly reduce animal welfare, it does not seem likely that it involves, or would lead to, the level of suffering that will typically be classified as severe. So, toe-clipping is unlikely to be ruled out on the basis of the third principle.

15.9 The Upshot

What's the upshot here? With respect to the first principle of animal research ethics, which enjoins minimization of harm to animals, the first of the 3Rs (replacement) neither counts for nor against toe-clipping, one (reduction) seems either neutral or slightly in favor of it, and the last (refinement) is difficult to assess, as it depends on how further research into the welfare impacts shakes out, the alternative marking methods available in any given situation, and the relevance of financial feasibility to the ethical assessment of research protocols. With respect to the second principle of animal research ethics, which focuses on balancing harms and benefits, many research protocols involving toe-clipping may have perfectly legitimate aims but be insufficiently likely to achieve them to justify the harm. Others, though, will pass this test. With respect to the final principle, toe-clipping looks to be in the clear.

So, it looks as though toe-clipping probably can be ethically justified in some cases, depending on how certain empirical and ethical questions are sorted out.

15.10 Conservationists' Concerns

Now, some conservationists may become concerned that the careful application of these principles, as we have tried to do above, might significantly restrict more invasive forms of wildlife research. Funk et al. (2005, p. 193), for instance, argue that "We believe it is less ethical to sit back and watch species slip into extinction than it is to use the best available methods to help to conserve them." Put another way, there's a view that invasive research techniques are sometimes inevitable, and that they are integral parts of animal research in the global pursuit of biodiversity conservation (McMahon et al. 2006). So, here there is an obvious conflict between animal welfare and conservation.

This is, by now, a familiar argument in conservation controversies: advocates for an approach that may compromise animal welfare defend it on the grounds that it may help to avoid further extinctions and/or support ecosystem flourishing. This view could be based on the belief that species or ecosystems have very high levels of intrinsic value, and that these deserve the strongest possible protections that should not be traded off against other goods, such as animal welfare. Or it could be a more consequentialist approach that weighs values – including animal welfare and species protection – against one another on a case-by-case basis. This approach allows trade-offs, and for that reason is likely to lead to significant animal welfare compromises where animal welfare is weighed much less heavily than species values. Both these views could accept something like the position Funk and colleagues advocate.

Surprisingly, perhaps, even some utilitarians, with the broad goal of maximizing good welfare over time, might accept toe-clipping and other more invasive research practices. It's at least possible that if the toe-clipping strategy really helped to protect a frog species, for instance by allowing the successful monitoring of a frog species reintroduction, then the pain undergone by the current generation of toe-clipped frogs could be outweighed by the good lives led by many more *future* members of the species, who would not have existed but for the toe-clipping of their ancestors. Taking a long enough view, then, it's possible that more individuals are benefited than harmed by toe-clipping. For this to work out, members of this frog species would, of course, need to have lives worth living in the first place.

Having said all this, and as we have pointed out several times, none of these invasive uses of animals would be accepted by defenders of animal rights. It also seems possible that advocates of compassionate conservation (see Chapter 8) would reject toe-clipping, as their guiding principle of "first, do no harm" may rule it out (Bobier and Allen 2022). So, even if there are utilitarian arguments to support toe-clipping, there will still be significant opposition from many others whose ethical focus is the importance of individual animals.

Conservationists may find much of what's been said in this chapter understandably frustrating, on the basis that different standards are being applied to wildlife research than to the ways other animals are treated across society. Earlier, we briefly mentioned seal branding (Figure 15.2). In the Southern Ocean, that practice became so controversial that the program was suspended indefinitely. The scientists who had been performing the branding argued that this suspension was unjustified, given that millions of cattle are branded each year (McMahon et al. 2006). Similar arguments might be made about amphibian toe-clipping. Millions of pigs in many countries are castrated and have their tails docked each year, mostly without the use of anesthetic; so, if that's justifiable for the sake of satisfying humans' preferences for meat, then it's surely justifiable to trim the digits of amphibians with the goal of understanding or tracking them better, in the hope of helping to protect species and ecosystems.

There does seem to be societal hypocrisy in holding wildlife researchers to ethical standards that are readily waived in agricultural and other contexts – a point that has been made by frustrated scientists (Hampton and Hyndman 2019). However, as we noted at the outset, wildlife researchers are members of a larger research community; they are not acting in isolation. Moreover, there appears to be ethical justification for the principles that the research community has adopted, including the 3Rs, cost benefit analysis, and a cap on suffering. A research community without those ethical guiderails might make some discoveries more quickly and with fewer financial resources, but it would also permit many studies that are now widely condemned as unjustified and cruel. So, as one researcher puts it, "As a sixth wave of mass extinction looms, conservation biologists desperately need the knowledge that comes from such field studies … however, there are good reasons why we need to think more carefully about some present practices" (May 2004, p. 403).

15.11 Conclusion

Toe-clipping of frogs to identify individuals reintroduced to the wild is an invasive research practice that harms frogs. On the other hand, it's also a practice that could, in some cases, contribute to saving the species of which the toe-clipped frogs are members. On some views, including many from within conservation biology, the importance of preserving biodiversity and species is likely to outweigh the harms to frogs – though this argument rests on toe-clipping (or any other form of wildlife identification) not biasing such studies. However, if the lives and welfare of *individual* frogs are taken seriously, ceasing such invasive research also deserves closer consideration, though this will depend on how the welfare of present and future frogs is weighed. Finally, it's possible that technology may come to the rescue: noninvasive ways of identifying even nonpatterned frogs may eventually become reliable and cheap enough to make the conversation irrelevant.

References

Arlettaz, R., Schaub, M., Fournier, J. et al. (2010). From publications to public actions: when conservation biologists bridge the gap between research and implementation. *BioScience* 60: 835–842.

Association of Reptilian and Amphibian Veterinarians (2009). Position statement: toe-clipping in amphibians. https://arav.org/wp-content/uploads/2018/04/Toe-clipping-position-statement.pdf

Australian Society of Herpetologists (2007). Position statement #1 – lizard toe clipping. www.australiansocietyofherpetologists.org/position-statements

Beauchamp, T.L. and Morton, D.B. (2015). The upper limits of pain and suffering in animal research: a moral assessment of the European Union's legislative framework. *Cambridge Quarterly of Healthcare Ethics* 24: 431–447.

Bee, M., Bernal, X., Calisi, R. et al. (2020). Guidelines for the treatment of animals in behavioural research and teaching. *Animal Behaviour* 159: I–XI.

Bloch, N. and Irschick, D.J. (2005). Toe-clipping dramatically reduces clinging performance in a pad-bearing lizard (*Anolis carolinensis*). *Journal of Herpetology* 39: 288–293.

Bobier, C. and Allen, B. (2022). The virtue of compassion in compassionate conservation. *Conservation Biology* 36 (1): e13776.

Brannelly, L.A., Berger, L., and Skerratt, L.F. (2014). Comparison of three widely used marking techniques for adult anuran species *Litoria verreauxii alpina*. *Herpetological Conservation and Biology* 9 (2): 428–435.

Brønstad, A., Newcomer, C.E., Decelle, T. et al. (2016). Current concepts of harm–benefit analysis of animal experiments – report from the AALAS–FELASA working group on harm–benefit analysis – part 1. *Laboratory Animals* 50: 1–20.

Du Sert, N.P., Ahluwalia, A., Alam, S. et al. (2020). Reporting animal research: explanation and elaboration for the ARRIVE guidelines 2.0. *PLoS Biology* 18 (7): e3000411.

Funk, W.C., Donnelly, M.A., and Lips, K.R. (2005). Alternative views of amphibian toe-clipping. *Nature* 433: 193–193.

Hampton, J.O. and Hyndman, T.H. (2019). Underaddressed animal-welfare issues in conservation. *Conservation Biology* 33: 803–811.

Hampton, J.O., Warburton, B., and Sandøe, P. (2019). Compassionate versus consequentialist conservation. *Conservation Biology* 33: 751–759.

Harlow, H.F., Dodsworth, R.O., and Harlow, M.K. (1965). Total social isolation in monkeys. *Proceedings of the National Academy of Sciences of the USA* 54: 90–97.

Heard, G.W., Scroggie, M.P., and Malone, B. (2009). Visible implant alphanumeric tags as an alternative to toe-clipping for marking amphibians–a case study. *Wildlife Research* 35 (8): 747–759.

Hursthouse, R. (2011). Virtue ethics and the treatment of animals. In: *The Oxford Handbook of Animal Ethics* (ed. T.L. Beauchamp and R.G. Frey), 119–143. New York, USA: Oxford University Press.

Langkilde, T. and Shine, R. (2006). How much stress do researchers inflict on their study animals? A case study using a scincid lizard, *Eulamprus heatwolei*. *Journal of Experimental Biology* 209: 1035–1043.

Machin, K.L. (1999). Amphibian pain and analgesia. *Journal of Zoo and Wildlife Medicine* 30–31: 2–10.

May, R.M. (2004). Ethics and amphibians. *Nature* 431: 403–403.

McCarthy, M.A. and Parris, K.M. (2004). Clarifying the effect of toe clipping on frogs with Bayesian statistics. *Journal of Applied Ecology* 41: 780–786.

McMahon, C., Bradshaw, C., and Hays, G. (2006). Branding can be justified in vital conservation research. *Nature* 439: 392–392.

Narayan, E.J., Molinia, F.C., Kindermann, C. et al. (2011). Urinary corticosterone responses to capture and toe-clipping in the cane toad (*Rhinella marina*) indicate that toe-clipping is a stressor for amphibians. *General and Comparative Endocrinology* 174 (2): 238–245.

Olsson, I.A.S., da Silva, S.P., Townend, D., and Sandøe, P. (2016). Protecting animals and enabling research in the European Union: an overview of development and implementation of directive 2010/63/EU. *ILAR Journal* 57 (3): 347–357.

Olsson, I.A.S., Nicol, C.J., Niemi, S.M., and Sandøe, P. (2019). From unpleasant to unbearable – why and how to implement an upper limit to pain and other forms of suffering in research with animals. *ILAR Journal* 60 (3): 404–414.

Phillott, A.D., Skerratt, L.F., McDonald, K.R. et al. (2007). Toe-clipping as an acceptable method of identifying individual anurans in mark recapture studies. *Herpetological Review* 38: 305–308.

Retnam, L., Chatikavanij, P., Kunjara, P. et al. (2016). Laws, regulations, guidelines and standards for animal care and use for scientific purposes in the countries of Singapore, Thailand, Indonesia, Malaysia, and India. *ILAR Journal* 57 (3): 312–323.

Schilthuizen, M. (2004). Don't touch my toes. www.sciencemag.org/news/2004/08/dont-touch-my-toes

Smith, A.J., Clutton, R.E., Lilley, E. et al. (2018). PREPARE: guidelines for planning animal research and testing. *Laboratory Animals* 52 (2): 135–141.

Wake, D.B. and Vredenburg, V.T. (2008). Are we in the midst of the sixth mass extinction? A view from the world of amphibians. *Proceedings of the National Academy of Sciences* 105: 11466–11473.

Zoonotic Disease: Bad Bats?

16

16.1 Introduction

Malaysia, 1998. Shortly after rural farmers discovered that their pigs were dying, the farmers got sick too. Extensive work from epidemiologists uncovered a hitherto unknown virus that they named after the village in which it was first detected: *Nipah*. All told, there were 265 human cases reported and 105 deaths from that first outbreak. It could have been worse: Nipah virus is as deadly as Ebola, with a human mortality rate of up to 75%. Unlike Ebola, which attacks blood vessels, Nipah attacks the brain and causes encephalitis (a symptom that inspired the 2011 disaster pandemic movie *Contagion*). And as we have indicated, humans were not Nipah's only victim; the outbreak also led to the death of more than one million domestic pigs. Some, of course, were killed by the virus. However, the vast majority were healthy pigs, culled by the government in an effort to stop the outbreak. So, in addition to the loss of human and porcine life, the economic impact of the Nipah outbreak was enormous: it led to the collapse of the once-thriving billion-dollar Malaysian pig-farming industry, as all the affected farms were shut down (Chua 2003).

How did the virus manage to infect both the pigs and the farmers? The story involves Nipah-carrying bats. In brief, the farmers had let their pigs forage under trees where

Wildlife Ethics: The Ethics of Wildlife Management and Conservation, First Edition. Clare Palmer, Bob Fischer, Christian Gamborg, Jordan Hampton, and Peter Sandøe.

bats had been feeding; this put the pigs in contact with the bats' bodily fluids. And the farmers, of course, were in contact with the pigs.

Bats have recently become notorious for carrying viruses that can affect people – *zoonotic pathogens* (in short, "zoonoses"). Many zoonoses have made their way from bats to humans in recent decades, including Ebola, Marburg, SARS, MERS, and Hendra virus. SARS-CoV-2, the virus that caused the COVID-19 pandemic, probably also evolved from a bat virus. The bats that were found to be the hosts of Nipah were not the tiny, shy, cave-dwelling bats that have been the focus of SARS-CoV-2 investigations; they were giant *Pteropus* bats, also known as "fruit bats" or "flying foxes" (Figure 16.1). So far, the only countries to have reported outbreaks are Malaysia, Singapore, Bangladesh, and India (and likely cases in the Philippines), all confined to southern Asia. However, the home range of the *Pteropus* bats that carry Nipah is large, extending as far as Madagascar to the west, Australia to the east, and China to the north. So, there is concern that Nipah outbreaks could occur in many more places.

The phenomenon of zoonoses originating in wildlife, exemplified by Nipah virus, reflects a disvalue of wildlife for humans that has been recognized for millennia, especially in the Global South, but which has been gaining much more attention recently in the Global North. In this chapter, we'll consider some key ethical issues relating to the threat of infectious disease spreading *from* wildlife. We'll also touch upon the less noticed reverse concern where diseases spread from humans *to* vulnerable wildlife populations. Ethical questions center on how much value wildlife populations or individuals have when weighed against human health – and how these values should be prioritized when they are in conflict.

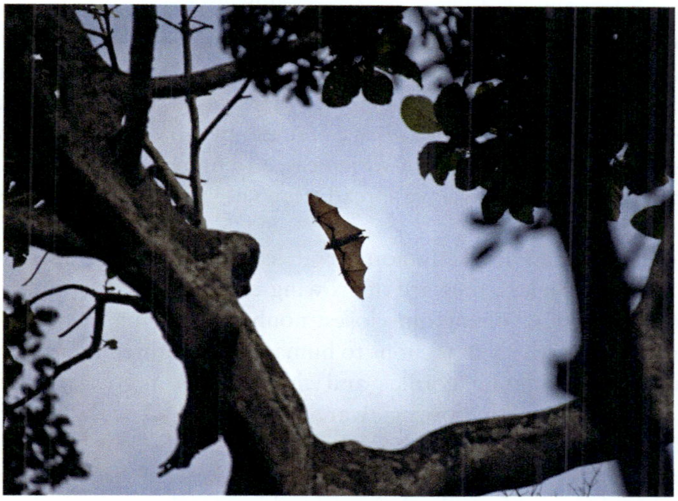

Figure 16.1 A fruit bat flying over a forest in Southeast Asia. *Source:* Keith Gentry/Dreamstime LLC.

We'll begin with a brief look at the relationship between wildlife health and human health and then move to one influential approach for dealing with such concerns, the so-called One Health approach (Gibbs 2014), which explicitly takes the health of humans, animals, and ecosystems to be connected. This will provide a framework for looking more closely at ethical issues raised by responses to the Nipah virus.

16.2 Wildlife Health, Human Health, and Zoonotic Disease

What's meant by the idea of *health* is much contested, though it's widely agreed that health is a general state of wellbeing, not just the absence of disease. The idea of *wildlife* health has already arisen in several places in this book: for instance, we discussed Aldo Leopold's contention that wildernesses are the healthiest kind of ecosystems in Chapter 3; the role of health in wild animal welfare in Chapter 5; and, in Chapter 7, we explained how arguments for sustainability can be framed as being about sustaining population or ecosystem "health." But none of these discussions focused on infectious disease. Due to the COVID-19 pandemic, however, concerns about preventing the spread of zoonoses have moved to the foreground.

Until recently, human diseases and animal diseases were generally understood separately. Recent global developments have, however, increased awareness of the threats that zoonoses pose to humans. There are also concerns going in the opposite direction: zoonotic diseases can also be transmitted from humans to animals. ("Spillover" is the colloquial term for zoonotic diseases passing from animals to humans; "spillback" is the term for zoonotic diseases passing from humans to animals [Daszak et al. 2000].)

One 2008 review estimated that, from 1940 to 2004, approximately 60% of all newly reported human infectious diseases globally had emerged from an animal reservoir. Approximately 72% of these came from wildlife, meaning that, as we noted in Chapter 2, zoonoses from wildlife accounted for approximately 43% of the 335 emerging infectious human diseases considered (Jones et al. 2008). One of the most famous such diseases is caused by the family of viruses that caused the last great human pandemic before COVID-19: AIDS, the disease caused by HIV or human immunodeficiency viruses (there are several), all of which came to humans from wild primates. (In fact, it's thought that HIV viruses have spread from wild primates to humans at least 12 times [Sharp and Hahn 2011].)

Spillback events are far less common, or at least far less well documented, than spillover events. Nevertheless, they are of growing concern. The best understood spillback processes are those involving our closest nonhuman animal relatives: great apes. Metapneumoviruses, relatively innocuous to humans, have caused fatal respiratory outbreaks in threatened mountain gorillas and chimpanzees in African national parks (Gilardi et al. 2022), leading to growing awareness of spillback within the conservation community. There are also concerns about spillback of SARS-CoV-2 to threatened species, including species of bat (Cox-Witton et al. 2021). Beyond viruses, there have been several documented cases of spillback from antibiotic-resistant bacterial strains into wildlife populations (Ramey and Ahlstrom 2020).

16.3 The Idea – and Reality – of the One Health Approach

One Health refers to an approach that recognizes the links between public health, animal health, and ecosystem health – and also disease. While this approach has been characterized in varying ways, an authoritative definition from the World Health Organization puts it thus:

> One Health is an integrated, unifying approach that aims to sustainably balance and optimize the health of people, animals and ecosystems. It recognizes the health of humans, domestic and wild animals, plants, and the wider environment (including ecosystems) are closely linked and inter-dependent. The approach mobilizes multiple sectors, disciplines and communities at varying levels of society to work together to foster well-being and tackle threats to health and ecosystems, while addressing the collective need for clean water, energy and air, safe and nutritious food, taking action on climate change, and contributing to sustainable development.
>
> (World Health Organization 2021)

The One Health movement started with a focus on poverty, endemic zoonoses, and livestock disease in developing nations. It gained global prominence after outbreaks of avian influenza ("bird flu") and SARS in southern Asia in the late 1990s and early 2000s. As the quoted passage indicates, the One Health approach "aims to sustainably *balance* and *optimize* the health of people, animals and ecosystems" (emphasis added). The commitment to *balancing* the health of people, animals, and ecosystems suggests that people ought to give at least *some* weight to the health of animals and ecosystems; it does not seem like a purely anthropocentric position. The commitment to *optimizing* the health of people, animals, and ecosystems suggests something even stronger: namely, that the goal is to make people, animals, and ecosystems as well off as possible. So, One Health does not seem to imply that human health should be optimized, whatever the cost to animals and ecosystems. Instead, it rather seems to suggest a *compromise* between the interests of humans, animals, and ecosystems – given the underlying aim of making them all as well off as humans can make them. This appears to be a kind of consequentialist approach that accepts health as a value (the health of humans, animals and ecosystems) and tries to bring about the best outcome overall, taking all these values into account.

There have indeed been situations where One Health approaches, at least at one level, seem to have yielded win–win situations for humans and animals. Take the handling of the Hendra virus (closely related to Nipah) in Australia, which also originated in bats but was transmitted to humans through domestic horses. There, neither bats nor horses were culled. Instead, a vaccine was developed for at-risk horses, allowing humans to yield health benefits without horses having to pay the price (Middleton et al. 2014). The bats, however, may still have lost out. The spillover event likely occurred because humans cleared land in the bats' habitat, thereby changing virus transmission patterns (Eby et al. 2023). So, creating a horse vaccine did not address the bats' loss of habitat (or the damage to that ecosystem), even if it did protect human and equine health.

More generally, though, the application of One Health from the outset was highly anthropocentric (Sandøe et al. 2014), with its initial implementation focusing on protecting humans from zoonoses. Essentially, One Health was used as an argument for recognizing a previously unappreciated instrumental value of ecosystems (see Chapter 7): namely, protection from spillover events or the idea of conserving nature to prevent the next pandemic. However, when human health is essentially all that's valued, animals, and flourishing ecosystems can be sacrificed. We've already described one example of domestic animals being sacrificed: namely, the healthy pigs on Malaysian farms that were culled to protect human health from Nipah (van Herten et al. 2019). This anthropocentrism has also been applied to wild animals, including culls of mammalian carnivores such as foxes to control rabies (Smith and Wilkinson 2003). So, a focus on preventing disease transmission to humans can, in many situations, come at the cost of both conservation and concern for the lives of the affected individual animals.

In Chapter 11, when discussing hyperabundant white-tailed deer in suburban US communities, we asked: "Hyperabundant for whom?" Here, in the same vein, we might ask: "Whose health matters?" As we have seen, the official One Health answer is that *everyone's* health matters, but it has not yet lived up to that ideal. However, we are going to assume the broader and less anthropocentric interpretation of One Health and use it to think about the ethics of different possible responses to the Nipah virus – while accepting that this is not the only existing or possible interpretation of One Health. First, though, we'll take a short detour to better understand one of the parties involved in the spread of the Nipah virus: bats.

16.4 Bats – The Bad and the Good

Bats have been so high-profile in recent spillover events that they have been termed the "supervillains" of zoonoses (Luis et al. 2013). This has begun to change the way in which many humans perceive bats, including in the Nipah story. Regardless of where they live in the world, "it's a bad time to be a bat" (Bittel 2020). Even before our dawning understanding of the disproportionate role they play in zoonoses, bats had a bad rap. Myths and legends have frequently associated bats with darkness and evil, cultivating negative attitudes toward them (Sieradzki and Mikkola 2022). The origin of these perceptions may lie in their nocturnal habits and relatively unusual physical form (for mammals, anyway). These preexisting biases against bats seemingly make it even easier for people to persecute bats when spillover events occur.

In the years 2020–2021, as the world struggled with the COVID-19 pandemic, a phenomenon began to be reported from diverse parts of the world: people were killing bats. Reports of bat-killing sprees came from Cuba, Rwanda, and Peru, among others. But the global region where this phenomenon was most pronounced was South and Southeast Asia, with mass killing of bats reported from India to Indonesia (Bittel 2020). Authorities in Indonesia culled hundreds of bats at an animal market at the early stages of the COVID-19 pandemic in a bid to curb the spread of the virus that causes the disease (Pinghui 2022), while in China, many people began requesting that hibernating bats in or near their houses be expelled (Zhao 2020).

Killing bats is not new. Bats have been a food item for subsistence wildlife harvesting for centuries and, more recently, have been culled to protect fruit production. But the *motive* unified many recent cases of bat killing: fear of bats as the hosts for viruses that may infect humans (Manenti et al. 2020). The presentation of bats as the culprits for spillover events, such as the Malaysia Nipah outbreak, has had repercussions for efforts to conserve their species (Rocha et al. 2021); it has also had implications for the welfare of individual bats. This type of wildlife killing is most akin to a practice that occurs when wild carnivores attack and kill humans or livestock, known as retaliatory killing (see Chapter 2). Given the extreme negative impact that COVID-19 had on human lives, unsurprisingly, many societies independently began to reevaluate their willingness to live in close proximity to wild bats.

But then there is also the *positive* value of bats. Beyond their possible intrinsic value as individuals or as species, there are instrumental reasons for humans to value bats, such as their contribution to ecosystem services (see Chapter 7). For example, they play a crucial environmental role in reduction of insect populations and thereby protect both crops and public health (since some of the insects are so-called disease vectors, spreading diseases to humans). Some analysis suggests that this role is so important that, for example, loss of bats in North America could lead to agricultural costs estimated at more than $3.7 billion/yr (Boyles et al. 2011). In addition, bats are critical to some locally important economic activities such as guano collection. Clearly, then, bats aren't all bad.

16.5 What to Do about Nipah?

With this background of the positive value, as well as the disvalue, of bats in mind, what can the people of Malaysia (and surrounding nations) do to mitigate the risk of further Nipah outbreaks? Let's consider the ethical implications of four possible options: culling bats; moving people or changing human practices; moving bats in non-lethal ways; and vaccinating people, livestock, and/or bats. We'll use the lens of the "ideal" One Health approach – the idea of "sustainably balancing and optimizing the health of people, animals, and ecosystems" to help think these through. (And obviously here we are just sketching the leading possible *ethical* options, rather than presenting costed alternatives evaluated for effectiveness.)

16.5.1 Culling Bats

Wildlife culling remains a mainstay of institutional responses to the risks of zoonoses (Degeling et al. 2016). While this option does not seem to have been officially considered in Malaysia or Bangladesh in the context of Nipah virus, other nations have been willing to contemplate mass culling of wildlife when human health is threatened. In Australia, for instance, culling of bats was discussed after only seven human cases of Hendra virus (Middleton et al. 2014).

However, mass wildlife culls seem to be problematic in at least three ways. First, they do not always work. In fact, they sometimes make zoonotic disease risks worse by changing host ecology and population immune status, for example by actually increasing disease transmission by enlarging the home ranges of reservoir species (Olival 2016). Second, in the case of Nipah at least, since most bats aren't clinically affected by Nipah, their welfare does not seem to be drastically affected by the disease itself so culls do not benefit the bats at all. Third, ecosystems may be negatively impacted by such culls.

Given this, while mass culls of bats could be justified from a wholly anthropocentric perspective (assuming the culls' effectiveness in protecting humans), they seem much less likely to be ethically acceptable from a One Health perspective that's attempting to optimize the wellbeing of humans, animals, *and* ecosystems. As we'll discuss below, this does not mean that culls are ruled out in principle from a One Health perspective, but they are certainly going to be more difficult to justify in this context than from approaches where only human wellbeing matters.

16.5.2 Moving People or Changing Practices

The second – and arguably the least anthropocentric – option would be either to reduce populations of humans and farmed animals in high-risk rural areas with dense bat populations, possibly in combination with mass reforestation projects to ensure that bats have adequate habitat, or to make significant changes to human practices in these areas.

There's a case to be made for both options, though both also raise similar problems. Human populations in many parts of the world, including Southeast Asia, are growing, increasing contact between people and wild animals. And other human activities may also be pushing wildlife into contact with people. Over the last two decades in particular, bats' forest habitats have been substantially reduced by deforestation. In 1997–1998, slash-and-burn practices resulted in the formation of a haze that blanketed much of Southeast Asia in the months directly preceding the Nipah virus disease outbreak in Malaysia. This was exacerbated by a drought driven by the severe 1997–1998 El Niño event, which was probably influenced by global climate change. This series of events likely led to a reduction in the availability of flowering and fruiting forest trees for foraging by fruit bats and culminated in their encroachment into cultivated fruit orchards. These anthropogenic events, coupled with the location of piggeries in orchards (Figure 16.2), allowed Nipah to jump to the human population (Chua et al. 2002).

This suggests that at least in this case, various anthropogenic factors may be driving Nipah's spillover into human populations, which is likely to be true of many other zoonoses. Some of these causes, such as land clearing, are obviously inconvenient to address (Coghlan et al. 2021). However, an argument could be made that since the causes are anthropogenic, it's also people who should pay the price, relocating to reduce the danger. (We'll discuss this kind of ethical argument shortly.) The case of Nipah also makes it clear that there are many more factors than the often maligned wildlife trade (Bezerra-Santos et al. 2021) involved in spillover events.

One difficulty here is that a line of argument that emphasizes moving people is in tension with most interpretations of environmental justice (see Chapter 8). Traditional peoples have been living in these areas for centuries, albeit at lower population densities (Ellis et al. 2021), raising livestock and trading wildlife without massive outbreaks of zoonotic disease (though historically, case detection capabilities were also low). Much of the deforestation is not the responsibility of these traditional peoples, nor is a changing climate. And on top of all that, many such peoples are relatively economically impoverished. To return to principles of One Health, while culling entire bat populations to solve anthropogenic problems seems unbalanced, so too does making traditional subsistence communities relocate to lower the risk of spillover.

An alternative strategy would be to change the riskiest practices rather than to move people. This is in fact what happened in Malaysia, where officials focused on ending pig farming in orchards in favor of other forms of animal agriculture. Similar strategies could

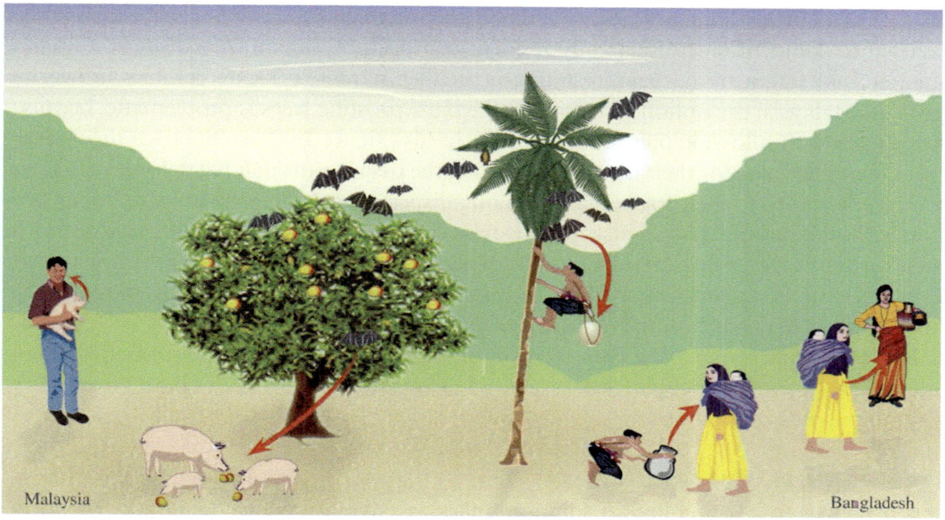

Figure 16.2 The Nipah virus transmission cycles in Malaysia and Bangladesh. Fruit bats are the natural reservoir, and the virus is transmitted to humans via contaminated fruit (Bangladesh) or via contact with farmed pigs that have been infected (Malaysia). *Source:* de Wit and Munster 2015/ John Wiley & Sons.

be employed elsewhere for Nipah, based on the route of transmission. In Bangladesh, for instance, bats infect people via raw date palm wine (Figure 16.2), so a solution would be encouraging people to refrain from that traditional activity (Islam et al. 2016). An even less invasive solution may be to protect trees being harvested for palm sap from fruit bats by constructing simple physical barriers (Khan et al. 2012). However, although the costs here are less severe than relocation, these are still significant changes to traditional life-ways, so this also appears to raise questions of environmental injustice.

In contrast to culling, bats and the ecosystems in which they live are relatively unaffected by strategies that require humans to move or change their behavior. However, the cost to human welfare may be very high. So perhaps neither of the strategies we have considered so far is "balanced" in the way One Health would suggest. A third strategy avoids killing bats but does not involve enormous human sacrifices.

16.5.3 Removing Bats

Rather than trying to move humans or to alter human behavior, people could instead make efforts to move bats or alter the bats' behavior. This could involve deliberately translocating whole bat colonies; alternately, it could involve what's sometimes called colony "dispersal" – scaring or harassing bats away from sites where they threaten people (Jeong and McCallum 2021). Alternatively, key bat roosting trees could be removed from villages or livestock farms.

This option seems promising from a One Health perspective. It looks relatively balanced: bats aren't killed and humans and pigs are protected from infection. However, being forced to move can be costly for the bats. If humans capture and translocate them, bats can be injured. Any kind of animal relocation, whether by translocation or dispersal, requires sufficient resources in the new location to support them and the bats are very likely to be exposed to competition from already resident conspecifics. Attempts to disperse colonies often end up fragmenting them, resulting in smaller, harder to locate colonies in nearby areas. In Malaysia, the option of removing the bats' roosting trees is problematic, because the farmers were allowing pigs to forage in orchards (Figure 16.2), so the trees themselves have economic value for their fruit. But retaining the trees means that bat colonies can later reunite and return to their former sites, making dispersal an ongoing process that may not do much to reduce the risk of disease transmission. (More positively, while there's often a question about the ecological impacts of moving animal populations, this does not appear to be an issue here; since the regions in question are already substantially modified by farmers, there may not be any additional ecological concerns.)

All told, while moving the bats seems more in line with One Health principles than culling bats or moving people, there are also reasons for concern about both practicality and the impacts on bat welfare.

16.5.4 Mass Vaccination

This brings us to a technological solution: mass vaccination, which could take the form of vaccinating people, livestock, or the bats themselves. Vaccinating people is the most common approach, though livestock vaccines have been developed to break transmission cycles (as in the case of horses and Hendra virus in Australia; Middleton et al. 2014). That said, vaccinating bats might not seem feasible. Even though there have been mass vaccinations of wild animals in the past, it's mainly been restricted to rabies. At present, no registered Nipah vaccines are available (for humans, bats, or pigs), which is a common problem for infectious diseases restricted to the Global South (known as "neglected tropical diseases"). However, vaccines are currently under development (Foster et al. 2022). If large-scale vaccination became feasible, it would likely be the best option from a One Health perspective. No one would be made worse off and humans and pigs would benefit. (Since bats do not appear to have symptoms of Nipah, they would not be directly benefited, but obviously they would no longer need to be culled or dispersed.)

If a Nipah vaccine becomes widely available, then, in principle, it should be possible to vaccinate both humans and livestock. Moreover, there are promising efforts to develop topical vaccines for rabies that transfer between wild bats which, if successful, could serve as a model for delivering other bat vaccines (Bakker et al. 2019). Still, vaccination is only a strategy for addressing known threats; it does not reduce the risk of new pathogens evolving and spreading from wild animals to domesticated animals or directly to humans. Moreover, the cost of mass vaccination – both in terms of R&D and implementation – is likely to be a significant hurdle, not to mention possible human social resistance to receiving it. So, while attractive from a One Health perspective, there are still some reasons against adopting vaccination as the main approach.

16.6 Ethical Views and One Health

We've now looked a bit more closely at how the broad principles of One Health work out in a particular case. Although it does provide basic principles for thinking through the case, One Health does not really give a lot of guidance as to how to go about balancing and optimizing the health of people, animals, and ecosystems. To be clear, this is not surprising or a fault of One Health: ethical investigation into this field is still developing (Coghlan and Coghlan 2018).

As an example, let us revisit the idea of culling. As noted above, the language of balancing and optimizing linked to the ideal of One Health sounds broadly consequentialist. But it is not straightforwardly *utilitarian*, as it includes ecosystem health alongside that of humans and animals. It also does not specify that balancing and optimizing should be carried out by giving *equal weight* to the interests of the many sentient creatures whose health is at stake. As a form of consequentialism, though, One Health shares with utilitarian approaches the idea that no solutions, including culling, are absolutely ruled out in principle (even though in practice there may be strong commitments regarding appropriate ways to treat humans). From both approaches, culling of bats *could* be the best way to balance and optimize the health of all sentient individuals, since the combined interests of people and farmed animals *could* outweigh the interests of the relatively few bats, even if the bats would have had good lives without a cull.

This inclusion of ecosystem health makes One Health an interesting kind of ethical hybrid between *individualist* forms of consequentialism, like utilitarianism, and *ecocentric* forms of consequentialism, like Aldo Leopold's Land Ethic (on both, see Chapter 6). Also, some individualists argue that there is reason to try to improve the lives of wild animals infected with debilitating diseases even where there is no obvious attendant human benefit, because suffering should be reduced when possible. We came across views like this in Chapter 8 (Horta 2017). Vaccination for infectious nonzoonotic diseases might be pursued on this view – assuming that infectious diseases cause welfare impacts in wild animals (Hampton and Hyndman 2019), that vaccinations would be feasible, and that it would yield outcomes that might be desirable.

Ecocentric consequentialists, on the other hand, would focus on attempts to optimize for *ecosystem* health. They would not advocate for welfare-improving medical treatment for wild animals independently of ecosystem gains and would oppose such treatments if reducing disease impacts were to lead to hyperabundant wildlife populations. But ecocentrists might support culling in the Nipah case, though of pigs rather than bats, as bats play significant roles in the ecological community. There are, for example, more than 530 species of flowering plants that rely on bats as either their major or exclusive pollinators (Fleming et al. 2009) and as noted earlier, bats also play a crucial environmental role in reduction of insect populations (Boyles et al. 2011).

There are some examples, however, where ecocentric and individualistic concerns might align – for instance, in the case of devil facial tumor disease in Tasmanian devils (McCallum and Hocking 2005), where large numbers of animals have been removed from wild populations into disease-free captive breeding colonies, but with a view to later wild reintroduction. However, such cases aren't that common. For One Health, the real difficulty is how to go about *balancing* the potentially competing interests of humans, sentient animals, and ecosystems, without any obvious "single currency" in which to convert these different values.

One Health, and other forms of consequentialism such as utilitarianism and ecocentrism, aren't the only frameworks for thinking about ethics and zoonoses. Other ethical approaches pick up on some different and important ways of thinking ethically about zoonotic disease transmission – in particular, the role of humans in creating the problem.

Thus, One Health has also in recent years given rise to the idea of One Welfare, a framework that aims to align interest in the welfare of humans, animals (including wild animals), and even the environment (Pinillos 2018).

16.7 Contextual Ethics and Anthropogenic Influence

The Nipah case brings out the possibility of human involvement in the spread of wildlife diseases – and therefore for both spillovers and spillbacks. If humans are at least partially causally responsible, then on *contextual* ethical views (see Chapter 6) they may have special moral responsibilities related to the harms they create. The issue here is not just about direct transmission of disease. It's also about changing environments in ways that make diseases spread more easily (between wild animals, as well as between humans and wildlife). Indeed, some critics of One Health suggest that the focus of disease investigations is too often on proximate animal causes for spillovers, especially where ultimate causes (e.g., land clearing) are inconvenient to address (Coghlan et al. 2021).

So, is there a significant anthropogenic influence on wildlife disease? In some cases of spillback, the answer is clearly *yes*, as when mountain gorillas directly contract metapneumoviruses from humans (Gilardi et al. 2022). In general, though, the short answer seems to be: *probably*, though often rather indirectly (Crozier and Schulte-Hostedde 2014). Some pathogens have clearly spread globally via anthropogenic means, such as the nonzoonotic chytrid fungus that has decimated the world's amphibian populations (Weldon et al. 2004). In other cases, human involvement is more complicated. The scientific consensus is that many factors are contributing to disease emergence, including climate change, globalization, and urbanization, and most of these factors are caused by humans (Lindahl and Grace 2015). As we have already seen, a series of human practices from farming to land clearing allowed Nipah to jump to the human population (Chua et al. 2002). A similar story emerged in Bangladesh, which has lost nearly three-quarters of its forest in the last three decades as the country's human population more than doubled, to 165 million. The point is that human habitat change in the form of deforestation is at least partly responsible for the spread of Nipah to humans (Islam et al. 2016).

If many wildlife disease events are, at least partly, anthropogenic, what does this mean from a contextual account of ethics? First, perhaps, it may suggest an increased focus on *prevention*, trying to mitigate the human activities that boost the risk of spillovers and spillbacks occurring, rather than banking on "end-of-pipe" treatment or containment options. This may also imply retreating from interaction with at-risk species (Gilardi et al. 2022). Second, it might provide a justification to refrain from harming wild (or domestic) animals in response to spillovers or, more positively, even to help them, since humans are to some degree causally responsible for disease emergence in the first place.

The general idea here is that spillovers aren't really ways that wild animals are harming people, but ways that people are harming wild animals and themselves. Accordingly, people should take responsibility. Having said all this, however, some caution is warranted; the origins of emerging diseases are complex, dynamic, and differ from place to place. So, we need to beware of *any* simplistic “origin narrative” for any particular zoonotic disease, let alone wildlife diseases in general.

16.8 Other Ethical Concerns

Beyond consequentialist and contextual views, animal rights theory would probably preclude culling any animals, whether wild or farmed. The exceptions would be cases where humans are truly acting in self-defense or where it would be better for the animals themselves to be culled, perhaps due to the suffering caused by the clinical effects of the disease. So, while there could still be an attempt to balance and optimize for the health of people, animals, and ecosystems, there would be strict constraints on the ways in which that goal could be pursued. And since animal rights theory does not assign rights to ecosystems, it would be acceptable to compromise ecosystem health to respect those constraints. So, if bat colonies could be dispersed in ways that harm the bats minimally but negatively affect flowering plants, then as long as there were not any other negative effects on other sentient beings (i.e., other rights holders, according to this view), that would be acceptable.

Similar points could well be made from the perspective of various wildlife management and conservation paradigms (Chapters 7 and 8). For instance, compassionate conservation would interpret balancing and optimizing in terms of finding ways for there to be “peaceful coexistence” between bats and humans (Wallach et al. 2018), which again seems to imply that bats should not be killed. A commitment to environmental justice, however, as noted, would likely insist that traditional and Indigenous peoples should not be excluded from areas where there is a high risk of spillover nor prevented from engaging in traditional practices, such as making date palm wine in Bangladesh (Figure 16.2). In addition, traditional and Indigenous peoples should not be left with the blame for spillovers significantly influenced by practices like forest clearing – practices that may be supporting the lifestyles of much more affluent others.

The perspective of virtue ethics may also be important here – and may, in fact, provide some support for adopting a One Health approach in the first place. Tom Hill (1983) argued that an important trait for developing environmental virtues is the recognition of one’s humble place in the universe. One Health, with its acceptance that human, animal, and ecosystem health are deeply entwined, undermines ideas of human superiority and exceptionalism; humans, like all animals, have bodies vulnerable to hazards and diseases. In this respect, it’s important to recognize that we are all in it together.

16.9 Conclusion

The spread of infectious diseases from wildlife to humans has been a long-term challenge associated with living around wild animals. Since the 1990s, cases such as the Nipah outbreak described in this chapter have become a global concern given high political priority. The framework of One Health has, over time, developed to deal with this concern, but it has also raised new ethical questions regarding how human societies can coexist with wildlife and the risks to our own health of doing so.

The idea of One Health – at least, in the terms in which we have discussed it – rests on the view that it is important to *try* to balance and optimize the health of people, animals, and ecosystems. That alone resists the most extreme forms of anthropocentrism and ecocentrism, which direct us to optimize for just one of the three concerns that One Health identifies. However, the idea of One Health also illustrates the difficult trade-offs involved when public health is in tension not only with the interests of wildlife, but also with what's good for ecosystems.

Important though this issue is, there has been relatively little written on ethics and wildlife disease thus far. Presumably, the COVID-19 outbreak will change this. A growing concern about wildlife-based zoonoses is going to raise vexing questions about our future interactions with wildlife. Will it be safe for people to be around wild (and in some cases, domesticated) animals? And will it be safe for them to be around us? The short answer is: Probably not. How humans manage these risks and the competing interests involved will, in part, come down to which values are prioritized.

It's worth pondering how other nations may have dealt with the situation in which Malaysia found itself in the 1990s. It's likely that some societies would have focused on removing bats rather than changing human livelihoods. Moreover, if spillover events continue to originate from this group of species, some human communities are likely to reassess their willingness to tolerate the presence of bat colonies around their settlements. We may not have to wait long to find out the answer to this question: there have been multiple outbreaks of Nipah virus reported in humans in India since 2018 (Aborode et al. 2022).

References

Aborode, A.T., Wireko, A.A., Mehta, A. et al. (2022). Concern over Nipah virus cases amidst the COVID-19 pandemic in India. *Journal of Medical Virology* 94 (8): 3488–3490.

Bakker, K.M., Rocke, T.E., Osorio, J.E. et al. (2019). Fluorescent biomarkers demonstrate prospects for spreadable vaccines to control disease transmission in wild bats. *Nature Ecology and Evolution* 3: 1697–1704.

Bezerra-Santos, M.A., Mendoza-Roldan, J.A., Thompson, R.A. et al. (2021). Illegal wildlife trade: a gateway to zoonotic infectious diseases. *Trends in Parasitology* 37 (3): 181–184.

Bittel, J. (2020). Experts urge people all over the world to stop killing bats out of fears of coronavirus.www.nrdc.org/stories/experts-urge-people-all-over-world-stop-killing-bats-out-fears-coronavirus

Boyles, J.G., Cryan, P.M., McCracken, G.F., and Kunz, T.H. (2011). Economic importance of bats in agriculture. *Science* 332 (6025): 41–42.

Chua, K.B. (2003). Nipah virus outbreak in Malaysia. *Journal of Clinical Virology* 26 (3): 265–275.

Chua, K.B., Chua, B.H., and Wang, C.W. (2002). Anthropogenic deforestation, El Niño and the emergence of Nipah virus in Malaysia. *Malaysian Journal of Pathology* 24 (1): 15–21.

Coghlan, S. and Coghlan, B.J. (2018). One health, bioethics, and nonhuman ethics. *American Journal of Bioethics* 18 (11): 3–5.

Coghlan, S., Coghlan, B.J., Capon, A., and Singer, P. (2021). A bolder one health: expanding the moral circle to optimize health for all. *One Health Outlook* 3 (1): 1–4.

Cox-Witton, K., Baker, M.L., Edson, D. et al. (2021). Risk of SARS-CoV-2 transmission from humans to bats–An Australian assessment. *One Health* 13: 100247.

Crozier, G.K.D. and Schulte-Hostedde, A.I. (2014). The ethical dimensions of wildlife disease management in an evolutionary context. *Evolutionary Applications* 7 (7): 788–798.

Daszak, P., Cunningham, A.A., and Hyatt, A.D. (2000). Emerging infectious diseases of wildlife – threats to biodiversity and human health. *Science* 287 (5452): 443–449.

Degeling, C., Lederman, Z., and Rock, M. (2016). Culling and the common good: re-evaluating harms and benefits under the one health paradigm. *Public Health Ethics* 9 (3): 244–254.

Eby, P., Peel, A.J., Hoegh, A. et al. (2023). Pathogen spillover driven by rapid changes in bat ecology. *Nature* 613 (7943): 340–344.

Ellis, E.C., Gauthier, N., Klein Goldewijk, K. et al. (2021). People have shaped most of terrestrial nature for at least 12,000 years. *Proceedings of the National Academy of Science USA* 118: e2023483118.

Fleming, T.H., Geiselman, C., and Kress, W.J. (2009). The evolution of bat pollination: a phylogenetic perspective. *Annals of Botany* 104 (6): 1017–1043.

Foster, S.L., Woolsey, C., Borisevich, V. et al. (2022). A recombinant VSV-vectored vaccine rapidly protects nonhuman primates against lethal Nipah virus disease. *Proceedings of the National Academy of Sciences* 119 (12): e2200065119.

Gibbs, E.P.J. (2014). The evolution of one health: a decade of progress and challenges for the future. *Veterinary Record* 174 (4): 85–91.

Gilardi, K., Nziza, J., Ssebide, B. et al. (2022). Endangered mountain gorillas and COVID-19: one health lessons for prevention and preparedness during a global pandemic. *American Journal of Primatology* 84 (4–5): e23291.

Hampton, J.O. and Hyndman, T.H. (2019). Underaddressed animal-welfare issues in conservation. *Conservation Biology* 33: 803–811.

van Herten, J., Bovenkerk, B., and Verweij, M. (2019). One health as a moral dilemma: towards a socially responsible zoonotic disease control. *Zoonoses and Public Health* 66 (1): 26–34.

Hill, T. (1983). Ideals of human excellence and preserving natural environments. *Environmental Ethics* 5 (3): 211–224.

Horta, O. (2017). Animal suffering in nature: the case for intervention. *Environmental Ethics* 39 (3): 261–279.

Islam, M.S., Sazzad, H.M., Satter, S.M. et al. (2016). Nipah virus transmission from bats to humans associated with drinking traditional liquor made from date palm sap, Bangladesh, 2011–2014. *Emerging Infectious Diseases* 22 (4): 664–670.

Jeong, J. and McCallum, H. (2021). Using stochastic modeling to predict the effect of culling and colony dispersal of bats on zoonotic viral epidemics. *Vector Borne and Zoonotic Diseases* 21 (5): 369–377.

Jones, K.E., Patel, N.G., Levy, M.A. et al. (2008). Global trends in emerging infectious diseases. *Nature* 451 (7181): 990–993.

Khan, S.U., Gurley, E.S., Hossain, M.J. et al. (2012). A randomized controlled trial of interventions to impede date palm sap contamination by bats to prevent Nipah virus transmission in Bangladesh. *PLoS One* 7 (8): e42689.

Lindahl, J.F. and Grace, D. (2015). The consequences of human actions on risks for infectious diseases: a review. *Infection Ecology and Epidemiology* 5: 30048.

Luis, A.D., Hayman, D.T.S., O'Shea, T.J. et al. (2013). A comparison of bats and rodents as reservoirs of zoonotic viruses: are bats special? *Proceedings of the Royal Society B* 280: 20122753.

Manenti, R., Mori, E., and Di Canio, V. (2020). The good, the bad and the ugly of

COVID-19 lockdown effects on wildlife conservation: insights from the first European locked down country. *Biological Conservation* 249: 108728.

McCallum, H. and Hocking, B.A. (2005). Reflecting on ethical and legal issues in wildlife disease. *Bioethics* 19 (4): 336–347.

Middleton, D., Pallister, J., Klein, R. et al. (2014). Hendra virus vaccine, a one health approach to protecting horse, human, and environmental health. *Emerging Infectious Diseases* 20 (3): 372–379.

Olival, K.J. (2016). To cull, or not to cull, bat is the question. *EcoHealth* 13 (1): 6–8.

Pinghui, Z. (2022). Do bats carry deadly viruses? Yes. Would a cull help? No. Here's why. www.scmp.com/news/china/science/article/3169976/do-bats-carry-deadly-viruses-yes-would-cull-help-no-heres-why

Pinillos, R.G. (2018). *One Welfare: A Framework to Improve Animal Welfare and Human Well-Being*. Wallingford, UK: CAB International.

Ramey, A.M. and Ahlstrom, C.A. (2020). Antibiotic resistant bacteria in wildlife: perspectives on trends, acquisition and dissemination, data gaps, and future directions. *Journal of Wildlife Diseases* 56 (1): 1–15.

Rocha, R., Aziz, S.A., Brook, C.E. et al. (2021). Bat conservation and zoonotic disease risk: a research agenda to prevent misguided persecution in the aftermath of COVID-19. *Animal Conservation* 24 (3): 303–307.

Sandøe, P., Palmer, C., Corr, S. et al. (2014). Canine and feline obesity: a One Health perspective. *Veterinary Record* 175 (24): 610–616.

Sharp, P.M. and Hahn, B.H. (2011). Origins of HIV and the AIDS pandemic. *Cold Spring Harbor Perspectives in Medicine* 1 (1): a006841.

Sieradzki, A. and Mikkola, H. (2022). Bats in folklore and culture: a review of historical perceptions around the world. In: *Bats – Disease-Prone But Beneficial* (ed. H. Mikkola), 3–21. London, UK: IntechOpen.

Smith, G.C. and Wilkinson, D. (2003). Modeling control of rabies outbreaks in red fox populations to evaluate culling, vaccination, and vaccination combined with fertility control. *Journal of Wildlife Diseases* 39 (2): 278–286.

Wallach, A.D., Bekoff, M., Batavia, C. et al. (2018). Summoning compassion to address the challenges of conservation. *Conservation Biology* 32 (6): 1255–1265.

Weldon, C., Du Preez, L.H., Hyatt, A.D. et al. (2004). Origin of the amphibian chytrid fungus. *Emerging Infectious Diseases* 10 (12): 2100.

de Wit, E. and Munster, V.J. (2015). Animal models of disease shed light on Nipah virus pathogenesis and transmission. *Journal of Pathology* 235: 196–205.

World Health Organization (2021). Tripartite and UNEP support OHHLEP's definition of "One Health". www.who.int/news/item/01-12-2021-tripartite-and-unep-support-ohhleps-definition-of-one-health

Zhao, H. (2020). COVID-19 drives new threat to bats in China. *Science* 367 (6485): 1436.

The Cost of Green Energy: Wildlife and Wind Power

17

17.1 Introduction

In 2021, Mongabay – a US-based nonprofit conservation and environmental science news platform – reported that conservationists in Brazil had "raised alarms" about the construction of a new wind farm (Camargo 2021). This wind farm, proposed by the French renewable energy developer Voltalia, was to be built in Brazil's northeastern Bahia state – a region that is also the last stronghold of an endangered species, an iconic blue parrot (Figure 17.1) called the Lear's (or "indigo") macaw (Camargo 2021). The Lear's macaw has been the target of conservation efforts since being discovered in the wild in 1978, when it had an estimated population of 60 individuals (Barbosa and Tella 2019), and it was listed as Critically Endangered in 1994. Thanks to concerted conservation work, by 2009 its numbers had expanded to around 1500 individuals, enough for the species to be downgraded to the status of Endangered. However, this was before the proposal to build a wind farm in its habitat. This proposal led to fierce opposition from groups such as the American Bird Conservancy, and to a Change.org petition ("Help save endangered Lear's macaws! Say no to wind farm complex!") that at the time of writing in 2022 had been signed by more than 82 000 people (Change.org 2022). What was the worry here?

Wildlife Ethics: The Ethics of Wildlife Management and Conservation, First Edition. Clare Palmer, Bob Fischer, Christian Gamborg, Jordan Hampton, and Peter Sandøe.

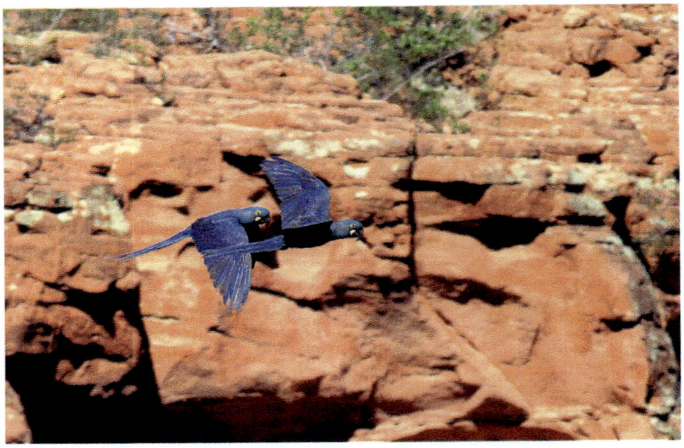

Figure 17.1 Two Lear's macaws flying in Bahia state, Brazil. *Source:* Rafael Cerqueira/ Dreamstime LLC.

It's well established that wind farms can harm and kill birds and bats, in particular from collisions with turbine towers and blades (Rehbein et al. 2020) (although, as we'll note later, bird deaths from wind turbines contribute only a fraction to total anthropogenic bird deaths). Lear's macaws appear to be at risk because they fly long distances each day to reach their feeding grounds; they fly in pairs or flocks, which increases the danger that one collision will kill many birds; and they fly at dawn and dusk when visibility is poor (Camargo 2021). In a 2017 study of bird and bat mortality from wind turbines, the Psittaciformes (parrots) were identified as one of the bird families more vulnerable to the construction of wind turbines (Thaxter et al. 2017). Of course, it's impossible to be sure about the effects on specific populations of Lear's macaws unless a wind farm was actually constructed. But given that the macaw population is not very large, were such collisions to turn out to be common, the impacts on the species would be very significant.

At the same time, environmentalists (among others) see wind energy as a sustainable and powerful weapon against climate change, as wind power is renewable and installed wind turbines produce electricity without producing carbon dioxide (CO_2). As such, wind power is a vital part of the current energy transition – and Brazil is well placed to contribute. Brazil's installed wind power capacity increased from 0.03 GW in 2005 to 20.1 GW in 2022, which makes Brazil seventh in the world in terms of installed wind energy (da Silva and Galvão 2022); in 2022, China was the leader with a capacity of 221 GW, or more than a third of the world's capacity. Nevertheless, Brazil has huge potential to expand its wind power production, especially in northeastern Brazil where winds blow steadily with little change in direction and speed, promising relatively clean, plentiful, and renewable energy far into the future.

This renewable energy versus wildlife dilemma is sometimes called a "green-on-green" environmental controversy (Warren et al. 2005), where there are environmental values driving both sides – in this case, reducing carbon emissions on the one side and protecting individual animals, species, and biodiversity on the other – as opposed to more familiar stand-offs between, say, reducing carbon emissions and promoting economic development.

The renewable energy versus wildlife dilemma is complicated further by the challenge of weighing short- versus long-term impacts and local versus global impacts (Straka et al. 2020). Wind turbine construction and operation has clear negative effects on some populations of animals currently living near the turbines. At the same time, it is likely to contribute to reducing global impacts from climate change, including to animals, far into the future and across the globe. So, even if the focus is only on wildlife concerns, there's still a dilemma between avoiding losses to *existing* wildlife, species, and ecosystems in this region of Brazil now, and reducing negative impacts in the *future* to species and ecosystems. And, as we'll discuss below, there are other ethical concerns here too, including those relating to impacts on individual animals, to environmental justice, and to human welfare over time.

Such challenging dilemmas force people to think more clearly about both values and moral priorities. We cannot resolve all green-on-green dilemmas in this chapter – or even resolve *this* one – but we hope, at least, to contribute to the ethical debate by providing a map of the kinds of values that are at stake and analyzing how different ethical theories would approach the case, to give a clearer sense of ways in which such a dilemma might be managed. We'll begin by describing the worries conservationists have about wind farms, move on to see what animal welfare issues might be at stake, discuss how different ethical perspectives would weigh in on these matters, and finally look at – in practice – how wind power developments might be handled.

17.2 Conservationists' Worries about Wind Farms

Humans are becoming more numerous and many societies are becoming more affluent. As a result, the demand for energy is increasing. Because of the threat of climate change, it's especially important to produce more energy from sources that do not produce greenhouse gases, unlike coal, oil, and natural gas.

Wind power – long used for sailing, for pumping water, and later for generating electricity – is one such source. Wind power development for electricity began in earnest in the 1970s energy (especially oil) crisis. Thereafter, the industry grew rapidly around the globe and, since the 1990s, capacity has doubled every three years. Despite the rise of solar energy, wind power remains the world's fastest growing energy sector. In fact, if development continues at this pace, wind energy will prevent nearly 23 billion tonnes of CO_2 being released into the atmosphere by 2030 from other energy sources (Diógenes et al. 2020). This figure should be seen in the light of about 43 billion tonnes of CO_2 being emitted into the atmosphere each year from human activities. However, with such growth in wind energy comes an increasing number of conflicts over wind power plants, including objections from conservationists.

These objections relate to different parts of the life-cycle of a wind farm, from mining the materials needed for construction, to disposing of waste at the end of the turbines' life. Clearing land to install wind turbines (and clearing corridors to build roads to service them and transmit the generated power) can destroy and fragment habitat, displacing animals in ways that amplify competition for now scarcer resources. There are also concerns in the case of off-shore wind farms for the impacts of underwater vibrations on aquatic species. But most prominently, as in the Brazilian case, conservation worries focus on the impacts of *operating* wind farms on volant (flying) species, primarily birds and bats.

Wind turbines cause fatalities through collisions. Many areas of high wind yield are located in areas with high bird and bat activity (Rehbein et al. 2020). Risks from collision with turbines vary by species, and are affected by factors including species' physiology and maneuverability, behavioral patterns, seasonality, topography, local weather, and the characteristics of wind farm design and operation (May et al. 2017). While there is variability in impacts across flying taxa, it remains the case that wind power production can exacerbate already serious problems for wildlife populations.

One Brazilian study, for instance, evaluated the composition of bird communities before and after construction of a wind farm. Of a total of 146 species recorded before construction, 32 species disappeared after construction and were not observed again at the site in the fouryears of the study (Falavigna et al. 2020). And injuries and deaths related to wind power aren't confined to birds. They are also a concern for bats – both in terms of individual animals and species-level conservation consequences (Willis et al. 2010).

The threat posed by wind farms to flying wildlife is certainly not confined to Brazil or South America. Not surprisingly, there's widespread concern about the wildlife mortalities caused by turbines globally, especially in Europe and North America (Breton and Moe 2009). Flying wildlife is often seen as so important that preservation has earned its own name: "aeroconservation" (Davy et al. 2017).

While population- and species-level impacts tend to be the focus of conservationists' concerns about wind power – which, broadly, we might understand as concerns about biodiversity – such development also threatens other environmental values we have explored in this book. For instance, turbines compromise the wildness of the spaces they occupy and, by extension perhaps, the wildness of the animals whose behavior is altered by human intervention in those spaces. Likewise, turbines compromise certain ecosystem values. Looked at from the perspective of the Land Ethic (Chapters 3 and 6), if wind power construction affects biodiversity, it might change the *integrity* and, if there are knock-on effects for other species, perhaps also the *stability* of the ecosystem. It's also likely to affect beauty, the third value Aldo Leopold mentions in the Land Ethic. Wind turbines – as prominent, dominating, anthropogenic objects with their large rotating wings – may be seen as negatively impacting the beauty of an ecosystem. Indeed, esthetic concerns – not only visual but also including sounds and vibrations – have long been one of the main sticking points for wind proposals in Europe and North America (Kempton et al. 2005). Although a seemingly sustainable source of energy, wind farms potentially threaten a wide range of ecosystem services, including those derived from cultural and esthetic, as well as ecological, values.

In addition, it's not just those who are concerned about conservation who have worries about the impacts of wind farms on wild animals. It's also those for whom animal welfare matters.

17.3 Wind Farms and Animal Welfare

Since wind turbines injure and kill birds and bats, all of whom are sentient, there's an obvious concern here about turbines' impacts on individuals from ethical perspectives stressing the value of sentient beings. Some concerns are more about killing than suffering, as it would seem reasonable to assume that death would often, although not always, be immediate for animals struck by a fast-moving turbine blade. Bats can also be injured by barotrauma, caused by depressurization (Baerwald et al. 2008), an effect that has until recently been an unknown hazard and may help explain high bat fatality rates on wind farms. Many bats may also be nonfatally but painfully injured through barotrauma effects. Estimating the extent of such welfare impacts is difficult, since so many impacts on wildlife, direct as well as indirect, probably go undetected (Fraser and MacRae 2011). While there's disagreement, as we saw in Chapter 5, about whether a quick, painless killing is a welfare issue, on some accounts at least, if the being had a good life ahead, premature death can be regarded as a loss of future good welfare. And suffering, such as from barotrauma, is a welfare issue on almost all accounts. So, wind farms certainly raise welfare issues for flying wildlife.

Given both conservation and welfare concerns, what are the major positive ethical considerations when thinking about the construction of wind power projects, such as the Brazilian proposal, with its potential impacts on bats and birds (such as the Lear's macaw)? So far, we have looked somewhat briefly at the local and short-term negative effects of such projects on wildlife. But of course, one major reason for pursuing these projects is for their *long-term* and *global* benefits to humans *and* to wildlife, that on some – but not all – ethical approaches could outweigh the costs of undertaking them. While there are many ways of thinking about this – corresponding to the ethical theories we explored in Chapter 6 – we'll focus on just two possible approaches here: a broadly consequentialist approach, on which ethical "costs" and "benefits" are weighed against one another, and a rights approach, where such weighing is not generally permitted.

17.3.1 Weighing Ethical Costs and Benefits

As we discussed in Chapter 6, dominant forms of consequentialism maintain that we should optimize the good, whatever that is defined to be – bringing about the best consequences overall. This case, however, shows how complicated it can be in practice to work out what this might mean.

First, a *plurality* of values is at stake here. We've already discussed conservation values relating to ecosystems, species, and wildness, and the value of animal welfare. Of course, direct effects on human welfare and other human values also need to be taken into account in any overall ethical consideration. Second, all these values need to be projected into the future, including the impacts of a wind power project over its lifetime, and beyond. And third – and we'll start here – strictly speaking, a consequentialist approach requires us to think about wind farms and *all* their possible alternatives in seeking an optimal outcome. But what does "all possible alternatives" mean – does it include possibilities that seem very unlikely to be realistic?

Let us look at this third complication more closely. Consequentialist approaches aim at optimizing, comparing *all* possible actions and looking for the set of actions that's likely to have the best outcome over time and all things considered. In this case, that might be taken to mean comparing building more wind turbines to the *best* thing people could do to generate green energy, assuming fossil fuels are to be replaced. But the best thing may in fact be to reduce energy consumption. After all, there's no need to assume that humans *must* continue to extract more energy from the environment, even if by relatively green methods; maybe it would just be best to use much less.

While in principle such radical changes in energy consumption are possible, in practice reductions of this kind are very unlikely. Including apparently attractive but highly implausible alternatives (given the way the world is currently set up) seems to fall into the category of what's sometimes called "ideal theory" – theory based on optimal assumptions about what's possible but that may not relate very closely to the real world. It's also not clear that a significant reduction in overall energy consumption actually *would* be optimific (producing the maximum good consequences), given that in almost all countries, at least some of the population lives with energy poverty, unable to access or afford the energy required for tasks associated with everyday living. Any reduction in energy access for these people would cause severe hardship, and so reduce wellbeing. Reductions in energy use therefore raise significant issues of what's called "energy justice" – here about the fair distribution of access to energy (Jenkins et al. 2016). For energy reductions to be fair, they would need to be targeted at those who are wealthier but these people likely have the greatest ability to resist them, making this possibility even less plausible.

An alternative approach is to limit the comparison to nearer, more plausible options, weighing the short- and long-term implications of producing energy via wind farms against producing similar amounts of energy via fossil fuels, these being the more realistic and likely alternatives. We could think of this weighing approach as a kind of *ethical cost–benefit analysis* (economists, notably, use cost–benefit analysis to appraise the economic, often societal, desirability of a given policy). As noted above, an ethical cost–benefit analysis would need to take into account multiple values, including wildlife populations and species, wildness loss, ecosystem values, and animal welfare. This could be understood in a broadly anthropocentric way, where all the nonhuman values are cashed out in terms of ecosystem services which would make calculation somewhat easier, or in more complex ways in which multiple values are weighed that cannot be cashed out in any single "currency."

However this kind of weighing is carried out, we think it will turn out in favor of building new wind farms, at least in many cases, despite the ethical concerns wind farms raise. To understand why, let's consider what's likely to transpire if future wind power developments in Brazil were successfully blocked (and reliance were instead placed on fossil fuels, at least for now, assuming that consumption is stable or growing). There would be benefits of a ban on wind power developments – most obviously, for the local flying wildlife. Further declines in endangered bat and bird species, such as Lear's macaw, from this source at least would be avoided, and the wildness and integrity of species and ecosystems would not be compromised in this particular way. However, there are many ethical costs too, especially looking into the future. Climate change will advance unabated (or slightly more quickly). Disadvantaged people will continue to be disproportionally impacted by climate effects. Significant numbers of wild animals globally will be negatively affected by higher temperatures and more frequent extreme weather events. In Chapter 18, for example, we discuss the plight of the polar bear, losing habitat and food due to polar warming. Other impacts from climate change already witnessed include bats dropping from tree roosts during extreme heat waves in Australia (Welbergen et al. 2008), and explosions in fatal winter tick populations on moose in North America in unseasonably warm winters (Jones et al. 2019).

What becomes clear here is that, even if we think about wildlife alone, refraining from building wind farms will not prevent harm. Instead, it will change *which* wild animals are harmed, *how* and *when* they are harmed, and even which individual animals actually *exist*. It will shift the harm from the present to the future, expand it from a local level to a global one, and extend the harm from (mostly) flying vertebrates to a broad suite of wild animals. Not using wind power may also increase the magnitude of effects, insofar as the impacts of climate change have ramifications far into the future. However, as we'll discuss below, this does not mean uncritical support for every proposed wind farm of any scale anywhere.

There are some possible ways of objecting to this conclusion. For instance, it might be argued that the interests of *present* generations (of humans and nonhumans) should be prioritized over the interests of *future* generations (for instance, if one does not buy into the concept of sustainable development; see Chapter 7). It could be argued that it's more important to avert harms to current populations, species, and ecosystems than future ones, even if all else is equal in terms of secondary effects, by *discounting* the future, as many forms of economic analyses already do. Given a high enough discount rate, current harms will matter far more, supporting the conclusion that efforts should be targeted toward preventing them.

There are three problems with this defense. First, it's very difficult to square with environmentalists' own views about the importance of the (distant) future. A main plank of traditional environmentalism is that it matters a great deal whether there are wild spaces and flourishing ecosystems many years from now. If that's true, then it would be strange for environmentalists to turn around and discount the very future they are otherwise determined to protect. Second, it's difficult to justify what's sometimes called a "pure time preference" (Anthoff et al. 2009) for present individuals over future ones. What reason could there be for prioritizing the value of existing lives and welfare over future lives and welfare, just because the future lives are in the future? If such a judgment were made over *distance* – for instance that Swedish lives are more important than Nigerian lives – this would generally be regarded as morally objectionable but it's not obvious why space and time are different in this regard. Indeed, this is the ethical foundation for sustainable development, requiring justice *within* and *between* generations. And third, climate effects on humans, wildlife, species, and ecosystems are already being felt. So, reducing the impacts of climate change is not just about the future; it matters for present generations too.

Another way to argue that such an ethical cost–benefit argument would not necessarily come out in support of the Brazilian wind project would be to reject the assumption that the construction of an extra wind farm will in fact have a noticeable impact on the negative effects of climate change. After all, it might be argued that a single wind farm is not going to make much difference to average global temperature. But deciding not to build an extra wind farm in eastern Brazil – say, the one in Bahia state – may make a big positive difference to the local population of Lear's macaw. So, the endangered species ought to be prioritized.

There are difficulties with this objection too. Causal inefficacy is not specific to one particular Brazilian wind farm; if one looks piecemeal at the consequences of constructing *any* individual wind farm, this argument is likely to be true. But then this would lead to the consequence that no wind farm is built and climate change accelerates, generating worse consequences overall than if wind farms had been built. So, a better way of thinking about this might be to consider the climate impact of gigawatts of energy produced by different means, including fossil fuels, rather than concentrating on the impacts of individual installations in isolation. In addition, it's not clear whether the absence of an extra wind farm in northeastern Brazil would save the local population of Lear's macaw or other endangered species. The loss of that population may be overdetermined, in that there may be too many other factors conspiring against that population for it to matter whether a new wind farm goes in (including climate change impacts on macaws). So, if environmentalists are genuinely focused on populations and species rather than individuals, there may not be much benefit at all of blocking new renewable energy development.

Of course, this does not mean that windfarm developments should ignore what's being discovered about mitigating harms to wildlife (in terms of location, technology, size of turbines, and so on) – for example, painting blades to increase visibility for diurnal birds or minimizing blade rotation in nocturnal periods of high collision risk for bats. Consequentialists carrying out such value weighing would, of course, defend such mitigation: better outcomes come from wildlife-sensitive developments. But nonetheless, they are unlikely to oppose wind farm developments altogether, even subject to the empirical uncertainties we have outlined here. However, wind farms look much more problematic from some other ethical approaches. Let's now consider a rights view.

17.3.2 Rights Approaches

Most consequentialist arguments make the fundamental assumption that costs and benefits can be traded off. However, for rights theories not all costs are equal: some are simply unacceptable, regardless of the benefits that might result from allowing them. If building wind turbines would violate rights, then it does not matter whether their creation would produce the most good overall; it is simply wrong to build them. But *do* wind turbine proposals, such as the proposal in Brazil, violate anyone's rights?

First, we need to think about whose rights might be at stake. One possibility is *human* rights. And certainly, some wind farm developments have been accused of violating human rights, especially where they are constructed on the lands of Indigenous peoples who have not been meaningfully consulted; recognition of the cultures and concerns of traditional and Indigenous peoples is an important issue of energy justice (Jenkins et al. 2016). However, human rights violation is not a *general* problem around windfarm construction, and does not seem to be an issue specifically in the Bahia case. A second possibility could be to argue that *species* or *ecosystems* have rights that can be violated (Pepper 2019). As discussed earlier in the book, however, there are significant difficulties with this idea, in particular where claims are made that species or ecosystems have identifiable interests that could ground their rights. Nevertheless, in some jurisdictions, laws have been developed that confer *legal* rights on specific rivers, forests, and mountains; some countries, such as Ecuador, have included the rights of nature in their constitution (see Chapter 9).

Let's think about this in the context of the Brazilian case. First, no legal rights of nature currently apply in this part of Brazil, so no legal protection of this kind exists. Second, even if different parts of nature supposedly have rights, this is not much help here because rights are likely to conflict in cases like this. So if rights are grounded in interests, while it may be in the best interest of the Lear's macaw species (if it is assumed reasonable to say that species have interests) for there *not* to be any wind power development, it may be in the interest of the *ecosystem* (again, assuming that this is seen as plausible) as a whole, in contrast, to have such development. After all, if the ecosystem could continue to function without the Lear's macaw, then its interests are likely to be best served by doing whatever reduces the threat of climate change. So, unless this argument is supplemented with a theory about how to handle conflicts among the rights of different parts of nature, there is not yet a clear case against wind farm development in general, or this case in particular.

More common than assigning rights to ecosystems or nature as a whole is giving *animals* rights (Chapter 6). While many conservationists have reservations about attributing rights to individual sentient animals, those who accept such rights might also object to wind farms. Most obviously, if sentient animals, such as birds and bats, have a right to life then being killed by turbines might violate that right. Moreover, if animals have a right not to have unnecessary suffering inflicted upon them, then turbines might violate that right as well (Pepper 2019).

However, this is not completely straightforward because it raises difficult questions about what *makes* a harm or a killing a rights violation. Must the harms be intended? Can accidental harms be rights violations? After all, no one intends to kill Lear's macaws by building a wind farm. In fact, everyone would probably prefer it if the wind farm did not kill the birds. Their deaths may be foreseen but they aren't intended.

This way of phrasing the issue invokes what is known in moral philosophy as the Doctrine of Double Effect – an idea that goes back to Thomas Aquinas, the thirteenth-century theologian and philosopher. Although there are different versions of the doctrine, most forms maintain that it may be permissible to cause harm when: (i) an action has two effects, a good effect and a bad effect; (ii) the good effect is intended while the bad effect is unintended; (iii) the good effect is otherwise morally permissible and sufficiently important; (iv) the bad effect does not follow from the good effect; and (v) the good effect cannot be produced without also producing the bad effect (McIntyre 2019). Applied to the Brazil proposal, this means that the wind farm would need to be important and morally permissible, and to have a good effect (let's say, producing electricity without carbon emissions), while the killing of Lear's macaws would both need to be a bad effect that even if foreseeable was unintended, and it would also need to be the case that the wind farm could not be built without potentially killing the macaws.

Do these conditions hold here? In a general sense, the positives seem to be present: building wind farms is important, they produce good effects, and they are morally permissible. The bad effect – killing bats and birds – is clearly not intended. But could the wind farm be built *without* killing the macaws? Meeting this condition would require all harm mitigation efforts to be explored and the possibility that other local locations might, for some reason, be better with respect to macaw mortality. While we cannot explore these questions here in any detail, it is by no means a trivial matter to meet the conditions specified by the Doctrine of Double Effect in this context. So, a commitment to animal rights may provide a case against at least some particular wind farm developments; but on the other hand, some may turn out to be permissible.

17.4 How to Handle Wind Power Developments

While animal rights defenders may reasonably be concerned about wind farm developments such as the one proposed in the Bahia and other parts of Brazil (Figure 17.2), we have so far found less reason for environmentalists to oppose such developments, given the long-term ecological benefits wind farms offer. However, this does not mean there is not a serious dilemma in cases like this. Given this dilemma, there are a couple of further points to mention here that seem to speak in favor of wind farms.

First, the number of birds and bats killed by wind turbines is relatively small compared to other human sources of bird and bat mortality and related threats to species and ecological functioning. In the US, windows in human structures account for the largest share of bird mortality, with estimates ranging from 97 to 976 million dead birds per year; transmission lines to conventional power plants account for another 175 million per year; domestic and feral cats account for 110 million deaths; poisoning from pesticides is responsible for 72 million deaths; and so on (Sovacool 2013). Wind turbines, by contrast, account for fewer than 700 000 bird deaths by any account. Obviously, accurate estimation of impacts, mainly fatality, is complicated as the impact of wind turbines on wildlife is highly variable and often species specific, as we discussed earlier in this chapter. Moreover, there are often serious limitations of estimates of fatality: few account for bird (and bats) species diversity. Still, these numbers suggest that of the anthropogenic threats to avian and bat populations, wind turbines are relatively low on the scale.

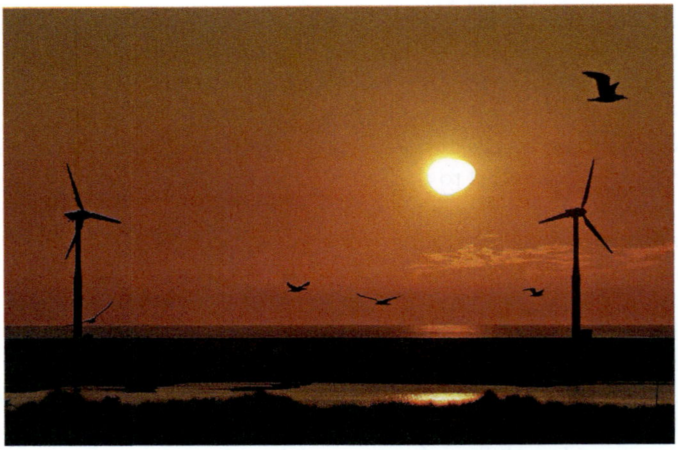

Figure 17.2 Wild birds fly close to the turbines of a wind farm at sunset. *Source:* Zlikovec/Dreamstime LLC.

Second, the wildlife/wind power issue is, like many issues in this book, a *wicked problem*. In 1973, design theorists Rittel and Webber coined this term (as opposed to so-called "tame" problems) for problems that are resistant to clear definitions and easily identifiable, predefined solutions, and that are generally characterized by their inherent complexity, a context of different values and norms, and the difficulty of seeing all the consequences of intervention (DeFries and Nagendra 2017). A wicked problem, then, should be seen as something to be *handled* rather than solved. With the wind power/wildlife problem, the aim is to determine what handling involves.

One part of such handling is to better *coordinate planning* of energy expansion and wildlife conservation measures, with an eye to reducing conflict between the two. However, since these conflicts will never be eliminated, one of the key questions to be answered by decision makers is where and how to set impact thresholds (Sinclair et al. 2018). Assessing risks to wildlife population is an inexact science, especially over time and at ecosystem level. There are no clear criteria on how to progress from individual to population to ecosystem-wide effects. Moreover, as is typical of wicked problems, there are profound disagreements at societal level about the values that should guide setting criteria and especially thresholds.

A tiered approach, then, may be helpful in trying to ensure that considerations about how to mitigate negative effects on wildlife (and the environment as such) are included before implementation. One such mitigation hierarchy, suggested by May et al. (2017), is informed by general environmental impact assessment procedures: (i) planning phase: avoid impacts prior to actual siting of wind turbines; (ii) design phase: if impacts are unavoidable then they should be seen to be minimized before construction; (iii) construction phase: further measures should be taken to limit impacts before operation commences; (iv) operational phase: residual impacts should be compensated; and finally, (v) decommissioning: the area should be restored after the end of the project. In other words, at least some negative impacts are not necessarily inevitable – there are recommendations for how wildlife impacts can be reduced through careful siting, pre-assessment impact studies, and mitigation. This may not satisfy those with animal rights views, but should significantly reduce the ethical costs weighed against the benefits of wind power.

Another significant aspect of trying to handle this green-on-green dilemma is by *engaging stakeholders* in adaptive wind power design, planning, construction, and implementation to try to determine trade-offs and thresholds in order to maintain a green energy transition while minimizing harm to wildlife (Straka et al. 2020). This involves the processes we described in Chapter 9, including building trust and sharing power between stakeholders as part of the process of trying to achieve procedural justice. Moreover, many conflicts over wind power and wildlife conservation tend to focus only on effects on wildlife in the here and now and in relation to single wind energy projects. By contrast, what may be required is a shift from looking (only) at regional to biogeographic levels. Additionally, replying to the mismatch between global and long-term environmental (climate) benefits and short-term environmental (wildlife) costs involves scaling such processes to accommodate intermediate spatial and temporal scales (Sinclair et al. 2018).

17.5 Conclusion

A shift to wind power, and other renewable sources of "green energy," is often claimed to be the most important change that humans can make to avoid the worst effects of the looming climate change crisis – a crisis that is projected to produce enormous harms not only to humans but also to wildlife, as well as damaging ecosystems and hastening the extinction of species.

Essentially, there is no harm-free type of energy; there is not a choice between harming wild animals or not harming them. All forms of energy, like all forms of food production, harm wild animals in some way or other (Fraser and MacRae 2011). If the global human community continues its trajectory of energy consumption but fails to expand its use of renewable energy sources such as wind farms, while some direct but unintentional impacts of flying wildlife will be avoided, other indirect negative impacts on biodiversity and individual wild animal welfare will be exacerbated into the future.

The choice here, then, is between a world where nearly all wildlife populations have been profoundly affected by climate change or an alternative future where some wild animals, species, and ecosystems suffer significant impacts around energy installations, but the longer term threats from climate change are reduced. From most ethical perspectives, choosing wind farms, despite their toll on wild animals, ends up looking like the best solution.

References

Anthoff, D., Tol, R.S., and Yohe, G.W. (2009). Risk aversion, time preference, and the social cost of carbon. *Environmental Research Letters* 4 (2): 024002.

Baerwald, E.F., D'Amours, G.H., Klug, B.J., and Barclay, R.M. (2008). Barotrauma is a significant cause of bat fatalities at wind turbines. *Current Biology* 18 (16): R695–R696.

Barbosa, A.E.A. and Tella, J.L. (2019). How much does it cost to save a species from extinction? Costs and rewards of conserving the Lear's macaw. *Royal Society Open Science* 6 (7): 190190.

Breton, S.P. and Moe, G. (2009). Status, plans and technologies for offshore wind turbines in Europe and North America. *Renewable Energy* 34 (3): 646–654.

Camargo, S. (2021). Lear's macaws threatened by planned wind farm in Brazil, experts warn. https://news.mongabay.com/2021/06/lears-macaws-threatened-by-planned-wind-farm-in-brazil-experts-warn

Change.org. (2022). Help save endangered Lear's Macaw: say no to wind farm complex! www.change.org/p/help-save-endangered-lear-s-macaw-say-no-to-wind-farm-complex

Davy, C.M., Ford, A.T., and Fraser, K.C. (2017). Aeroconservation for the fragmented skies. *Conservation Letters* 10 (6): 773–780.

DeFries, R. and Nagendra, H. (2017). Ecosystem management as a wicked problem. *Science* 356: 265–270.

Diógenes, J.R.F., Claro, J., Rodrigues, J.C., and Loureiro, M.V. (2020). Barriers to onshore wind energy implementation: a systematic review. *Energy Research and Social Science* 60: 101337.

Falavigna, T.J., Pereira, D., Rippel, M.L., and Petry, M.V. (2020). Changes in bird species composition after a wind farm installation: a case study in South America. *Environmental Impact Assessment Review* 83: 106387.

Fraser, D. and MacRae, A.M. (2011). Four types of activities that affect animals: implications for animal welfare science and animal ethics philosophy. *Animal Welfare* 20 (4): 581–590.

Jenkins, K., McCauley, D., Heffron, R. et al. (2016). Energy justice: a conceptual review. *Energy Research & Social Science* 11: 174–182.

Jones, H., Pekins, P., Kantar, L. et al. (2019) Mortality assessment of moose (*Alces alces*) calves during successive years of winter tick (*Dermacentor albipictus*) epizootics in New Hampshire and Maine (USA). Canadian Journal of Zoology 97 (1), 22–30.

Kempton, W., Firestone, J., Lilley, J. et al. (2005). The offshore wind power debate: views from Cape Cod. *Coastal Management* 33 (2): 119–149.

May, R., Gill, A.B., Köppel, J. et al. (2017). Future research directions to reconcile wind turbine-wildlife interactions. In: *Wind Energy and Wildlife Interactions* (ed. J. Köppel), 255–276. Cham, Switzerland: Springer.

McIntyre, A. (2019). Doctrine of double effect. In: *The Stanford Encyclopedia of Philosophy* (ed. N.Z. Edward). https://plato.stanford.edu/archives/spr2019/entries/double-effect.

Pepper, A. (2019). Adapting to climate change: what we owe to other animals. *Journal of Applied Philosophy* 36 (4): 592–607.

Rehbein, J.A., Watson, J.E., Lane, J.L. et al. (2020). Renewable energy development threatens many globally important biodiversity areas. *Global Change Biology* 26 (5): 3040–3051.

da Silva, V.P. and Galvão, M.L.d.M. (2022). Onshore wind power generation and sustainability challenges in Northeast Brazil: a quick scoping review. *Wind* 2 (2): 192–209.

Sinclair, K., Copping, A.E., May, R. et al. (2018). Resolving environmental effects of wind energy. *Wiley Interdisciplinary Reviews: Energy and Environment* 7 (4): e291.

Sovacool, B.K. (2013). The avian benefits of wind energy: a 2009 update. *Renewable Energy* 49: 19–24.

Straka, T.M., Fritze, M., and Voigt, C.C. (2020). The human dimensions of a green-green-dilemma: lessons learned from the wind energy-wildlife conflict in Germany. *Energy Reports* 6: 1768–1777.

Thaxter, C.B., Buchanan, G.M., Carr, J. et al. (2017). Bird and bat species' global vulnerability to collision mortality at wind farms revealed through a trait-based assessment. *Proceedings of the Royal Society B* 284: 1862.

Warren, C.R., Lumsden, C., O'Dowd, S., and Birnie, R.V. (2005). 'Green on green': public perceptions of wind power in Scotland and Ireland. *Journal of Environmental Planning and Management* 48 (6): 853–875.

Welbergen, J.A., Klose, S.M., Markus, N., and Eby, P. (2008). Climate change and the effects of temperature extremes on Australian flyinge-foxes. *Proceedings of the Royal Society B* 275 (1633): 419–425.

Willis, C., Barclay, R., Boyles, J. et al. (2010). Bats are not birds and other problems with Sovacool's (2009) analysis of animal fatalities due to electricity generation. *Energy Policy* 38: 2067–2069.

Climate Change Interventions: Feeding Polar Bears?

18

18.1 Introduction: Climate Change and the Polar Bear

Warming global temperatures are already having significant impacts on wildlife. Some animals are benefiting, their populations increasing in abundance as more food or habitat becomes available. Others are losing out, many being threatened by rising temperatures on land or in the water, by exposure to new parasites and infectious diseases, and by more intense weather events. Wild animals respond to these threats in many ways. Some shift their range toward the cooler poles, move to higher altitudes, or occupy new parts of the oceans. Others shift the timing of key seasonal activities (Parmesan 2006), such as migration or laying eggs, or change their behaviors or their diets. And there's even evidence, in some species, of natural selection at work. For instance, selective pressure from intense hurricanes appears to be driving change in a species of anole (a small lizard) living in the Turks and Caicos Islands in the Caribbean, enlarging their front toe pads (used for clinging) and shortening their hind limbs (Donihue et al. 2018).

However, some wild animal species cannot adequately respond to rapid climate change, especially where the species, or some populations of the species, require a very specific set of environmental and/or dietary conditions to flourish. In these cases,

Wildlife Ethics: The Ethics of Wildlife Management and Conservation, First Edition. Clare Palmer, Bob Fischer, Christian Gamborg, Jordan Hampton, and Peter Sandøe.

populations decline and individual species members are likely to face – or, in some cases, are already facing – very severe welfare problems.

Polar bears provide a vivid example. Across the Arctic, there are currently around 26 000 polar bears in total, with 19 subpopulations across Norway, Alaska, Greenland, Russia, and Canada. Polar bears use sea ice as the base from which to ambush ringed seals, their main prey and food source (Figure 18.1). When there's no sea ice, which is the case for some polar bear populations over the summer, such ambush is impossible and the bears mostly fast, living on their own stored fat plus whatever they can scavenge. It's because of this dependence on Arctic sea ice that they are vulnerable across their circumpolar range, but especially in the Canadian Arctic Archipelago (Wiig et al. 2015).

Due to climate change, the sea ice on which bears depend is melting out earlier and re-forming later; in fact, scientists estimate that the Arctic is warming at least two to three times faster than any other region on Earth. As a result, bears have to fast for longer while they wait for the sea ice to form again. This has already resulted in significantly worse body conditions of bears in some populations (Stirling and Derocher 2012). Bears scavenging on land for food has other impacts too: human fatalities and injuries occur from bear attacks across the species' range; nutritionally stressed adult male polar bears are the most likely to pose threats to human safety (Wilder et al. 2017). In the Hudson Bay area of Canada, where this problem is especially acute, human–polar bear conflicts have more than tripled over a 30-year period, resulting in bears threatening human life and property and some bears being killed (Towns et al. 2009). But it's not just that polar bears eat people; people also eat polar bears. The species is valued as a hunting resource by some of the Indigenous peoples of the Arctic, such as the Canadian Nunavut (Regehr et al. 2017). Changes in polar bear abundance and distribution have the potential to affect many groups' ability to engage in a culturally important practice (see Chapter 13).

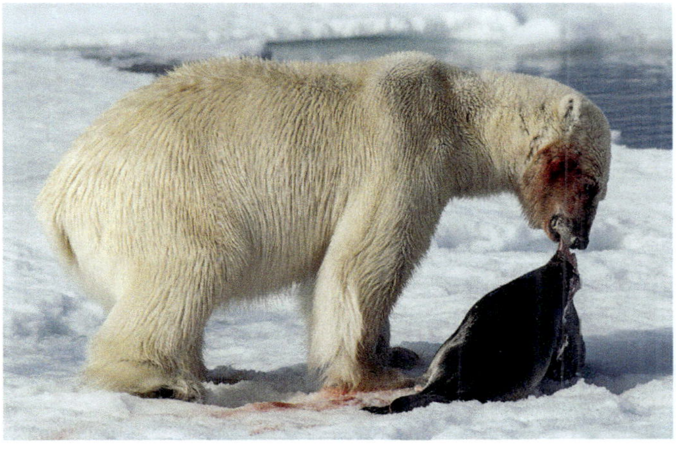

Figure 18.1 A polar bear preying on a seal on the ice in Svalbard, Norway. *Source:* Vladimir Seliverstov/Dreamstime LLC.

As the Arctic continues to warm, the sea ice will eventually melt out too early and re-form too late for some bears to survive the summer, however much they try to scavenge on land. Because of the way the climate has changed, polar bears will probably starve. So, should humans intervene if (or when) polar bears face starvation? If so, what does that suggest about what humans should do more generally? After all, polar bears aren't alone in this predicament: a number of large carnivore species (especially those that are more ecologically specialized) are likely to confront the loss of their natural prey – that is, loss of food resources – due to significant environmental change (Parsons et al. 2022).

As we approach the end of this book, we turn our attention to a large and thorny question: What responsibilities do humans have to wild animals in the wake of anthropogenic climate change? Let's begin by considering some general considerations in favor of intervening to help polar bears. Then, we'll consider the available kinds of interventions. Finally, we'll consider the ethical pros and cons of the various options.

18.2 Ethical Arguments for Intervention

In this section, we'll consider four arguments for human intervention. The first is that the increase in human–bear conflicts is bad for *human* welfare. Hungry bears scavenging in or near local human communities (Figure 18.2) are clearly problematic for those who live there (Smith et al. 2022). So, there is a straightforward anthropocentric argument for intervention.

Second, there are some broadly ecological values at stake. Even though the whole polar bear species is not currently at risk, particular populations might have ecological value, as might the ecosystems that are partially constituted by these threatened bear populations. In addition, losing those populations reduces the genetic diversity of the

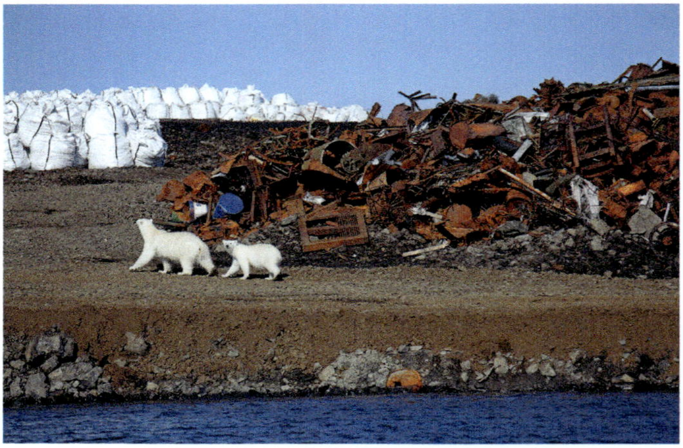

Figure 18.2 Polar bears scavenging in a highly modified environment in the summer in the Arctic. *Source:* Vladimir Melnik/Dreamstime LLC.

polar bear species and so makes the whole species more vulnerable. This means there's an ecological reason to try to preserve particular polar bear populations.

Third, there may be a justice-based concern at the level of species and populations, at the level of individuals, or both. After all, human greenhouse gas emissions are what's causing such dramatically negative impacts on these animals. For at least 30 years, the likely impacts of anthropogenic greenhouse gas emissions have been well known and energy policies could have been pursued that would have curbed these emissions. But for a host of political and economic reasons, greenhouse gas emissions have nonetheless increased. Massive cuts in greenhouse gases *now* (unlikely as they are) would take a while to change the current climate trajectory – and meanwhile, the chance of polar bears starving rises. And it is not as though polar bears have benefited from the production of the fossil fuels that have led to climate change. Indeed, some individuals may have been harmed in other ways by oil and gas extraction or transportation. So, the severe impacts of climate change on bears look like an *injustice*: climate change threatens bear populations and inflicts significant harms on sentient beings who have gained nothing from the process that produced the harms. If humans have any collective responsibilities, then they probably have collective responsibilities for these effects (Nolt 2011). (This does not imply that every *individual* human has equally strong reasons to act on behalf of polar bears; individual responsibility for climate change is, obviously, complex and uneven.)

Fourth, even if the bears aren't victims of an injustice, their welfare alone might provide sufficient reason for action. As noted in earlier chapters, some ethicists insist that suffering matters regardless of whose suffering it is. As Oscar Horta (2015, p. 29) puts it, the moral relevance of suffering "gives us reason to conclude that we should intervene in those cases where it is feasible, in order to reduce the disvalue suffered by nonhuman animals," though only in "cases in which we can reduce [suffering] as a whole, not in some isolated way that reduces disvalue for some in ways that trigger processes that result in more suffering elsewhere."

It's important to recognize, though, that these four arguments for intervention in general might not necessarily justify the same interventions in practice. This should not be surprising; a purely anthropocentric argument for intervening is likely to support different actions than an ecological- or welfare-oriented argument. Moreover, however strong these arguments are, there may also be stronger reasons *not* to intervene. In the next two sections, we consider both kinds of complications.

18.3 What Forms of Intervention are Possible?

Some leading polar bear scientists have already explored whether and how to intervene to help this species. Andrew Derocher et al. (2013, p. 368) examined several possible "proactive conservation and management options" in the event of "sudden negative population-level events." It's worth noting that the focus of their 2013 paper wasn't the welfare of *individual* polar bears (though occasionally this worry is suggested in the paper), but rather the persistence of polar bear *populations* and the avoidance of human/bear conflicts that may threaten human safety. However, and this may often be true in climate change cases generally, the strategies to protect species also appear to be the only plausible ones available to assist individual bears. We'll now outline the leading possible strategies.

- *Diversionary feeding*: Offering food in locations that reduce the incentive for bears to approach human communities and industrial facilities where they may otherwise scavenge.
- *Supplemental feeding:* Providing bears with sufficient short-term energy to help individuals survive periods of food deprivation. By doing so, polar bears can continue to live in environments where their populations probably would not otherwise be able to persist. (Although Derocher et al. [2013] do not actually propose it, presumably these first two strategies could be combined, allowing supplemental feeding to be offered in ways that divert bears from human communities; though, as we'll discuss later, there are other problems with this strategy.)
- *Translocating animals and temporary or long-term captivity*: Several interventions have a common feature: namely, capturing and moving bears. This can take different forms. One involves short-term local captivity, which keeps people safe by preventing bears from entering human communities until ice forms, though this does not address conservation and animal welfare concerns. Another option is to move bears to zoos, though this would not be feasible for more than a few bears and raises issues about keeping wild animals in captivity (see Chapter 14). A third option is translocating bears to new wild habitat, which is risky for the bears, not least because most suitable habitat that would be able to sustain the translocated bears is already occupied (as with the translocation of fruit bats discussed in Chapter 16).
- *Intentionally reducing bear populations:* This could mean increasing bear "harvest" (Regehr et al. 2017), culling bears both for human safety and to make a more viable small population, or through euthanizing starving bears when it's judged this would produce better animal welfare outcomes than to let them starve. All these strategies might result in fewer opportunities for polar bear hunting by Indigenous peoples of the Arctic (Regehr et al. 2017), unless they were involved in culling of bears. These lost opportunities potentially raise issues of environmental justice, though opportunities are likely to decline regardless of whether humans act.

Derocher et al. (2013) are largely negative about translocating animals due to its risks, the difficulty of scaling, and its low likelihood of success, so let's set that aside. The leading options for intervention, then, are either feeding bears or euthanizing bears and reducing bear populations. The alternative, of course, is taking no action at all – the *laissez faire* approach where bears are left to starve, letting "nature take its course."

As mentioned in the previous section, the four arguments for intervention might not justify the same interventions. So, for instance, confining bears until the ice forms or increasing bear culls might respond to anthropocentric worries about human safety, but they would not do much for worries about conservation or nonanthropocentric justice. Likewise, intentionally reducing bear populations might be justified based on ecological considerations, while being objectionable from an anthropocentric perspective, at least insofar as Indigenous hunters may want population levels preserved.

However, supplemental feeding in a way that's also diversionary has the potential to respond to all the concerns. It moves bears away from people; it helps populations to persist (which is potentially important both ecologically and for local Indigenous communities); it responds to demands of justice, since it assists bears in adapting to a problem for which humans are responsible; and it reduces the suffering from hunger that bears may feel. So, is that what should be done?

18.4 Ethical Concerns about Feeding Bears

We've suggested that there may be good ethical reasons for offering bears supplemental and diversionary feeding. But there are also significant ethical concerns. To understand these concerns, we need to look more closely at what such feeding would actually require. The case we have in mind is a sudden starvation event where, for at least one bear population, sea ice forms so late that bears will not make it through the summer. Initially, it's likely that such an event will be short; it will not happen every year and only some populations of bears will need feeding for a week or two. In this case, food could be air-dropped to the bears on a one-off basis. However, given continuing sea ice loss, supplemental feeding will eventually require a commitment to more populations, every year, for increasingly long periods. In principle, it could work out that many or even all bears in some populations would need feeding for several months each year.

Once this longer term commitment comes into focus, so do some of the difficulties involved. When we factor in *all* the animals affected – humans and nonhumans – does feeding bears over the longer term cause more net suffering than not feeding them? If so, then feeding them would not improve overall welfare nor, if bears suffer more, would it repair an injustice. Furthermore, this kind of intervention clearly represents a movement away from more hands-off, preservation-oriented traditional approaches to conservation. In particular, intervening could be perceived as reducing *wildness* value, especially in a situation where what's created is what Derocher et al. (2013) call "semi-managed bear parks."

18.4.1 Welfare: Will Feeding Harm Animals?

The issue here is the net effect of what's known as "human intentional supplemental feeding." Studies of this practice across a range of wild species show mixed benefits to wild animals' welfare, with the balance of benefits and risks depending on the nature and purpose of the supplemental feeding and how consistent and well controlled it is. In a wide-ranging review of publications on supplemental feeding, Sara Dubois and David Fraser (2013) argue that supplemental feeding can be hazardous to the animals being fed (e.g., by spreading infectious diseases; see Chapter 16), as well as leading to potential harms to other animals and to people. In particular, opportunistic and uncontrolled feeding, especially where it's associated with tourism, can have wide-ranging negative effects on the welfare of members of the assisted populations. Still, Dubois and Fraser (2013) think these problems can be avoided, at least in principle, if supplemental feeding is only undertaken in cases where it can be carefully controlled, is intended to benefit populations, and may improve animal welfare. This sounds like what supplemental feeding of polar bears would look like, so perhaps these worries do not apply to this case.

However, there would still be risks to the bears (and humans). An obvious risk is conflict with human beings, at least if feeding brought bears into humans' orbit, increasing threats to people. But that's just an argument for ensuring that feeding is suitably *diversionary*, not just supplemental – i.e., it would need to be located away from human communities to avoid generating human/bear conflict, such as being delivered to remote areas by helicopter (DeRocher et al. 2013). In some Arctic communities, diversionary feeding of bears is already occasionally used and ways of preventing conflict between bears, and between bears and other species, have been devised so this risk is probably manageable. Another risk is that infectious disease could spread between bears at feeding stations and while this risk can be minimized, it cannot altogether be eliminated. There have been examples of disease spread in this way elsewhere: a feline leukemia outbreak in endangered Iberian lynx was connected back to feeding stations (see Palomares et al. 2011) and it's also a common problem at garden bird feeders.

Another worry may be that while feeding bears has the short-term effect of reducing their suffering and keeping them alive, in the longer term it may make the fed bears no longer able or willing to hunt for themselves, or lead to selection for sedentary bears (Smith et al. 2022). Such a change in bears' behavior could reduce their welfare, since without supplemental feeding these bears will starve and die (van Dooren et al. 2023). That said, if the bears are starving *now*, their suffering is acute and their need is urgent. So, while there may be welfare worries down the road, in this desperate situation feeding may still be better for the bears' welfare than not feeding them.

But perhaps it's not all about bears; what about the other animals involved? Polar bears are predators, indeed "the most carnivorous of the extant species of bears" (Wiig et al. 2015, p. 6). They are adapted to eat extremely high levels of fat – much more so than most other carnivores – and they eat very little plant matter. They will scavenge on whale carcasses and sometimes eat fish, walruses, or birds' eggs, but their primary food source is ringed seals (and to a lesser extent, bearded seals). If, for instance, seals are killed and then air-dropped in areas that are accessible to the bears, which is one of the more plausible ways that bears might be fed, this surely raises questions about harm or injustice to the *seals*.

In conservation terms, ringed seals are classified as being of "least concern." So, from an ecocentric perspective, they are of less significance than the bears. But in terms of welfare, issues of consistency are raised here. If polar bears ought to be fed because humans are morally responsible for their suffering, or simply because it's good to reduce suffering as such wherever it's found, then surely such reasons cannot be species specific. Impacts on, and the suffering of, the members of other species need to be considered too.

So, should seals be fed to bears? This would require killing ringed seals. Being killed prematurely can be seen as harmful on views that take welfare seriously (Chapter 5) and over time, more than one seal per bear would need to be killed. On most rights views, killing wild seals to feed bears would be unacceptable because it involves violating the rights of the seals. In addition, killing seals to feed bears could be interpreted as attempting to address an ongoing injustice to one group of animals by harming or carrying out an injustice to a second group of animals to benefit the first group. This same concern has been raised about attempts to cull wolves to protect caribou herds threatened by anthropogenic processes in Canada (Harding et al. 2020).

Moreover, recent research suggests that populations of ringed seals are also threatened by climate change. They give birth in lairs protected by snow roofs so that bears cannot easily see them. However, as snow and ice melt out earlier due to climate change, the snow roofs on ringed seal lairs are collapsing, exposing pups to bear attacks. Although bears kill these exposed seal pups, the pups are still too small to have much nutritional value to the bears, and sometimes bears do not even eat them (Stirling et al. 2008). Climate change, then, is making ringed seal pups more vulnerable to attack and preventing many female seals from successfully raising pups. So, it's reasonable to say that ringed seals are *also*, like bears, being harmed by anthropogenic climate change, and perhaps that they are also victims of injustice. And it certainly seems ethically problematic to try to compensate one set of victims of injustice by killing another set of victims of injustice. Derocher et al. (2013, p. 372) may in fact be gesturing at this by commenting – somewhat elliptically – that "There are also ethical questions around killing one marine mammal species to supplement the diet of another."

In principle, bears could be fed something else: say, the bear chow that's used in zoos. That, of course, is also made from animals, albeit different ones. Current commercial chow, formulated especially for polar bears, includes fish meal and a high proportion of extruded pork fat and bone meal. The fish meal is made from menhaden, wild fish high in fat, normally used for fish oil and fishing bait. The pork fat and bone meal in the chow are almost certainly derived from parts of pigs that humans do not eat, rendered into animal by-product and which would otherwise be used for fertilizer or feeding pets. While feeding bears commercial chow is not a great solution, there are no great solutions here. As long as so many people and pets are eating fish and pork, perhaps it's unfair to refrain from feeding polar bears because they cannot be vegans – especially since humans have put them in a situation where they cannot feed themselves.

But this is not the end of the seal story. Suppose the bears are fed for a period of time, the ice re-forms, and the bears then go back out hunting again – that is, back to killing ringed seals. By intervening to feed the bears, are the harms to the seals now a human responsibility? If the focus is on preventing injustice, then there does seem to be a concern here, especially as the ringed seals are already suffering negative effects of climate change. Had the bears not been fed, these seals would not have been preyed on. In his book *Just Fodder* (2022), Josh Milburn argues that in cases like these – for instance, where predators are rehabilitated – they should not be released back into the wild to continue predation, as humans would then be responsible for an injustice. An alternative argument, from a justice approach, would maintain that the return of bears to hunting is just a resumption of the status quo, with the bears resuming their prestarvation predation trajectory. So, there's still room for debate about what justice would look like here.

But suppose the worry here is that wild animal suffering is *in general* a concern. Then the bears' continued predation is a specific example of a more general problem: namely, the harms that *all* predators cause prey. Some, like Tyler Cowen (2003, p. 174), go so far as to say that "we should count negative impacts on carnivores as *positive* features of … human policy" (our emphasis) and reject subsidizing "the propagation of carnivorous wild animals." From positions like Cowen's, then, helping predators is in principle unacceptable, since predators will inevitably go on and cause suffering. On such a view, the best option is to euthanize the bears and end their suffering while, at the same time, preventing them from causing suffering to seals by future predation. (Of course, Cowen's view raises very puzzling questions about how ecosystems could function without predators.)

There's one final complication about seals: namely, that it is not certain that euthanizing polar bears would actually reduce seal suffering, as the effects of removing members of one predatory species are unpredictable. Seals may suffer from other causes or become too abundant for available resources and, in any case, seals are *themselves* predators causing suffering. Trying to estimate the broad-range effects of euthanizing polar bears rather than feeding them to reduce overall suffering thus runs into huge difficulties in terms of lack of knowledge: the net effects of the actions aren't always clear. So, it may be that in this case, from the suffering reduction view, it's just best to look at the *immediate* suffering with which one is faced – the starving bears – and deal with that particular problem, rather than trying to work out what the down-the-line impacts on wild animal suffering overall would be.

Again, depending on the argument offered for intervening, some of these harms and potential injustices will be more relevant than others. However, welfare and justice aren't the only concerns here; there are also questions about naturalness and wildness. We turn to them now.

18.4.2 Naturalness and Wildness: "Semi-Managed Bear Parks"

One of the issues raised by Derocher et al. (2013) is that a supplementary feeding program might result in commitment to a "semi-managed bear park" model if habitat conditions continue to decline. Wouldn't the existence of such "bear parks" diminish wildness value, both of the bears themselves and of the Arctic landscape in which they are located?

Let's start by getting a bit clearer about the value at stake. Consider Ned Hettinger's (2018) idea of "respect for independent nature," which is one paradigmatic statement of this view (discussed in Chapter 4). Hettinger (2018, p. 68) says that naturalness "involves an overall judgment of the degree of independence of an entity from humans, that is, of the extent to which a being is autonomous vis-à-vis humanity." Clearly, anthropogenic climate change has reduced naturalness in this sense. Still, it has not entirely eliminated it so that anything goes; wildness comes in degrees. The Arctic is still wild to a high degree, and polar bears are still wild animals. Some ways of treating them reduce their wildness or "naturalness," and the wildness of Arctic landscapes, more than others. Hettinger notes:

> For example, that anthropogenic climate change has dramatically increased the rate of interbreeding between grizzly bears and polar bears does not mean there is no naturalness left to protect in our treatment of them or their ecosystems. This impact would not undermine the unnaturalness of relocating polar bears from the Arctic to Antarctica, even ignoring the negative consequences this would have on penguins and other southern species.
>
> Hettinger (2018, p. 78)

Would feeding the bears undermine naturalness, so understood? To answer this question, it's important to note that Hettinger's concern is about what's likely to protect naturalness best *overall*. A temporary intervention where the human influence would "wash out" over time could be a good thing overall. However, feeding the polar bears is unlikely to be temporary; that's why there's a concern about semi-managed bear parks. Some bears may become dependent on people indefinitely. This does look like a significant loss of naturalness value, suggesting that if naturalness value is a priority, polar bears should not be fed, quite independently of any concerns about the food they'd actually be given.

However, Hettinger (2018) does mention one case that leaves the door open – if only slightly – to justify feeding starving polar bears on the basis of naturalness or wildness value. When discussing an (imagined) case of genetically modifying members of the American pika (a small, rodent-like relative of rabbits) in order to prevent extinction from climate change impacts, Hettinger (2018, p. 69) notes that if the pika *were not* modified, "it is arguable that it [the extinction] would give us a much greater impact on nature than we would have with our rescue attempt." So, the impact of anthropogenic species loss on naturalness value *could* be greater than the impact of a human intervention to save the species, even a long-lasting intervention like genetic modification.

Reasoning in a similar way, it could be maintained that feeding polar bears is one way of keeping bears on the landscape. An Arctic landscape that retains polar bears may be regarded as wilder or more natural than an Arctic landscape that lacks them, even if human intervention is required to keep them there. This, however, may depend on the distinction we explored in Chapter 4 – whether landscape naturalness is understood more in terms of *composition* (what kinds of things are present) than *history* (how things got to be or to remain on a landscape).

However, the bear case does seem potentially more likely to undermine naturalness than the (imagined) American pika one. First, the pika intervention aimed to avoid extinction of the whole species but here we are talking about feeding some individual bears in some populations (although certainly particular bear populations in particular places could be lost, and this would be a big human impact on *those* landscapes). And second, the idea of modifying the pika was to allow them to go on living their normal pika lives, not to live in semi-managed pika parks. It is not clear what semi-managed bear parks would look like, but if they involved human structures (beyond feeding stations), human populations, tourists, etc., then they are likely to undermine naturalness values more significantly. In this sense, while a short-term intervention for a couple of weeks, preventing bears from starving and helping them back out onto the ice is likely to *enhance* naturalness value overall; if feeding becomes long term and institutionalized, and bears can no longer hunt from sea ice much at all, feeding bears is likely to *diminish* overall naturalness value.

18.5 Conclusion

Of course, even if feeding bears undermines their wildness or naturalness and the wildness of Arctic landscapes or seascapes (at least to some degree), there still remains an open question about how important naturalness is relative to concerns about justice and harm. On some views, including many from within traditional conservation biology, the importance of protecting naturalness is likely to outweigh these other goods. That said, these views may grant that if climate change were threatening the whole species, rather than some populations, intervention would be appropriate.

However, if the lives and welfare of individual bears are taken seriously, especially as humans are responsible for their plight, feeding bears deserves closer consideration. Even from this perspective, it is not *obvious* that feeding is the right option, partly due to the knock-on effects that feeding bears would have on bears themselves and other sentient animals (such as the ringed seals) and partly due to concerns about the long-term sustainability of any supplementary feeding operation. So, we should not be too quick to rule out euthanasia as the best option (which is not to say that it's a *good* option).

The hungry bears case is in some ways unique. It's urgent, it's dramatic, it's likely inescapable, and it's going to afflict individuals who are members of one of the most charismatic species on earth. But it's also just one example of a case where climate change will require us to make difficult choices between unpalatable alternatives, where whatever is done, some sentient animals are going to suffer. Moreover, it's a case where interventions will compromise wildness values over time. For this reason, it's particularly important that we think about these issues in advance (LeDee et al. 2021). As Derocher et al. (2013, p. 370) plausibly argue: "it is critical to contemplate and discuss options ahead of the need to respond … Although some of the topics may seem radical … future conditions may be well outside the range of past circumstances and necessitate very different actions than today. The success of interventions will be partly determined by the degree of advanced planning."

References

Cowen, T. (2003). Policing nature. *Environmental Ethics* 25 (2): 169–182.

Derocher, A.E., Aars, J., Amstrup, S.C. et al. (2013). Rapid ecosystem change and polar bear conservation. *Conservation Letters* 6 (5): 368–375.

Donihue, C.M., Herrel, A., Fabre, A.C. et al. (2018). Hurricane-induced selection on the morphology of an island lizard. *Nature* 560: 88–91.

Dubois, S. and Fraser, D. (2013). A framework to evaluate wildlife feeding in research, wildlife management, tourism and recreation. *Animals* 3: 978–994.

Harding, L.E., Bourbonnais, M., Cook, A.T. et al. (2020). No statistical support for wolf control and maternal penning as conservation measures for endangered mountain caribou. *Biodiversity and Conservation* 29 (9): 3051–3060.

Hettinger, N. (2018). Naturalness, wild animal suffering and Palmer on laissez-faire. *Les Ataliers de'l'Ethique* 13 (1): 65–84.

Horta, O. (2015). The problem of evil in nature: evolutionary bases of the prevalence of disvalue. *Relations* 3: 17–32.

LeDee, O.E., Handler, S.D., Hoving, C.L. et al. (2021). Preparing wildlife for climate change: how far have we come? *Journal of Wildlife Management* 85 (1): 7–16.

Milburn, J. (2022). *Just Fodder: The Ethics of Feeding Animals*. Montreal, Canada: McGill-Queens University Press.

Nolt, J. (2011). Non-anthropocentric climate ethics. *WIREs Climate Change* 2 (5): 701–711.

Palomares, F., López-Bao, J.V., and Rodríguez, A. (2011). Feline leukaemia virus outbreak in the endangered Iberian and the role of feeding stations: a cautionary tale. *Animal Conservation* 14: 242–245.

Parmesan, C. (2006). Ecological and evolutionary responses to recent climate change. *Annual Review of Ecology, Evolution, and Systematics* 37 (1): 637–669.

Parsons, M.A., Newsome, T.M., and Young, J.K. (2022). The consequences of predators without prey. *Frontiers in Ecology and the Environment* 20 (1): 31–39.

Regehr, E.V., Wilson, R.R., Rode, K.D. et al. (2017). Harvesting wildlife affected by climate change: a modelling and management approach for polar bears. *Journal of Applied Ecology* 54 (5): 1534–1543.

Smith, T.S., Derocher, A.E., Mazur, R.L. et al. (2022). Anthropogenic food: an emerging threat to polar bears. www.cambridge.org/core/services/aop-cambridge-core/content/view/DD849697E0358BA466D52B4C1A8CB33B/S0030605322000278a.pdf/anthropogenic_food_an_emerging_threat_to_polar_bears.pdf

Stirling, I. and Derocher, A. (2012). Effects of climate warming on polar bears: a review of the evidence. *Global Change Biology* 18 (9): 2694–2706.

Stirling, I., Richardson, E., Thiemann, G.W., and Derocher, A.E. (2008). Unusual predation attempts of polar bears on ringed seals in the southern Beaufort Sea: possible significance of changing spring ice conditions. *Arctic* 61 (1): 14–22.

Towns, L., Derocher, A.E., Stirling, I. et al. (2009). Spatial and temporal patterns of problem polar bears in Churchill, Manitoba. *Polar Biology* 32 (10): 1529–1537.

van Dooren, T., Price, C.J., Banks, P.B. et al. (2023). The ethics of intervening in animal behaviour for conservation. *Trends in Ecology and Evolution*. Online now.

Wiig, Ø., Amstrup, S., Atwood, T. et al. (2015). Ursus maritimus: e.T22823A14871490, The IUCN Red List of Threatened Species. www.iucnredlist.org/species/22823/14871490

Wilder, J.M., Vongraven, D., Atwood, T. et al. (2017). Polar bear attacks on humans: implications of a changing climate. *Wildlife Society Bulletin* 41 (3): 537–547.

Conclusion: Wildlife Ethics – The Future

19

19.1 Wildlife Management and Ethics

Poisoned possums, dehorned rhinos, toeless frogs, starving polar bears, infectious bats, endangered wildcats. This book has explored a wide range of wildlife controversies, the conflicting values behind them, and the ethical perspectives that shape them. These perspectives often aren't made explicit in decision-making about wildlife, nor when the significance of wildlife is debated by communities, wildlife professionals, citizens, or other stakeholders. Such values and ethical theories nonetheless influence much of what happens to wild animals.

In this book, we have introduced broadly anthropocentric approaches, where human lives and welfare matter most (or exclusively) and where wildlife is valuable – or otherwise – insofar as it impacts on human lives. We've also looked at several nonanthropocentric approaches, including ones where whole wild animal species, the ecosystems in which wild animals live, and/or the wildness they manifest are valuable in themselves or alternatively where the lives and welfare of individual wild animals are given priority. We've explored different ethical theories, including theories on which outcomes, rights, relationships, and virtues matter most – each of which may help us think through what we value, why we value it, and how to handle such values. And we

Wildlife Ethics: The Ethics of Wildlife Management and Conservation, First Edition. Clare Palmer, Bob Fischer, Christian Gamborg, Jordan Hampton, and Peter Sandøe.

have also considered the ways in which these different values and ethical theories are embedded in a variety of wildlife management and conservation frameworks.

These ethical resources can inform decision making about wildlife management and conservation in particular cases. Such decisions can be straightforward when different values and ethical perspectives reinforce one another – for instance, where both human-centered and ecocentric perspectives point to the same policy in practice. Frequently, though, there are significant tensions and conflicts *between* values (as many of the case studies in the second part of this book indicate) and so very different actions will be described as "ethical" depending on the approach people assume. This diversity of ethical approaches means that general calls for "ethical wildlife management" can be empty unless they specify what kind of ethic is actually being called for or what amount of agreement between ethical views is needed to guide management (Hampton et al. 2019).

With this variety of ethical approaches in mind, we'll turn to some concluding reflections on the future of wildlife ethics – the ethics of wildlife management and conservation.

19.2 Human Threats to Wildlife and Wildlife Threats to Humans

At the macro level, wildlife ethics will be shaped by increasing planetary-scale threats to wild animals. Many of the most severe threats will not be new, though they'll continue and intensify. In particular, overexploitation of wildlife through (for instance) hunting, fishing, and trade will continue to threaten whole species (Figure 19.1). A 2016 study found that, of the species listed as threatened or near threatened on the IUCN Red List, 72% were currently overexploited for commerce, recreation, or subsistence (Maxwell et al. 2016), a pattern likely to continue. According to the same study, agricultural activity, including the production of crops, livestock, timber, and aquaculture, is also a major threat to wildlife. Both sets of threats will be exacerbated by rising human population levels, at least in some parts of the world, and pressure for more affluent lifestyles almost everywhere. Relatedly, habitat loss and fragmentation through land clearing for housing, transport, energy production, and other industrial uses will constitute further ongoing threats, as will negative impacts from introduced infectious diseases and plant and animal species.

In total, current global estimates of terrestrial vertebrate species indicate that 41% of amphibians, 26% of mammals, 21% of reptiles, and 13% of birds are threatened with extinction; more than 80% of these threatened species are affected by more than one major threat (Global Change Data Lab 2022). In addition, existing threats can be expected to expand in new directions. For instance, while pollution from agriculture, mining, and industry has long posed problems for wildlife, concerns about the impacts of microplastic pollution and "forever" chemicals are now growing (Wilcox et al. 2015). Climate change will also compound existing threats to wildlife such as habitat change and the emergence of infectious diseases; it will drive more dramatic weather episodes, including more intense heat, drought, flooding, and ice melt. Many of these processes arise from anthropogenic disturbances to the balances and processes of nature, rather than from intentional human actions (Fraser 2019). Some highly adaptive wild animal generalist species (e.g., many rodents; Chapter 12) are likely to survive or even

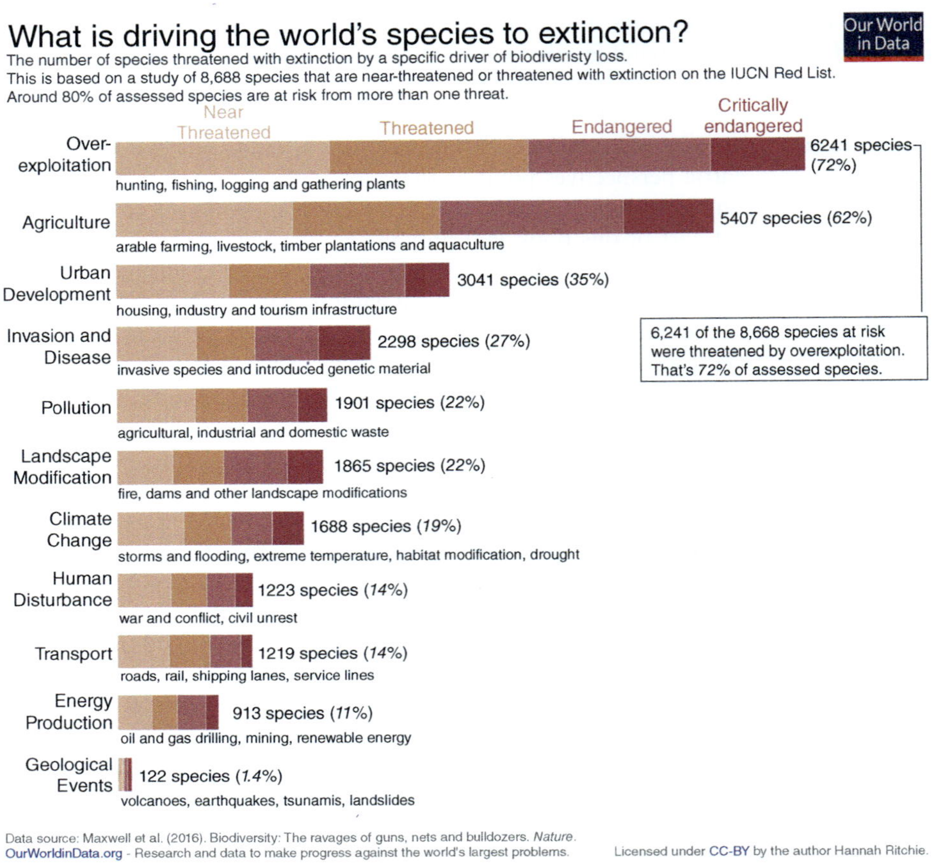

Figure 19.1 Global threats to wildlife. The underlying data were derived from Maxwell et al. (2016). *Source:* Hannah Ritchie, CC BY 4.0.

thrive; other, more specialized species (e.g., alpine frogs; Chapter 15) will struggle due to changes in habitat linked to human development, extreme weather, and loss of food resources (see Chapters 17 and 18).

Many of these wildlife challenges can be captured in the language of planetary boundaries, a framework developed by international scientists in 2009 (Steffen et al. 2015). The nine proposed planetary boundaries have standardly been conceived as "boundaries within which humanity can continue to develop and thrive for generations to come" while crossing these boundaries risks "large-scale, abrupt, and irreversible environmental changes" (Stockholm Resilience Centre 2022). However, the planetary boundaries need not be interpreted only in terms of what works for *human* thriving. Most (though not all) wild species – in particular, most sentient vertebrates, the focus of this book – have also evolved to thrive within these same boundaries. The boundaries provide a "safe operating space" for all and exceeding them threatens both human beings *and* wildlife.

What does moving out of this "safe operating space" for wildlife mean for the future of wildlife ethics? The challenges here are so extensive that global conversations will be needed about large-scale priorities. Not all wildlife species can be saved, much less all wildlife populations. So what should humans protect – and why?

Moreover, as we have discussed in this book, such threats aren't all one way: wild animals will pose more real and perceived threats to humans in the coming years. These include, most obviously, threats from emerging infectious diseases, including variants of Nipah virus (see Chapter 16), influenza, and other yet unknown spillover diseases that could have major global impacts. More locally, conflicts between humans and wildlife are likely to intensify as human populations expand further into wildlife habitat, where land is rewilded and species are reintroduced around human settlements, and where loss of "wild" habitat forces humans and wildlife to share more spaces.

In these situations, wild animals may raid crops and prey on livestock and pets; increase road danger from collisions; and introduce unwanted noises, smells, and sights into urban and suburban areas. In the most confronting sense, rewilding involving large predators will also lead to them preying on humans in places that were previously considered safe, providing a test for a commitment to living with wild animals. In the 1970s, for example, northern Australia stopped culling saltwater crocodiles; since then, there has been a 23-fold increase in crocodile attacks in the neighboring island nation of Timor-Leste (Brackhane et al. 2018). This change in management strategy has also increased the risk of crocodile attacks on northern Australian beaches (Figure 19.2). Similar challenges are emerging with large mammalian carnivores as rewilding efforts bring these species close to densely populated human settlements (Davoli et al. 2022). These issues will raise particularly challenging questions for wildlife ethics.

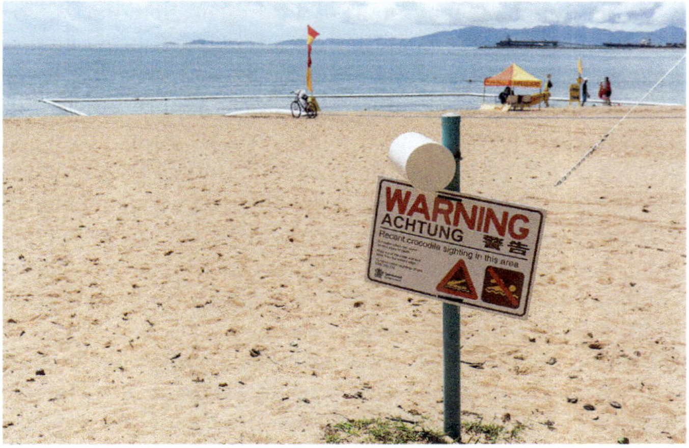

Figure 19.2 A sign warns human beach visitors against swimming due to the presence of saltwater crocodiles in north Queensland, Australia. *Source:* SherSS/Shutterstock.

19.3 Changing Values and Ethical Conversations

Conversations about how to minimize human threats to wildlife – and wildlife threats to humans – are ethical conversations. Some of them may be relatively easy, as there's bound to be some degree of ethical convergence in the future. For instance, reducing microplastic pollution is good for both people and wildlife (Wilcox et al. 2015) so, arguably, people ought to make efforts to reduce it. As this book has maintained, however, there's likely to be significant disagreement and divergence in many other cases.

In the case of climate change, even anthropocentric ethical policies diverge, as shown by the fact that human rights approaches to climate policy are rather different from consequentialist ones. Likewise, different wildlife value priorities are likely to lead to different policy responses – for instance, climate policies that emphasize protecting *wildness* will look different from those aiming at protecting *species*. The prospects for resolving conflicts that are driven by these differences will depend on multiple factors. One factor is the shift in value orientations toward wildlife (Chapter 8) – that is, how people imagine ideal human–wildlife relationships. As we have noted, there's evidence in some countries of a move toward "mutualist" perspectives (where wild animals are seen as individuals that could be part of human social networks and for whom care and concern are appropriate) and away from domination perspectives (where wildlife is understood primarily as being for human use and benefit; Manfredo et al. 2020). If this shift continues, then there might be a higher tolerance of wildlife *disvalues* in the future, especially among urban populations where these shifts in orientation are most prominent. Accordingly, there may be fewer conflicts between people over local wildlife management decisions. At the same time, such shifts may make it easier for people to accept more porous boundaries between humans and wildlife – for instance, by moving away from the idea that wildlife does not belong in cities (see Chapter 11). It will be interesting to see if such trends extend to large predators and rewilding, especially if that requires tolerating increases in fatal attacks from wildlife.

However, other developments may point in a different direction. There are already cases where concerns about wild animal impacts on human health and disease seem to trump wildlife mutualism – for instance, in calls for culls of suburban white-tailed deer because of links to Lyme disease (Connors and Short Gianotti 2021). Fear of disease spillover could easily lead to public support for mass wildlife culls in future. This is particularly likely for people who live close to bats (Chapter 16). Mutualism might also be challenged in times of severe economic hardship. There's significant evidence that alongside underlying value orientations, contextual factors – including existing habits, social norms, and economic stressors – play important roles in shaping behaviors (Nilsson et al. 2020). These factors may affect willingness both to forgo benefits from exploiting wildlife and to tolerate wildlife disvalues.

All this suggests that the future will contain many divergent views about how wild animals should be regarded and managed. Successful wildlife management, then, will be more about finding ways of recognizing and respecting such diversity, not necessarily aiming at resolving conflicts but rather at transforming situations to make progress (see Chapter 9). At the same time, disagreement about values and ethical theory needn't preclude agreement about what to do in particular situations.

19.4 Changing Technologies

Not only will there be changes in threat patterns, value orientations, and the ways conversations about wildlife are structured, there will also be significant changes in wildlife *technologies*. Given their profound effects on wildlife management and conservation (Sandler 2020), these will be increasingly relevant to wildlife ethics discussions.

We've mentioned several new technologies throughout the book, including immunocontraceptive vaccines for fertility control in hyperabundant native species in Chapter 11, the concept of gene editing for eradicating introduced species in Chapter 12, and transponder tags for animal identification in Chapter 15. Technologies related to wildlife include the use of GPS, cameras, thermal imaging, drones, and bioacoustics for monitoring, tracking, and surveillance; the use of cloning, artificial insemination, hormone implants, and immunocontraception to control breeding; and gene banks, gene editing, and "genetic rescue" to preserve species and biodiversity.

Alongside the very specific ethical questions raised by the use of particular technologies in particular cases, the "technologization" of wildlife management and conservation raises broader questions about the meaning of conservation. As Ron Sandler (2020) argues, the widespread adoption of new technologies may not involve just the use of a tool but a change in "form of life": technology can shape what's seen as a problem, how problems are understood and tackled, how people understand themselves in relation to other people and nonhumans, how they relate to the world around them, how activities and institutions are organized, and structured, and so on. (Just think how the smartphone – with apps like eBird and iNaturalist, allowing on-the-hoof wildlife photography, ID, and uploads – has changed human societies.)

One important conservation-related case is the set of technologies enabling "deextinction" programs. The idea that technology can be used to bring species back puts a question mark at the end of the adage that extinction is forever – and could have the effect of fundamentally shifting attitudes toward extinction (Jørgensen 2013). Whatever the benefits of the technologies, such attitudinal shifts may also be a kind of "moral hazard" – akin to the one raised by the idea of "perfect" ecosystem restorations (Chapter 3). If species and ecosystems can be recreated, how far should an effort be made to prevent their destruction in the first place?

The use of genetic technologies also raises broader questions about what's meant by "conserving a species" and what would actually count as species extinction. Christopher Preston (2021, p. 9), for instance, asks whether a genetically modified black-footed ferret whose genome has been reworked to "include a sequence of nucleotides designed on a computer" is of the same species as the wild black-footed ferrets of the past. He suspects not: "sometimes, it would appear, you do not have to be dead to be extinct" (Preston 2021, p. 9).

People may also worry that technological interventions are "unnatural" in ways that are ethically objectionable. Sometimes such worries focus on the unknown and potentially negative consequences of technological interventions (for instance, of releasing gene-edited organisms into the wild; Sandler 2020). Other concerns are independent of these technologies' consequences, arising instead from particular interpretations of human virtues and vices – for instance, arguments that the development or use of genetic technologies in the wild is arrogant or hubristic.

But perhaps the biggest concern is related to the balance between wildness values and other conservation values, especially the protection of species. This issue arose in several chapters of this book, especially in the case of supplementary feeding for polar bears (Chapter 18). It's also relevant for thinking about the ethics of assisted migration (that is, the translocation of populations outside their historic range, as climate change or introduced disease makes their historic habitat inhospitable; McLachlan et al. 2007). The development of gene editing and the potential use of gene drives (which substantially increase the likelihood that a particular set of genes will propagate through a population – see Chapter 12) raise these questions even more acutely. Would the use of these techniques make "the wild" into something more like a garden or a zoo? And would it matter if it did? Emma Marris (2015), for instance, argues that it might not, contending that humans should "sometimes give up our beloved wilderness and wildness to save other species."

That said, not all interventions *necessarily* reduce wildness. Take, for example, the case of the Hawaiian honeycreepers, a group of passerine bird species threatened by avian malaria, an infectious disease carried by nonnative mosquitoes. These mosquitoes can now reach honeycreepers' mountain habitats because climate change is warming the mountains. Suppose it's possible, as has been proposed, to gene edit the relevant mosquito species to produce "self-limiting" mosquitoes – mosquitoes who reproduce but whose offspring cannot survive into adulthood (Samuel et al. 2020). This could mean that the mosquito population concerned would become extinct in Hawaii. Would eliminating that mosquito population, and so protecting honeycreepers from malaria, really be a wildness-reducing intervention? Or, by eliminating a human influence (the nonnative mosquito), would it actually be wildness *restoring*? Wildlife ethics still has a lot to untangle here.

Changing technologies also raise questions about the value of individual animals' welfare and their rights. As we have maintained throughout this book, individual animals' welfare is becoming an increasingly important issue in wildlife management, a trend that's likely to continue. Indeed, one of the claimed advantages of technologies like fertility control and gene drives is that they can improve the animal welfare outcomes of wildlife control practices, reducing the need for killing or causing suffering. Instead, they prevent unwanted animals (unwanted by humans, that is) from being born in the first place (Chapter 12). (Of course, the development of these technologies is likely to involve research animals, raising its own suite of ethical questions about wildlife research; see Chapter 15.)

More recently, some philosophers and legal scholars have argued that wild animals may have an interest in *privacy*, a protected zone around wild animals that's part of what it is to be wild, which should protect them from constant surveillance. For instance, Henry Lininger and Tom Lininger (2017, p. 207) claim that "there's a public interest in protecting the privacy of wildlife" and Angie Pepper (2020) maintains that nonhuman animals have a *right* to privacy. Since almost all forms of wildlife technology could be argued to violate privacy, these arguments could open up new debates about the ethical costs of wildlife technology.

We've just scratched the surface here, not least because history suggests that it's often difficult to anticipate the technologies that emerge in the future. Subsequent generations may face tensions between values that we cannot anticipate, as we cannot imagine the technological context that gives rise to them. Clearly, this will be a growing area for future wildlife ethics.

19.5 In Conclusion

The world is changing rapidly for wildlife. At the same time, human understanding of wildlife is developing rapidly. Both sets of changes raise ethical challenges for traditional management and conservation goals and the strategies people adopt to achieve them.

First, traditional ethical justifications for conservation goals focused on ecological preservation and restoration. Due to climatic and other ecological changes, these objectives no longer make sense in many places (Sandler 2013). Anthropogenic influences will be at work however much land is set aside; species will be driven toward extinction even if humans refrain from overexploiting them or converting their habitat to farmland. This situation is one of the biggest challenges facing wildlife ethics. Should the goals of conservation, as discussed in Chapters 7 and 8, take the more traditional route of preserving habitats, populations, ecosystems, species, and biodiversity? Or should conservationists shift their focus to other values like ecosystem flourishing, even if the flourishing ecosystems are largely novel? Or should the focus be on key ecosystem services, as Sandler (2013) suggests?

Second, conservation strategies are updating in response to increased awareness that wild animals are sentient, complex, and often social *individuals*, not just members of populations, species, and ecosystems (Wallach et al. 2020). This change is ethically significant both in itself and instrumentally. Such ethical change in itself, by seeing sentient animals as individuals, complicates hyperabundant and introduced species control, as we saw in Chapters 11 and 12 respectively. Instrumentally, however, understanding the agency and adaptability of individual animals may also help researchers to better predict the outcomes of conservation interventions (Edelblutte et al. 2022).

As we contemplate the future of wildlife and ethical reflection about wildlife, it's worth remembering that almost whatever humans do, there will be wildlife on this planet. Indeed, there will probably be wildlife long after humans are gone. Debates about wildlife management and conservation, then, are primarily about what *kinds* of wildlife will accompany humanity into the future, not about whether there will be any wildlife at all. In a sense, this is a comforting thought: humans and their domesticated animals are unlikely to be alone. There will always be beings "out there," living their own lives, sometimes oblivious to human existence. What's uncertain is whether most of these animals will belong to adaptable, currently thriving species like "feral" domestic cats (Chapter 4), brown-headed cowbirds (Chapter 6), white-tailed deer (Chapter 11), and ship rats (Chapter 12). Put another way, will there still be a place for members of species now facing headwinds, like Sumatran tigers (Chapter 2), black rhinos (Chapter 10), orange-fronted parakeets (Chapter 12), alpine tree frogs (Chapter 15), and Lear's macaws (Chapter 17)? The answer will depend, to a significant degree, on the wildlife conservation and management policies adopted. We hope, in this book, to have made a contribution to developing debates about the ethical underpinnings of such significant wildlife policies.

References

Brackhane, S., Webb, G., Xavier, F.M. et al. (2018). When conservation becomes dangerous: human-crocodile conflict in Timor-Leste. *Journal of Wildlife Management* 82 (7): 1332–1344.

Connors, J.P. and Short Gianotti, A. (2021). Becoming killable: white-tailed deer management and the production of overabundance in the Blue Hills. *Urban Geography* 2021: 1–23.

Davoli, M., Ghoddousi, A., Sabatini, F.M. et al. (2022). Changing patterns of conflict between humans, carnivores and crop-raiding prey as large carnivores recolonize human-dominated landscapes. *Biological Conservation* 269: 109553.

Edelblutte, É., Krithivasan, R., and Hayek, M.N. (2022). Animal agency in wildlife conservation and management. *Conservation Biology* 37 (1): e13853.

Fraser, D. (2019). Why we need a new ethic for animals. *Journal of Applied Animal Ethics Research* 1 (1): 7–21.

Global Change Data Lab (2022). Our world in data: share of species threatened with extinction. https://ourworldindata.org/grapher/share-threatened-species

Hampton, J.O., Warburton, B., and Sandøe, P. (2019). Compassionate versus consequentialist conservation. *Conservation Biology* 33 (4): 751–759.

Jørgensen, D. (2013). Reintroduction and de-extinction. *BioScience* 63 (9): 719–720.

Lininger, H. and Lininger, T. (2017). Unlocking the virtual cage of wildlife surveillance. *Duke Environmental Law and Policy Forum* 207: 207–263.

Manfredo, M.J., Teel, T.L., Don Carlos, A.W. et al. (2020). The changing sociocultural context of wildlife conservation. *Conservation Biology* 34 (6): 1549–1559.

Marris, E. (2015). Handle with care. https://orionmagazine.org/article/handle-with-care

Maxwell, S.L., Fuller, R.A., Brooks, T.M., and Watson, J.E. (2016). Biodiversity: the ravages of guns, nets and bulldozers. *Nature* 536 (7615): 143–145.

McLachlan, J.S., Hellmann, J.J., and Schwartz, M.W. (2007). A framework for debate of assisted migration in an era of climate change. *Conservation Biology* 21 (2): 297–302.

Nilsson, D., Fielding, K., and Dean, A.J. (2020). Achieving conservation impact by shifting focus from human attitudes to behaviors. *Conservation Biology* 34 (1): 93–102.

Pepper, A. (2020). Glass panels and peepholes: nonhuman animals and the right to privacy. *Pacific Philosophical Quarterly* 101 (4): 628–650.

Preston, C.J. (2021). Extinct and alive: towards a broader account of loss. *Philosophia* 50 (5): 2221–2234.

Samuel, M.D., Liao, W., Atkinson, C.T., and LaPointe, D.A. (2020). Facilitated adaptation for conservation – can gene editing save Hawaii's endangered birds from climate driven avian malaria? *Biological Conservation* 241: 108390.

Sandler, R. (2013). Climate change and ecosystem management. *Ethics, Policy and Environment* 16 (1): 1–15.

Sandler, R. (2020). The ethics of genetic engineering and gene drives in conservation. *Conservation Biology* 34 (2): 378–385.

Steffen, W., Richardson, K., Rockström, J. et al. (2015). Planetary boundaries: guiding human development on a changing planet. *Science* 347 (6223): 1259855.

Stockholm Resilience Centre (2022). Planetary boundaries. www.stockholmresilience.org/research/planetary-boundaries.html

Wallach, A.D., Batavia, C., Bekoff, M. et al. (2020). Recognizing animal personhood in compassionate conservation. *Conservation Biology* 34 (5): 1097–1106.

Wilcox, C., Van Sebille, E., and Hardesty, B.D. (2015). Threat of plastic pollution to seabirds is global, pervasive, and increasing. *Proceedings of the National Academy of Sciences* 112 (38): 11899–11904.

Index

Wildlife Ethics: The Ethics of Wildlife Management and Conservation, First Edition. Clare Palmer, Bob Fischer, Christian Gamborg, Jordan Hampton, and Peter Sandøe.